PENGUIN
ARKANA

AYURVEDA

Robert E. Svoboda graduated from the Tilak Ayurveda College
of the University of Poona in 1980 as the first and, until today,
only Westerner ever to become a licensed Ayurvedic physician.
Since then he has travelled extensively, lecturing and conducting
workshops on Ayurvedic subjects. Among his writings on
Ayurveda are two books, *Prakruti: Your Ayurvedic Constitution* and
The Hidden Secret of Ayurveda, and a self-study programme, *The
Ayurvedic Home Study Course*. His book *Aghora: At the Left Hand
of God* introduces some of the little-known Tantric traditions of
his teacher, Vimalananda. He is on the staff of the Ayurvedic
Institute in Albuquerque, New Mexico, and divides his time
principally between North America, Hawaii and India. In India,
where he has lived for more than a dozen years, he continues his
research into Ayurveda and other ancient sciences.

ROBERT E. SVOBODA

————————

AYURVEDA

LIFE, HEALTH AND LONGEVITY

ARKANA
PENGUIN BOOKS

ARKANA

Published by the Penguin Group
Penguin Books Ltd, 27 Wrights Lane, London W8 5TZ, England
Penguin Books USA Inc., 375 Hudson Street, New York, New York 10014, USA
Penguin Books Australia Ltd, Ringwood, Victoria, Australia
Penguin Books Canada Ltd, 10 Alcorn Avenue, Toronto, Ontario, Canada M4V 3B2
Penguin Books (NZ) Ltd, 182–190 Wairau Road, Auckland 10, New Zealand

Penguin Books Ltd, Registered Offices: Harmondsworth, Middlesex, England

First published 1992
5 7 9 10 8 6 4

This book is a reference work based on the Ayurvedic system of medicine.
The information it contains is in no way to be considered a substitute for
consultation with a duly licensed health professional.

Typeset by DatIX International Limited, Bungay, Suffolk
Printed in England by Clays Ltd, St Ives plc

CONTENTS

ACKNOWLEDGEMENTS

————————

Vimalananda; Judy P. Allyn and Sevyn Galambos;
Kathy Araki and Don Beaucage, Ayumi and Kiyomi;
Pamela and Larry Barinoff and Nathan Yogesh;
Robert Beer and family; the city of Benaras;
the city of Bombay; Steven Brothers and Jeff Roger;
the island of Hawaii and Pele;
Dr V. D. Lad and the Ayurvedic Institute; Vaidya B. P. Nanal;
Roshni Panday and family; the city of Pune;
Launette Rieb and Naomi Serrano; Virginia and Doug Shilson;
Fred and Kathy Smith and family;
Laura and Edwin Svoboda and others of my family;
Robin Waterfield. Special thanks to Nature.

AYURVEDA: THE ART OF LIFE

Materialist philosophies existed even in the ancient world, but only since Descartes and Newton has materialism gained acceptance as an accurate model of reality. Our modern world-view assumes that we live in an objective universe that can be explored by objective observation, that only the physically observable is real, that a whole can be known by a study of its parts, that one cause produces one effect, and that mind and body are totally independent of one another. The early scientists who made these assumptions probably did so in good faith, based on their own observations and inferences, but because they also concluded that their postulates were incontrovertibly true, never subject to re-evaluation, we have been living with the consequences of these assumptions ever since.

Early researchers concentrated, cause by cause and effect by effect, on discovering the physical mechanisms of health and disease. Armed with the pathogen theory of disease, our science has triumphantly eliminated or controlled most of the epidemic and endemic infectious diseases that have ravaged human society for centuries – or so it seems. The evidence actually suggests that infectious diseases yielded to control less because of medical intervention and more because of economic development, which provided more and better food and improved sanitation to human populations, encouraging improved personal hygiene and a fall in the birth rate. Though modern science, convinced that the body is nothing more than a well-engineered machine, still believes that history, culture and personality have no effect on medicine, we really have modern civilization rather than modern science to thank for our improved health, such as it is.

Those of us who enjoy the benefits of living in modern civilization also suffer all its disadvantages: pollution of our air, water and food by chemicals and radiation, pollution of our minds by noise and information overload, pollution of our humanness by automation, specialization and the pressure of deadlines, and pollution of our emotions by loneliness, alienation and the breakdown of the family. These and other traumas produce in us the host of degenerative diseases that make it difficult for us to enjoy the high-tech pleasures that, we are told, make life worth living, pleasures we have accepted in exchange for the sort of pleasures enjoyed by more 'primitive' people.

In the remote parts of the world where civilization has not yet fully infiltrated, human beings live long and healthily. Centenarians credit a variety of factors for their longevity: good food, hard work, even cigars and brandy. In one area of China, which has dozens of citizens aged 100-plus, the people swear by a medicinal wine whose ingredients include local lizards. Perhaps there is some secret substance in the apricots of Hunza or in well-brewed lizard wine that is the biological equivalent of the fountain of youth, but it is more likely that the nectar of pure water, pure air and pure food, the satisfaction of directly reaping the fruits of their labours, and the support and enjoyment of their families and friends lengthen the lives of those who are privileged to live in these regions.

Civilization is quite a recent development in human history, and as our societies become more complex we move further away from the environment in which we evolved. Some contend that because humans have only lately learned how to live together in concentration we have not yet evolved an innate, instinctual ability to adapt to the artificial environments we have created for ourselves. Animals evolve along with their environments, but we humans have allowed our technological advances to run ahead of our capacity to integrate them into our lives. The crowding together of humans into towns and cities first caused epidemic infectious diseases, which we learned how to control, and now causes the epidemics of heart disease, cancer and other modern maladies that we are unable to control. In the pre-industrial environment patients were chronically predisposed to infection because of malnutrition and overcrowding; in the post-industrial environment we suffer instead because of overnutrition and isolation.

Most of the money and energy we spend to study these 'diseases of civilization' are misspent because these facts do not agree with the assumptions of modern science. For example, most scientific studies on the sorts of disease experienced by 'normal' populations of people ignore the crucial reality that modern life is anything but normal! The powerful stresses, avoidable and unavoidable, that we each experience daily accumulate within us and sicken us, and because we cannot adequately adapt to our artificial environment we cannot conceive of any sort of health other than the temporary alleviation of the degenerative conditions that our environment causes. And even that alleviation is fraught with peril; roughly one out of every four patients who enter a hospital today develops an iatrogenic disease, a disease caused by medical procedures. Death rates actually decreased in 1976 in Los Angeles and Bogotá and in 1973 in Israel when doctors went on strike! In its anxiety to destroy the reality of 'objective' disease modern medicine has lost sight of the 'subjective' reality of the patient, forgetting the Hippocratic dictum 'first do no harm'.

Our problems are less a result of such physical factors themselves than of our inability to cope with them, an inability that is, in turn, a result of the failure of our guiding philosophy to provide direction to our culture. For many years now we have tried to use scientific knowledge to control the environment, rather than live in harmony with it as most 'primitive' peoples have attempted to do, because the scientific world-view has become our religion, scientists its priests, and universities and institutes its monasteries. Scientists celebrate arcane rituals that they alone can comprehend to gain access to Reality; they then interpret that Reality for the benefit of the uninitiated masses.

In many ways science has become an institutionalized orthodoxy that often obstructs our progress toward truth as effectively as the Church in the Middle Ages delayed the development of modern science by forcing the Galileos of the world to deny the evidence of their senses. Today the pendulum is stuck at the other extremity of its course, and many scientists deny, often imperiously, any reality other than that supported by sensory evidence. Dedication to a harsh system that supports a black–white vision of reality promotes intellectual intolerance toward opinions that do not jibe with one's preconceived conclusions.

Just as we do not expect an instrument to interpret its observations for us, so we should not force science, an excellent tool with which to examine the universe, to serve either as our religion or our world-view. An instrument must remain separate from its object in order to observe impartially, but our current dedication to separation and impersonality has led us to become alienated little islands in the stream of observable life events. Objectivity applied to human relations has enhanced, not reduced, the divisive tendencies of humankind, allowing us the freedom to make existence on our planet so tenuous that we bid fair to destroy ourselves through impersonal environmental catastrophe if we succeed in avoiding our deliberate destruction through hi-tech war.

When scientists institutionalized the mind–matter disjunction to provide them with the objectivity they needed to be apart from the systems they study, they inadvertently institutionalized a dysfunctional doctor–patient relationship. Medicine is, has always been and will remain intimately associated with the religion of the society it serves, and so today for most of us it is our doctors who intercede for us at the scientific altar. Shamans are the doctors in primitive societies, and no matter how effective a mechanic of the human body a good doctor may be, he or she will always remain a sort of shaman. So long as 'objectivity' forces our society's shamans to distance themselves from their patients, there will continue to be crisis in our medicine.

Ironically, even though the classical assumptions of physics and chemistry that sparked the development of scientific medicine have now been turned upside down by the work of Einstein and his contemporaries, the medical establishment persistently retains an unswerving allegiance to the world-view of Newton and Descartes, refusing to recognize that the objectivity possible in the macrocosmic world disappears when we enter the microcosmic world, where mind and matter continually interact. Werner Heisenberg's Uncertainty Principle ushered relativity right into science's parlour by demonstrating that the laws of nature deal not with elementary particles but with our knowledge of those particles, that is, with the contents of our minds, making the separation of observer, observed and observation impossible.

The idea that the world is made up of objects that are independent of human consciousness conflicts with both the theories of quantum mechanics and with experimental fact. Far from being divorced from physical reality, ideas have a material impact on reality. The assumptions that underpin modern science and its medicine are such reality-impacting ideas, and only revolutionary change in these assumptions can solve the problems they create. Consider the case of Sir Francis Bacon, who was King James I's prosecuting attorney at the witch trials of his day. Sir Francis, apparently no more benignly disposed toward Mother Nature than to her votaries, the witches, openly stated that the aim of science was to make nature into a 'slave', and to 'torture nature's secrets from her'. Here is a reality-forming idea, one whose violence has persisted in science to the present day, empowering those who gladly rape the planet for profit scientifically.

Another of the reality-forming ideas that shape our world is the idea of progress. Linear progress, the belief that the old should be progressively replaced by the new, is a concept that has developed over only the last two hundred years or so. Its extreme forms include the totalitarian materialistic dogmas such as Communism, but even its milder incarnations have often been pernicious. For decades 'enlightened' scientists believed that breast milk provided nothing more to new-born children than could be provided by an artificial formula. We now know how false this belief was, but in the interim millions of children were, in the name of progress, denied the passive immunity they could have obtained from their mother's milk, the sense of security that comes from being held closely to the mother's breast and the intimate mother–child bonding that is essential to the maintenance of a society.

A progress that blindly assumes the inherent superiority of the new creates new and unforeseen problems. Here is an example: in India legumes are usually cooked with something sour to make them more digestible. In the southern state of Andhra Pradesh tamarind (*Tamarindus indica*) has been used for this purpose since time immemorial. About four hundred years ago the Portuguese introduced the tomato into India, and many Indians now use tomatoes in preference to their traditional 'sours' because of taste and because the tomato is more 'modern'. When whole villages in

5

Andhra Pradesh came down with fluorosis, a disease in which excess fluoride enters the bones, causing permanent, crippling deformities, research determined that the drinking water in these areas contains large amounts of naturally occurring fluoride. Tamarind binds this fluoride, preventing it from entering the body; tomato cannot. Those villagers who changed from tamarind to tomato absorbed more fluoride than before and developed the disease. Real progress here would have involved preservation, not elimination, of the tamarind tradition.

None of these observations invalidates the very real and perceptible benefits that modern medicine has provided to millions of people all over the globe, but given the obvious negative impact of these and other scientific reality-forming ideas, medicine must change. 'Holistic', 'environmental' and 'behavioural' medicine have developed as 'alternatives' to mechanistic medicine but, as certain sagacious thinkers have shown, such medical countermovements fail because they are too influenced by the biomedical legacy, the embedded bias of the language, which reflects the mechanistic paradigm. This paradigm, or pattern of thinking, reinforces the system and is reinforced by it, enabling both to resist substantive change. While these new medical models claim to be alternative paradigms, and have introduced significant insights, they still do not challenge the implied assumptions of modern science, which define disease and its causation in purely biological terms.

For example, there is now a wide appreciation of the difference between the disease a doctor perceives and the illness a patient experiences, which has led reformers to propose that all treatment be composed of both medical intervention, or cure, and individual support for the sufferer, or care. However, these distinctions between cure and care, disease and illness perpetuate an invidious presupposition that purely physical disease and treatment are possible, when a really new approach would actually integrate both perceptions into one. Until the fundamental misconception that the cause, pathology and cure of disease are all limited to the physical plane is overthrown no new paradigm will develop in modern medicine. We need a totally different perspective on life and health that can suggest to us ways in which to proceed.

Ayurveda, the ancient medical system of India, is one such perspective. The Ayurvedic paradigm shows how body, mind and spirit interactions can be predicted, balanced and improved to enable us to live gracefully, harmoniously. Ayurveda has already donated the drug reserpine and the discipline of plastic surgery to modern medicine, and most scientists who are interested in Ayurveda for other than historical or anthropological reasons see it as a potential source of new therapies. Ayurveda's greatest treasures, however, are its theories of health and disease, which are remarkably compatible with the models espoused by 'post-modern' medical thinkers. This book is an attempt to display some of the salient Ayurvedic assumptions and to show how they have metamorphosed into therapeutic modalities. It is not intended to be a simplistic use-herb-A-in-disease-B handbook, but an introduction to the Ayurvedic way of thinking and an exposition of some of its own reality-forming ideas about health and disease.[1]

Though today's Ayurvedic students study the remnants of the classical Ayurvedic system, Ayurveda survives because it remains a living tradition, practised by living people. Modern scientists often object that if Ayurveda is such a wonderful medical system, why is it that India is renowned for its masses of poor, diseased people? It is, in fact, because competent Ayurvedic doctors are no longer to be found in much of India that this situation obtains. And, of course, one may ask, 'If modern medicine is such a wonderful thing, why is it that modern industrial and post-industrial societies are so filled with unhealthy people?'

Translation of Ayurvedic wisdom into a form that presents an organically complete, comprehensible and accurate image is difficult. Like the blind men who described the parts of an elephant without ever grasping its totality, those who grope about in ancient medical lore always risk mistaking a part for the whole. The only answer is to have a guide, and I have been blessed with many such guides, including Shri K. Narayana Baba, who was the inspiration for my staying in India to study Ayurveda, and Vaidya B. P. Nanal and Dr V. D. Lad, who made the difference between success and failure for me at the Tilak Ayurvedic College. I respectfully offer this book to my teachers, to their teachers, and to all the teachers who have gone before. I salute everyone who has helped me to learn, most of all the Aghori Vimalananda. All insights in this work have come from my mentors; all errors and misstatements are mine and mine alone. May this book brighten the lives of everyone who reads it.

1

HISTORY

No one knows exactly when civilization developed in India; all dating is arbitrary until the time of Gautama Buddha (563–483 BC). The earliest culture about which we have any useful data is that of Harappa, the Indus Valley civilization, which arose around 3000 BC and lasted for perhaps 1,500 years. Successors to Neolithic settlements of 5,000 years previously, the Harappans built large cities, such as Mohenjo-daro, and traded with foreign lands via Lothal, their seaport. Their cities had wide, paved roads, aqueducts, public baths and extensive drainage systems. With such attention to sanitation, they almost surely also possessed a system of medicine, though no firm evidence yet exists to support this conjecture except for the discovery in Harappan remains of substances such as deer antler and bitumen, which are used in classical Ayurveda.

The Harappan civilization seems to have collapsed between 2000 and 1500 BC. Natural disasters may have been to blame, or the Harappan downfall may have been caused by nomadic Aryans from Central Asia, who, Indologists maintain, have frequently invaded the Indian subcontinent. The Aryans brought with them the Vedas, their ancient books of wisdom and sacrificial ritual. The Vedas took on their current form at some point during the second millennium BC, though this version, which has been carefully preserved by India's priests, the Brahmans, is derived from much earlier versions, which are now lost. From the youngest of the Vedas, the Atharva-Veda, developed Ayurveda, probably with the help of residual Harappan knowledge. At the turn of the first millennium BC the treatise now known as the *Charaka Samhita*, the first and still most important of all Ayurvedic texts, appeared. Although Ayurveda's most famous surgical text, the *Sushruta Samhita*, was also compiled around this time, the development of surgery being spurred by the

9

need to treat injuries sustained in warfare, the version that has come down to us dates from much later.

Indian culture entered its Golden Age during this period and learning flourished. By the sixth century BC a 'university' had been established at Takshashila (Taxila), near what is now Rawalpindi in Pakistan. This institution apparently had no true campus but was rather a concentration of scholars and their disciples, who lived near one another to facilitate debate and the exchange of ideas. One of Takshashila's products was Jivaka, the royal physician of King Bimbisara of Magadha (now part of the state of Bihar), who was appointed by the King to personally supervise the health of Gautama Buddha and his followers.

Ayurvedic medicine was already extensively developed by the time of the Buddha, a result, at least partly, of politics. Because the health of the king was equivalent to the health of the state, the services of a royal physician were essential to the state's political stability. The physician had to protect his royal patron from poisoning, cure him of wounds accidental and military, and ensure the regal fertility, the queen's safe pregnancy and delivery, and the royal progeny's healthy development. The Buddha, who taught compassion for all beings, supported both the study and the practice of medicine, and was himself sufficiently aware of medical theory and practice to once speak of a disturbance of the humours in his own body and to ask Jivaka for a purgative to set himself right. He allowed his monks almost all the therapeutic measures advised in classical Ayurveda, including surgery (except for fistula, the operation for which is often unsuccessful and which is better treated by other means).

Jivaka was so famous that at one point most of the citizens of Magadha joined the Buddhist community solely to be able to avail themselves of his treatment; the Buddha consequently prohibited anyone who was ill from being accepted into the fold. Many are the stories of Jivaka's amazing cures, and his studentship at Takshashila was apparently no less amazing. After seven full years of studies there, his guru handed him a spade and sent him out for his final examination: to search within a radius of several miles for any plant bereft of all medicinal value. Jivaka passed his exam when he returned unable to find any such substance, and it is still an article of faith in Ayurveda that nothing exists in the world that cannot be used as a medicine.

In 326 BC Alexander the Great invaded northern India. Though it is likely that Indian medical knowledge had already found its way to Greece before then, this was the first documented exposure of the two cultures to one another. Alexander was sufficiently impressed by Ayurvedic practitioners that he ordered all cases of poisoning to be treated by them alone. He carried some of these doctors away in his retinue on his departure.

In the third century BC Ashoka, the emperor of most of northern India, became a convert to Buddhism. Motivated by compassion for all sentient beings, as Buddha taught, Ashoka built charitable hospitals, including specialized surgical, obstetric and mental facilities, for both humans and animals throughout his realm. Numerous rock-cut edicts around India attest to this, and to the embassies and Buddhist missionaries he sent to many neighbouring countries. These emissaries carried Indian science with them, which is probably how Ayurveda reached Sri Lanka. The Ayurveda now existing in Sri Lanka is almost identical to that in India except that it has been adapted to the requirements of the island and reflects basic Buddhist philosophies, as it might still in India had Buddhism not been exterminated there almost a thousand years ago.

Medical missionary activity continued long after Ashoka, as documented by the Bower Manuscript, written in the fourth century AD and found in Central Asia, where the missionaries had carried it. It contains recipes for various medicines and a long panegyric on garlic. In the later empires of the Guptas and the Mauryas state-employed and private practitioners seem to have coexisted, and village physicians were maintained by the government through gifts of land and payment of salary. The state also planted medicinal herb gardens, established hospitals and maternity homes, and punished quacks who tried to practise medicine without imperial permission.

During this period of intellectual flowering three more famous Ayurvedic texts appeared. *Ashtanga Sangraha* (probably seventh century) and *Ashtanga Hrdaya* (about a century later) are both ascribed to one Vagbhata, though they were almost certainly written by two different people. These two texts are condensations of the works of Charaka and Sushruta, with some new diseases and therapies added.

The eighth century also saw the appearance of the *Madhava Nidana*, a treatise on diagnostics. The Buddhists, who supported all forms of learning, set up true universities to teach Buddhism, Vedic lore and more secular subjects such as history, geography, Sanskrit literature, poetry, drama, grammar and phonetics, law, philosophy, astrology, astronomy, mathematics, commerce and even the art of war, as well as medicine. The most famous of these universities was that of Nalanda, also in Bihar, which was established during the fourth century AD and flourished until about the twelfth century.

Students came from all over the world to study at these universities. The best accounts we have of Nalanda are those of two Chinese travellers who visited India as students in the seventh century. We learn from them that only 20 per cent of all applicants could pass the entrance examinations, that instruction was free to all, that senior students acted as teaching assistants and that teaching went on day and night. Some graduates elected to stay on as research scholars at Nalanda, whose campus covered half a square mile, housing as many as 10,000 pupils and 1,500 teachers at a time, with numerous cooks and support staff. 'Nalanda brothers' even had the same kind of old-boy network that old Etonians or alumni of Harvard enjoy today.

The Golden Age ended when waves of Muslim invaders inundated northern India between the tenth and twelfth centuries. Buddhism had developed as a reaction against the meaningless ritualization with which many of the members of the Vedic priestly class, the Brahmans, had polluted the Vedic religion. While the Hindus had responded to this reaction with both isolated violence against Buddhist temples and monasteries and a widespread reformist movement of their own, the Muslims slaughtered the monks wholesale as infidels, destroyed the universities and burned the libraries. Those who could escape fled to Nepal and to Tibet, where Ayurveda had first penetrated in the eighth century AD. Some Ayurvedic texts are thus preserved today only in Tibetan translation.

In spite of these catastrophes and of the import into India by the Muslim conquerors of their own medicine, *Unani tibbia*, Ayurveda survived. *Unani* (the word means 'Greek') was created by Arabic physicians by combining Greek medicine with Ayurveda, which they learned from texts translated into Persian in the early years of the modern era when the Sassanian dynasty controlled part of northern India. *Unani* medicine is thus closely related to Ayurveda, and while India's Muslim rulers tended to support *Unani*, Ayurveda also prospered. In the thirteenth or fourteenth century a new treatise on medicine, the *Sharngadhara Samhita*, appeared, introducing new syndromes and treatments. During the sixteenth century Akbar, the greatest Mogul emperor and a remarkably enlightened ruler, personally ordered the compilation of all Indian medical knowledge, a project that was directed by his finance minister, Raja Todar Mal.

For centuries Europe had coveted Indian spices, which were used to preserve meat and to mask the taste and odour of putrefied meat. During the sixteenth and seventeenth centuries, with the opening of secure trade routes to the East to ensure a steady flow of spices, a European fascination for things Indian developed. An Indian massage therapist named Sake Deen Mohammed, known as the 'Brighton Shampooing Surgeon' (the Hindi word for massage, *champana*, metamorphosed into the English word 'shampoo'), became the toast of that resort town in the late eighteenth and early nineteenth centuries with his 'Indian Vapour Bath and Art of Shampooing'. Lords and ladies flocked to him for both treatment and preventive care, and odes were written to his expertise.

The Europeans brought to India syphilis, which was first described in Ayurveda in *Bhavaprakasha*, a sixteenth-century text, under the name of 'the foreigners' disease' in honour of the Portuguese, who imported it. They also imported their own intellectual bigotry, which gradually superseded their fascination. Sir Praphulla Chandra Ray in his *History of Hindu Chemistry* cites an essay by a Briton in which the author endeavoured to prove that the entire Sanskrit literature as well as the Sanskrit language itself was a 'forgery made by the crafty Brahmans on the model of Greek after Alexander's conquest'. This denigration of traditional wisdom reached its zenith in 1835, when Lord Macaulay settled the controversy over whether the government should support indigenous or Western learning by ordering that European knowledge should be exclusively encouraged in all areas governed by the East India Company.

Before 1835 Western physicians and their Indian counterparts exchanged knowledge; thereafter only Western medicine was recognized as legitimate, and the Eastern systems were actively discouraged. Since living traditions are lost when experts die without being able to teach others, vast quantities of indigenous expertise evaporated during the next several decades. Even during these years of persecution, however, Ayurveda generously contributed to modern medicine. During the nineteenth century the Germans translated from Sushruta's treatise details of an operation for repair of damaged noses and ears. This operation, which now appears in modern textbooks as the pedicle graft, led to the development of plastic surgery as an independent speciality, and today Sushruta is regarded by plastic surgeons around the world as the father of their craft. Skin grafting and operations for cataract and bladder stone were still being performed by Ayurvedic surgeons in India as late as the eighteenth century.

Many writers on Ayurvedic history decry the evident decline of Ayurvedic surgery after the Classical Age, often blaming the Buddhists and their doctrine of non-violence for discouraging wilful injury to the body. It is more likely, though, as Debiprasad Chattopadhyaya argues in *Science and Society in Ancient India*, his excellent study of Ayurveda's struggle in the Vedic and Classical eras, that it was the ritual 'impurity' involved in surgery, the close physical contact that a surgeon must have with blood and other bodily substances, that discouraged its practice, since the Buddha himself did not object to surgical intervention when it was necessary.

With the assertion of Indian nationalism at the dawn of this century, interest in Indian art and science was reawakened and Ayurveda began a gradual renaissance. Today it is one of the six medical systems in India that are officially recognized by the government, the others being allopathy (also known as modern, cosmopolitan or biomedical medicine), homeopathy, naturopathy, *unani, siddha* (a variety of Ayurveda practised by the Tamils of southern India) and yoga therapy. The practitioners of these six systems must compete for patients with each other and with a profusion of practitioners of other medical skills, including itinerant tonic sellers, pharmaceutical representatives, village curers, bone-setters, midwives, exorcists, sorcerers, psychics, diviners, astrologers, priests, grandmothers, wandering religious mendicants, and experts in such maladies as snakebite, hepatitis, infertility and 'sexual weakness'.

Today's developmental planners, who often seem to be Lord Macaulay's spiritual descendants, tend to think of traditional systems like Ayurveda as archaic and dysfunctional, and so non-progressive (all the while ignoring the clear evidence of obsolescence and dysfunction in the practice of biomedicine). Believing, as do many foreigners, that 'traditionalism' has kept India backward, they would prefer for most ancient traditions, including the medical ones, to disappear. Many practising allopaths agree, ostensibly because traditional medicine is not 'scientific', but practically because elimination of alternative medical systems would reduce their competition. Social scientists have noted that allopaths derive their social status less from their medical ability than from the culture of modernity and 'progress' that they represent; when in distress, most Indians seek out any practitioner of any system who can cure them, and many allopaths use Ayurvedic preparations and dietary or lifestyle advice in their own practices.

Political patronage has been an important factor in the spread of allopathy in India, and the government of India spends more money on allopathic medicine than on all other systems of medicine combined. Politics is not foreign to Ayurveda – like other colleges my alma mater, the Tilak Ayurveda Mahavidyalaya in Poona, was founded as a direct result of a political agitation – and there is still an ongoing tussle between those who support the practice of 'pure' Ayurveda and those who wish to integrate Ayurveda into allopathy. In Sri Lanka the term 'Ayurveda' has already come to signify 'integrated' medicine; the pure form of Ayurveda exists there under a different name. Though this is not yet the case in India, the majority of students who study in and graduate from Indian Ayurvedic colleges do, desiring enhanced social status and income, go on to practise a sort of medicine that is basically allopathic in nature.

VEDA AND AYURVEDA

Ayurvedic doctors have been struggling for respect ever since they began to professionalize, well before 1000 BC. Ayurveda is the *upaveda*, or accessory Veda, to the Atharva-Veda. Though all four Vedas are collections of hymns written by seers called rishis, the

Atharva-Veda differs in subject matter from the other three Vedas (the Rig-Veda, Yajur-Veda and Sama-Veda), being basically a manual of magic. Atharvan hymns fall into two main groups: those that are meant to cure disease and create peace and prosperity, which we might call white magic, and those that are meant to wreak havoc, which is sorcery, or black magic. Some writers believe that many of its incantations were adopted by the Aryans from the natives of their new homeland, incantations that were, perhaps, left over from the civilization of the Indus Valley.

There are a few references to treatment in the other Vedas, like a charm in the Rig-Veda for chasing consumptive disease from all parts of the body, and an entire hymn in praise of medicinal herbs, invoking their healing power and comparing the physician to a warrior. The god Rudra is invoked in yet another hymn as the ablest of physicians, preparing medicine for all with his beautiful hands. One of the most famous of the Vedic hymns, the 'Rudra Adhyaya' of the Yajur-Veda, praises Rudra as the first physician, and mentions many medicinal plants.

Most of the Vedic healing verses occur in the Atharva-Veda. Over one hundred of its hymns are devoted to conditions as varied as fever, leprosy, consumption, dropsy, heart disease, wounds, headache, parasites, eye and ear diseases, poison, rheumatism, madness and epilepsy. Charms, plant and animal juices, natural forces like the sun and water, and human contrivances were all used therapeutically in Vedic times. The medicinal substances mentioned were used as amulets, most of the references to diseases and their treatment being incantations for use in expelling the disease from the patient. One treatment for jaundice, for example, requests the body's yellowness to flow out of the patient into yellow birds, turmeric roots and other yellow things.

The health of the body, rather than the cure of disease, is the subject of another hymn:

May I have breath in my nostrils, voice in my mouth, sight in my eyes, hearing in my ears, hair which does not grey, teeth that are not discolored, and much strength in my arms. May I have power in my thighs, swiftness in my legs, steadfastness in my feet. May all my limbs remain unimpaired and my soul unconquered.

MEDICAL POLITICS

As cultural rigidity increased, the social hierarchies that developed when the previously nomadic Aryans settled down and established kingdoms in India were formulated into what is now called the caste system. The older portions of the Rig-Veda, the oldest of the four Vedas, are filled with a freeness of spirit and a broadness of perspective in which the caste system finds no place. This spirit becomes narrowed in the Riga-Veda's later hymns, and in the other Vedas, which reflect society's stratification into four layers, with the Brahmans, the priestly caste, at the apex. Second to them came the nobility, next the merchants and agriculturalists, and finally the labourers.

The basis for this stratification was apparently 'purity', arising from the human tendency to brand our transitory physical existence 'impure' and the ethereal world of the spirit 'pure', and to advocate worship of pure spirit extricated from all association with base physical existence. Historically, the religions that glorify the feminine, fecund aspect of existence exemplified by the Earth goddess have often suffered subordination to the austere, masculine religions of the sky-gods. Jehovah is such a sky-god; so is Jupiter, whose name is cognate with the Sanskrit *dyaus-pita*, the sky-father, who is lord of the upper atmosphere.

The priests of the post-nomadic period reorganized the Vedic religion to ensure a leading role for themselves in the emerging social organization by mandating that the degree of one's ritual purity is determined by the extent to which one is involved in the physical world on a daily basis. Brahmans were regarded as the purest of mortals since they (supposedly) spent most of their days in worship, away from the polluting realities of everyday life. Kings and queens must deal with the world, but by virtue of their exalted positions they are greatly insulated from it and so come next in purity. Tradespeople, who follow, must involve themselves in the buying and selling of commodities, items of commerce created out of physical matter, but do not have to go out and get their hands dirty as labourers do. Only the first three castes are allowed initiation into Vedic studies; because they are 'reborn' through this initiation they are called the 'twice-born' castes.

Those who advocated minimizing contact with the physical aspects of life disapproved of the Atharva-Veda's emphasis on mundane magic. Many authors, in fact, speak of the 'three Vedas', refusing even to extend Vedic status to the Atharva. Such disrespect for medicine and magic extended also to the Ashvin twins, the physicians of the gods, who are highly respected in the Rig-Veda, where they are mentioned over four hundred times, particularly with regard to the miraculous cures they achieved. Though the Ashvins also play an important role in the *Mahabharata*, one of India's two epic poems, by the time of the Yajur-Veda they have been reduced to begging for a share of the sacrificial libations, and are alloted a share only after the other gods grudgingly purify them. In this context the Yajur-Veda specifically states that a Brahman must not practise medicine, because a physician is impure, unfit even to attend a sacrifice.

Clearly only the practice of medicine, and not medicine itself, was objected to, for all students of the Vedas were expected to learn some medicine, particularly the daily and seasonal health maintenance routines, just as they were expected to learn astrology, grammar and the other accessory subjects needed to live a Vedic life. Medicine is mentioned as a seemingly honourable profession in the Rig-Veda:

Various are the thoughts and diverse the callings of men. The carpenter seeks what is broken, the physician the diseased, the priest the Soma-presser. . . . I am a poet, my father is a physician, my mother throws the corn on the grindstone. We pursue wealth and follow our callings as the herdsman his cattle.

After the time of the Yajur-Veda, however, Brahmans were discouraged from selecting medicine as a profession. This was reinforced by the codification of religious law in the middle of the first millennium BC. Several lawgivers assert that it is as bad to eat food offered even as alms by a physician or surgeon as it is to eat the food of 'defiled' people like hunters, fowlers, whores and eunuchs. Manu, the most important among these Solons, opines that the food of a doctor is as vile as pus, and reiterates that doctors should never be allowed to attend sacrifices. Because Sushruta advises surgeons to get their instruments made of good iron from a good blacksmith, Manu also asserts that the food offered by a doctor is as filthy as that given by a blacksmith.

Manu dictated that no twice-born Hindu should ever earn his living from the practice of medicine, logic or 'poison removal', except in dire straits of penury, because these forms of knowledge are 'non-Vedic', meaning that they belong to the Atharva-Veda and not to the three approved Vedas. The Maitri Upanishad went so far as to brand the practitioners of poison removal as heretics unfit for heaven, and warns kings against listening to them. The lawgivers alloted the practice of medicine to those born of mixed marriages, specifically those between Brahman males and females from the mercantile caste.

Although pressured by the priests to conform to their theology, Ayurvedics refused to compromise on truth. Charaka advises that should anyone ask a physician which Veda he follows, he should proudly answer, 'The Atharva-Veda, because it advocates the treatment of disease'. In a section entitled 'In Praise of Physicians', Charaka writes regarding the respect paid to the Ashvins in the Rig-Veda:

If the Ashvin twins, by virtue of their office as healers, are thus held in honor by the very gods, what need then is there to say that physicians can never be honored too much by mere mortals?

As if to upbraid the Brahman lawgivers he continues:

On the completion of his studies the physician is said to be 'reborn' and acquires the title of 'physician'. For no one is a physician by right of birth. On the completion of his studies, the spirit of revelation or inspiration of the truth descends into the student. It is by reason of this initiation, then, that a physician is called a 'twice-born'.

The study of medicine is thereby placed on a par with the study of the Veda, and physicians, of whatever caste, become as 'twice-born' as Brahmans.

Professionalized medicine suffered another onslaught with the arrival of the Upanishads, which are records of discourses on the import of Vedic passages; collectively they are termed Vedanta, the 'end of the Veda' or the logical conclusion of Vedic philosophy. The composers of the Upanishads believed strongly that the only knowledge that is worthwhile is knowledge of the soul, and that all other learning, however useful, is merely a form of ignorance. They therefore had little use for medicine, since to them the body is itself merely a disease, a millstone around the neck of the immortal spirit within. Some of the Yoga Upanishads speak of human physiology and of the varieties of prana, the life-force, in the organism, but their purpose is to instruct the spiritual practitioner in how to identify and control the movements of his own prana in order to disengage his consciousness from his body and mind rather than to integrate body and mind with spirit, which is Ayurveda's goal.

The Vedas suggest that a human life be divided into four parts: the first for study, the second for working and raising a family, the third for retirement and the fourth for renunciation of the world in order to meditate continuously. Those who took Vedanta as the beginning instead of the end of the Vedic path began to advise renunciation as a way of life. Renunciates need medicine as much as anyone else, but disdain its practice for money. A new tradition of Ayurveda therefore developed in which medical knowledge was passed down from renunciate gurus to renunciate disciples for their own treatment, and for free treatment of any sick person who might come to them.

Part of the general disdain for professional doctors also arose from a visceral aversion to the commercialization of any kind of knowledge. This passage appears in the *Charaka Samhita*:

He who practices medicine out of compassion for all creatures rather than for gain or for gratification of the senses surpasses all. Those who for the sake of making a living merchandise medicine bargain for a dust-heap, letting go a heap of gold. No benefactor, moral or material, compares to the physician who by severing the noose of death in the form of fierce diseases brings back to life those being dragged towards death's abode, because there is no other gift greater than the gift of life. He who practices medicine while holding compassion for creatures as the highest religion is a man who has fulfilled his mission. He obtains supreme happiness.

Even today the general public in India, in Sri Lanka, and elsewhere in Asia revere doctors who have entered the medical profession in order to serve humanity, not to make money.

TEXT AND TRADITION

In spite of, or perhaps because of, these many forces discouraging the development of professionalized medicine in India a professional form of Ayurveda arose early and persisted. The texts of Charaka and Sushruta were written to train doctors to treat kings, princes and captains of industry, for then, as today, once fame was achieved, wealth did not lag far behind. These texts thus reflect the philosophies and goals of physicians who consciously aimed to become experts in order to succeed in life. Why no female physicians are mentioned in them is unknown. Since female seers appear in the Vedas, and since there are charms in the Atharva-Veda for attracting men, which were obviously specifically meant for use by women, the lack of female doctors is puzzling. It is possible that just as some Vedic gurus refused to accept female pupils, women were deliberately excluded by male doctors intent on preserving the 'purity' of their profession. Whatever the reason, all the renowned physicians of the Classical Age were male.

Charaka's book explains that 'women are by nature unsteady, tender, wavering, easily disturbed, and generally delicate, weak and dependent on others', but they have an Ayurvedic tradition of their own, a tradition of herbal first-aid for common childhood diseases, transmitted from mother to daughter, which is known in the region near Bombay as 'grandmother's purse' in honour of the medicinal herbs grandmothers used to keep in purses on the kitchen wall. While this medical tradition, like those of the renunciates and of special-interest groups such as bone-setters and *vaidus* (lower-class practitioners who know a few specific herbs, minerals and animal products for use in a few specific diseases), remains mainly oral, the vast majority of Ayurvedic texts belong to Ayurveda's Classical or professional tradition.

Unlike its ritual counterpart, the medical tradition has never been particularly resistant to change. Over the centuries mainstream Ayurvedic beliefs and practices have deviated substantially from those of the ancient texts. Indian spiritual tradition, and everything that has been derived from it, has always been dynamically balanced between orthodoxy and innovation, between the primacy of the mainstream and the legitimacy of individual experience. Whenever a trend becomes petrified, a counter-trend appears to shake it out of its smugness.

Often charismatic individuals codify their experience into theories and practices, and if enough followers are attracted, this individual system becomes a sect and develops its own orthodoxy, as did Buddhism. There have been many systems and schools of Ayurveda, though only a few have survived to the present day. Actually, because Ayurveda is such an individualized science, there should be as many schools as there are physicians; ideally, each doctor carves out his own niche in the world of therapeutics. This personalization of medical theory extends to patients as well; each doctor was and is expected to tailor a different treatment for each sufferer. Such detailed individual care does not often occur in practice today, and may never have been common, but the intent is clear.

Despite the great changes that have refashioned Ayurveda since its genesis, the ancient texts remain the best guide to what is or is not Ayurvedic. Of these texts, a verse states: 'Madhava is best in diagnosis, and Vagbhata in aphorisms. Sushruta is superior in anatomy, and Charaka excels in internal medicine.' Madhava and Vagbhata wrote nearly two millennia later than Charaka and Sushruta, and were greatly indebted to the two older works. Vagbhata's *Ashtanga Hrdaya* is the text of choice for many modern Ayurvedic physicians precisely because it is a concise condensation of the essence of the earlier texts. Sushruta differs from Charaka mainly in his argument that surgery is the best medicine because it produces instantaneous actions and immediate results, and on certain technical points. Charaka, who clearly states that he believes surgery to be as important as internal medicine, has a rather more evenhanded approach to his subject.

The *Charaka Samhita* is truly the primary Ayurvedic text, though it is difficult to know how much of Charaka's original has survived the ministrations of the various editors and revisers. Drdhabala, who lived some time during the early centuries AD and was the major reconstructor of Charaka's text says, 'The reconstructor creates anew an ancient treatise', and there is certainly nothing to prevent such an individual from altering the text wherever he thinks fit while attributing the changes to the original author.

Treatises in other disciplines have been shown to have been amended by interested parties, and it is likely that both the *Charaka* and *Sushruta Samhita* have also been tampered with.

For example, when we find a passage like this in the *Sushruta*: 'Ayurveda with its eight limbs is revealed by Brahma as a discipline subsidiary to the Veda. Hence the doctor, aware of his own role, must act in subservience to the priest', we can be relatively sure that this is an interpolation. And when we read in the *Charaka* that seeing Dravidas and Andhrakas, who are inhabitants of southern India, in a dream is as inauspicious as seeing vultures, owls, dogs, crows, demons, ghosts, women and untouchables, there is little doubt that this was written by a bigoted northern Indian Brahman attempting to extend his bigotry to doctors, who were, however, expected to view all their patients, regardless of race or caste, with an equal eye.

Official orthodoxy undoubtedly forced some ancient Indian scientists to write conformity into their texts, but every reference to the other-worldly is not a later addition, and one can only speculate on which was which. Was it fear of reprisal that made Brahmagupta, a renowned Indian astrologer, repeat at the beginning of his treatise the myth that eclipses are created when a cosmic serpent tries to swallow the sun or the moon, before quietly tucking into the body of his work formulae for the calculation of those very eclipses? Or did he perhaps include the myth to provide continuity with previous treatises or to remind his readers of hidden esoteric meanings, or did all these considerations weigh upon his mind? There is little way to be sure. As Charaka himself puts it, 'Many are the ways in which an author expresses his ideas, so the meaning of a text can be determined only after due appreciation of the context of the particular place and time in question, the intention of the author and the technicalities of the science.'

Whoever the author and whatever the interpolations, the *Charaka Samhita* is a monumental work, being about three times in bulk what survives of the corpus of Hippocratic medicine. Its 120 chapters are grouped into eight sections, or *sthana*.

I *Sutra* ('aphorism') *Sthana*   Thirty chapters on Ayurveda's origin, general principles, philosophy and theories.

II *Nidana* ('diagnosis') *Sthana* Eight chapters on the causes and symptoms of diseases.

III *Vimana* ('measure') *Sthana* Eight chapters on many subjects, including physiology, methodology and medical ethics.

IV *Sharira* ('body') *Sthana* Eight chapters on anatomy and embryology, and on metaphysics and ethics.

V *Indriya* ('sense organ') *Sthana* Twelve chapters on prognosis.

VI *Chikitsa* ('treatment') *Sthana* Thirty chapters on therapeutics.

VII *Kalpa* ('preparation') *Sthana* Twelve chapters on pharmacy.

VIII *Siddhi* ('success') *Sthana* Twelve chapters on purification therapy.

THE TRAINING OF A PHYSICIAN

In an essay called 'The Risks of Being Treated by a Quack' Charaka emphasizes that only a well-educated physician approved by the guild of physicians should be allowed to treat one's person. Ideally, people look after their own health, but when imbalances beyond their ability to manage develop, patients are advised not to be led astray by the exaggerated claims of smooth operators who, having accidentally cured one patient, treat every other patient with precisely the same therapy, loudly trumpeting their successes and quietly burying their failures. Quacks were apparently plentiful 3,000 years ago, just as they are today.

In that era the process of preparing expert physicians began with self-examination. An intelligent individual weighed the difficulties and obligations of medical practice against the rewards obtainable therefrom, and if he found himself suitable for the study of medicine, he then selected a text for study. Charaka observes that there are many medical treatises current in the world, and that all texts are not equal. Thinking perhaps of the strengths of his own volume, he suggests that only that treatise should be chosen that is widely popular, approved by the wise, comprehensive, fit for all students no matter how intelligent they might be, revealed by a seer, well and logically arranged and authenticated without repetition, free of vulgar usages and obscure terms, relevant, filled with definitions and illustrations, and concerned mainly with elucidating the true nature of things.

Ayurvedic texts like the *Charaka Samhita* are not the compendia of exhaustive detail that are modern medical texts; rather, they are books of sutras, pithy aphorisms that encapsulate the essence of the lore in a minimum of words, with 'memorial' verses at the end of each chapter to recapitulate the teaching and reaffirm its authority. These sutras and memorial verses are mnemonics, memory-enhancing devices, which are often couched in simple poetic metre to make their memorization easier. The sutras of the Ayurvedic texts are florid compared with those of other subjects, whose writers dedicated themselves to cramming the maximum information into the minimum words. It is said that a sincere sutra writer would rather lose one of his own sons than add a single syllable to one of his sutras.

Because the text itself is so spare, it is always studied with a commentary written by an expert that elucidates the meanings of its cryptic passages; for example, the most famous commentator on Charaka's compilation was the eleventh-century writer Chakrapani. Charaka's text itself is a commentary on the sutras of Atreya, which were collected, compiled and probably commented upon by Agnivesha. In the text-commentary system the bare facts of the science become laminated with layers of interpretation by eminent physicians from century to century, preserving their expertise and permitting the tradition to grow and change to keep pace with growth and change in the external environment.

Traditionally, Ayurvedic study follows the Vedic method of learning: memorization of the text and study of its commentary, with further glosses and practical hints added by the teacher. Until recent times the Vedas were never written down; they existed only in the memories of the Brahmans. The Vedic system of education is advantageous in the Ayurvedic context because medical knowledge is vast and the human mind is limited in what it can recall quickly under pressure. When a physician diagnoses a patient and mentally repeats the sutras relating to the disease and its treatment, that memory provides access to everything else on the subject the physician has ever learned. It is an elegant and effective way to index information.

After selecting the text, the prospective student began his search for an expert to teach him how to understand its import. 'Weapons, learning and water are wholly dependent for their merits and demerits on their holder', observes Charaka. 'Hence it is the understanding that should first of all be rendered immaculate and worthy of holding the knowledge of medicine.' Elsewhere he adds,

The whole of suffering which cleaves to mind and body has ignorance for its basis and, conversely, all happiness is founded in clear scientific knowledge. However, this very knowledge of mighty import is no illumination to those who are devoid of understanding, as is the sun to those who have lost their eyesight.

Charaka writes that a good teacher is skilful, upright, pure, a knower of human nature, free from self-conceit, envy and irascibility, endowed with fortitude and affection toward his pupils and able to clear all the disciple's doubts because of his special insight into the science. It is not surprising that this definition is almost identical with the definition of a good physician given elsewhere in the text, for only a good physician knows how to teach medicine.

Once the pupil settled on an instructor, it became the guru's turn to test. During a six-month period of probation the teacher identified the student's strengths and weaknesses and ensured that he was peaceable, noble, persevering, intelligent, devoted to truth, modest and gentle; free of egotism, irritability, addictions of any kind, covetousness and sloth; pure, skilful, courteous, single-minded in devotion to knowledge, desirous of the welfare of all creatures, obedient to all the instructions of his teacher and devoted to his mentor. If the disciple was found fit, he was then ritually initiated. The lengthy oath of initiation emphasized the importance placed on individual inquiry: 'There is no limit at all to the Science of Life. . . . The entire world is the teacher to the intelligent and the foe to the unintelligent.'

The guru–disciple relationship was thus originally marked by a high degree of mutuality. At the outset each tested the other; once instruction began, each taught the other, the guru learning more about humans and human nature with each student taught. The bond between guru and disciple was much stronger than the bond that exists today between teacher and student, because today instruction has become an article of commerce. In the past the disciple was expected to respect the guru as much as, or more than, his own parents, because the guru caused the disciple to be 'reborn'. Often the disciple lived in the preceptor's home like one of his children; the word for a teacher's academy, *gurukula*, literally means 'guru's family'. By tradition, all teaching was free of charge, but at the end of the many years of study the disciple was expected to offer *guru dakshina*, any gift that his guru might request, in exchange for the gift of knowledge.

The intense emotional relationship between guru and disciple made it easier for knowledge to be transmitted from the one to the other, and discouraged the student from indulging in idle pastimes. The strict but affectionate discipline that the guru instilled was easier to tolerate than that imposed by an impersonal authority, and it exemplified for the disciple the attitude of loving firmness with which a physician was expected to treat his patients.

The guru also elucidated for the disciple the spiritual aspects of the study. The study of any branch of knowledge is traditionally considered a *sadhana*, a spiritual practice, which, if followed sincerely and persistently, takes one to 'the peace which passeth all understanding'. A good disciple respects his or her own guru like God, and extends this respect to the other members of the guru's lineage. One family in Kerala, whose hereditary vocation has for centuries been the practice of medicine, still performs ritual worship to Vagbhata, whose book, *Ashtanga Hrdaya*, is their Ayurvedic bible.

The student recited text and commentary, and the guru solved difficulties and transmitted trade secrets. On occasion the disciples would sit together with the guru to ask questions, and he would respond by expounding on the various points of view that had previously been proposed by other authorities, concluding with the point of view he felt worthiest. Experts also used to meet together for seminars on specific subjects; Charaka preserved the proceedings of a few of these conferences in his tome. Sometimes debates were organized between proponents of opposing views. Debate reinforced the students' facility with the laws of rhetoric and so helped to clarify their understanding, and provided them with opportunities to learn new things from opponents. Winning a debate improved one's reputation. These disputations were conducted according to strict rules including, as in modern debate, the definition of numerous fallacies that would immediately defeat one's case.

Debates between physicians were restricted to three subjects: medicine, sacrificial ritual and spiritual philosophy. The use of arguments from one context in a different context was prohibited, in consonance with the doctors' view that idle spiritual theorizing should not intrude in questions of therapeutics. Students were advised not to assault the wise with casuistry, but rather to demolish those pretentious fellows who pose as experts with any appropriate quibble:

One should not suffer foolish, obstreperous disputants of little learning, not from any consideration of oneself but with a view to keeping the light of the knowledge unobscured. Those whose compassion for all creatures is great and who are devoted to truth are ever zealous to put down false doctrines.

Religious doctrines are handed down from on high; Ayurvedic doctrines arise from the fertilization of empirical observation by theory. A false doctrine is one that works against the healing forces of Nature: 'A science, if badly handled, destroys its user like a poorly handled weapon destroys its inept user, while the same science or weapon when rightly handled becomes a source of succour.'

Debate was encouraged to help create inquiring minds willing to rebel against dogma that could not be substantiated in fact, because a scientific system of medicine must be based on logical reasoning. Says Charaka, 'Any success achieved without the exercise of reason is indeed success resulting from chance.' Boastful opponents deserved to meet defeat in debate because they lacked the skill in treatment that sets the well-trained physician apart from the quack. Idle questioning without practical value was, however, permissible solely to discomfit such charlatans; as the seer Atreya admonished his fellow sages after one seminar:

Truth is hard to find by taking sides in a debate. Those who advance arguments and counter-arguments as if they were finalities never arrive at any conclusion, going round and round like the man who sits on an oil-press. Letting go of this wordy warfare, then, apply your minds to the essential truth.

A doctor should think for himself, using tradition as a spring-board from which to plunge into new researches rather than slav-ishly following previous usages. A doctor's highest responsibility is the health of his patients, and a lifelong willingness to learn new theoretical approaches and therapeutic techniques is his greatest obligation. To use a 3,000-year-old Ayurvedic metaphor, just as a bird needs two wings to fly, the 'bird' of medicine requires the two wings of theory and practice. To learn the fundamental principles of a lore and then to master one of its aspects is to achieve two 'wings', two dimensions of knowledge. The third dimension, the 'tail' of the bird of medicine, which steers it through the air, is the relationship the disciple develops with his guru, which, hopefully, becomes the model for all his future relationships. The image these three dimensions define grows and matures with time and the fledgling's own experiences until it manifests as competence.

Ayurveda requires both logic and hands-on experience, two of the practices the lawgivers found most reprehensible, because it follows a path in which empirical knowledge is the most important proof of a postulate. Logic alone is insufficient for therapeutic success; Sushruta declares: 'A learned physician must never try to examine on grounds of pure logic the efficacy of a medicine, which is known by direct observation as having by nature a specific medical action.'

The word 'surgery' comes from the Greek word meaning 'manual operation', and Sushruta emphasizes that of all surgical instruments the hand is the most important, because all other instruments are useless without it. For the purpose of creating skilled hands students dissected human corpses to learn about anatomical structures, and practised the arts of surgery, such as extraction and incision, on dummies, melons, animal bladders, cadaver skin, dead animals and lotus stems. Sushruta describes in detail the method of corpse dissection. You take a corpse that is not missing any of its parts, is not superannuated and did not die of poisoning or chronic disease. After removing its bowels and their contents, you wrap the corpse in a shroud and soak it in a swiftly flowing stream for seven days. Then you scrub it slowly with a brush to display all the under-lying structures. Knowing corpse dissection to be an essential part of medical training, Sushruta courageously advocated it despite inevitable opprobrium, since the lawgivers regarded the touch of a corpse as supremely defiling.

Ayurvedic students also learned other practical arts, such as cookery, since diet was an essential aspect of treatment; the preparation of medicines, including the brewing of medicinal wines; horticulture, with grafting; the purification and preparation of minerals as medicines; and the various methods of combining ingredients into drugs. Doctors were expected to be wanderers, taking the assistance of forest-dwelling tribals and cow-, sheep- and goatherds to identify and collect medicinal substances personally, for which purpose they had to know the characteristics of the various types of soil (which affect the characteristics of the herbs grown there), the time when each plant should be collected and the parts to collect. While all students learned the basics of all the various divisions of Ayurveda, each usually specialized in one of Ayurveda's eight 'limbs': internal medicine; surgery; eye, ear and nose; gynaecology, obstetrics and paediatrics; psychology; toxicology; rejuvenation; and virilization.

At the end of the period of study, whether in a university, the guru's home or a jungle, the disciple was thoroughly tested, sometimes comprehensively, as in Jivaka's case, sometimes more randomly. At Mithila in the thirteenth century the student stood before examiners who used a probe to skewer one of the pages of the text and asked questions on the subject matter on it. After passing his exam, a young physician was entitled to call himself *vaidya*, the Sanskrit word for physician, which literally means 'one who knows'. He then sought the king's permission to practise, and when this was granted, the Physician's Oath was administered. The Ayurvedic Physician's Oath reads much like the Hippocratic Oath; it is a list of the rules of conduct a physician is expected to follow, among them being: 'Better to suffer the effects of snake venom or to be burned by hot iron rather than to demand money from a poor person as a condition for treatment.' The guru, recluses, sages, Brahman priests, the helpless and one's friends were always to be treated free.

Although upwardly mobile Ayurvedic physicians of the classical era ministered mainly to the affluent, most probably regarded medicine as a sacred calling. When Ayurveda lost official government patronage in most of India after various invasions, it was kept alive mainly by Brahman families, who, despite the strictures of the lawgivers, were, and are, proud of their spiritual and professional traditions, often trying to reconcile their caste and their calling by such strategems as refusing to touch the patient themselves so as to retain some of their purity, leaving the execution of their instructions to technicians of lower caste.

THE MODERN AGE

India's people daily talk, knowingly or not, in the Ayurvedic idiom. Even the most illiterate resident of the most remote village knows that yoghurt causes phlegm to accumulate in the chest, and everyone makes regular use of simple herbs like vetiver (cuscus), which removes 'heat' from the body and makes life during the hot season a little more bearable. I have casually debated whether castor oil is 'hot' or 'cold' in the office of a Bombay lawyer, and have received unsolicited dietary and therapeutic advice from total strangers. Ayurvedic thought is part of the conceptual universe of every Indian who thinks like an Indian, and has been part of India's collective consciousness since, probably, prehistoric times.

One of the few scholars who has understood something of the impact of Ayurvedic reality on southern Asian culture is Carolyn Nordstrom, who has studied Ayurveda on the island of Sri Lanka. Nordstrom finds that in Sri Lanka, as I have found in India, people use the Ayurvedic 'humours' or metabolic forces to describe themselves and their society. Some compare the political system to a body, and the political parties to the body's humours. As with a human body, as long as these humours are balanced, all will be well in the body politic, but when one humour gains ascendancy and begins to dominate, abuses are inevitable, resulting in a disease. A 'cancer on society' is more than a simile; it is an expression of a deeper-than-usual reality, a statement that cancer in a human and cancer in a human organization ultimately proceed from the same sort of causes and are curable by the same sort of methods.

Such metaphors pervade the speech of even those who are completely ignorant of the system of Ayurveda *per se*. Nordstrom explains why:

The basic philosophies of Ayurveda provide a series of metaphors that are applicable to any major conceptual system characterized by balance and disorder, health and disease. Thus Ayurveda does/ not exist simply as a medical tradition, nor is it confined solely to the discourse of medicine. On one level, this popular body of knowledge provides a mechanism for integrating the various traditions of health care into a coherent encompassing framework for patients. In addition, the impact of Ayurveda extends beyond issues of illness and health . . . to provide an explanatory framework capable of synthesizing the many facets of Sri Lankan life, and concepts drawn from this body of theory are used to explain that life itself.

Ayurvedic metaphors have persisted because they help to illustrate reality on every level, not merely on the level of physical health. Ayurveda is more than a medical system; it is a state of mind. Only one who understands the internal reality of Ayurvedic thought can fully appreciate the words of the Sri Lankan woman who, seeing rain fall after a long drought said, 'Look, it is health.'

Medicine in India is not now and never has been the exclusive province of physicians, though physicians have often attempted to arrogate that privilege to themselves. Even today there are thousands of otherwise non-medical people all over India who have somehow learned a diagnostic or treatment method and regularly use it to alleviate suffering. For example, one man who used to sell fruit on a Bombay street was also well known in our locality for his ability to diagnose disease by just looking at a sample of the patient's urine. Another man in a different part of Bombay brews up a single product, a decoction used in liver ailments, and dispenses it free to everyone who asks for it.

Most of today's professionalized Ayurvedic doctors have become wholly body-oriented; one study showed that villagers in the state of Maharashtra often knowingly or unknowingly describe mental illness in Ayurvedic terms but rarely even think of approaching an Ayurvedic physician for its treatment. Ayurveda remains a living tradition because it is itself alive, a living being that integrates into the consciousness of living beings, flowing from guru into disciple. To learn the details of the science without first having the tradition awakened and enlivened within yourself is to try to practise 'the science of life' with dead knowledge.

The fate of Ayurveda is distinct from the fate of those who aspire to employ it in practice. Physicians come and go, but Ayurveda is eternal; it is the universal healing art, which has always existed and will persist until the destruction of the universe. While its manifestations arise and disappear, the living tradition remains. In spite of doctors who do not want to practise it and patients who do not want to be treated by it, Ayurveda persists in the lives of the people, living on even in those who are unaware of it, flourishing whenever physicians appear who make its tradition theirs, because its existence is independent of those who wield it.

2

BASIC PRINCIPLES

As the science of life, Ayurveda is applicable to every living thing. While modern science has limited the definition of life to embodied beings, the Vedic sciences recognize that many more beings in the universe possess life than most of us realize, one of them being Ayurveda itself. While modern researchers have finally begun to realize that Earth behaves like a living organism, the Vedic seers went even further, maintaining that, like Earth, every planet and every star is a living, conscious being, and that all natural forces – wind, fire, death, and the like – are living, conscious beings.

The foundation of Vedic thought is the conviction that the entire cosmos, manifested and unmanifested, is part of one singular Absolute. This Absolute Reality cannot be accurately described in human language, because it contains everything and possesses all possible qualities; all representations of this singularity represent only part of its totality, just as the various blind men could only comprehend portions of that elusive elephant. 'Truth is singular; the wise speak of it in various ways,' says a Vedic proverb, and all disciplines are varied paths that lead ultimately to this common point of origin, the unity of all existence.

One of the ways in which the Vedic seers attempted to describe their experience of the indescribable was to call it *satyam*, *rtam*, *brhat*: 'the true, the harmonious, the vast'. Reality exists (it is true); it has a natural order or rhythm, which is self-perpetuating and self-correcting (it is harmonious); and it is all-pervasive, extending beyond the farthest reaches of the human imagination (it is vast). Even the gods must act in accordance with this cosmic order, and when they do not, they too suffer; the universe does not play favourites.

According to the Law of the Microcosm and Macrocosm,

everything that exists in the vast external universe, the macrocosm, also appears in the internal cosmos of the human body, the microcosmic universe of 50–100 million million cells, which, when healthy, is harmonious, self-perpetuating and self-correcting. Charaka says, 'Man is the epitome of the universe. There is in man as much diversity as in the world outside, and there is in the world as much diversity as in man.' When the individual becomes aligned with the universe, the lesser cosmos functions as a harmonious unit of the greater.

This perspective is no abstraction to the people of southern Asia; it is a fundamental plank in their personal reality. Most do not draw sharp philosophical distinctions between themselves as individuals and the environment in which they live because in their societies individuals are not distinguished as parts that can be isolated from the whole. This is as true of that grand society of stars and planets that is the universe as it is true of any human society; both are made up of, and continually redefined by, their constituent parts. A healthy system is made up of healthy units functioning together in a healthy relationship, and so the well-being of a particular individual cannot be separated from the well-being of the community, the land, the supernatural world or the cosmos. There is no individual so individual that he or she does not interact with the environment.

Because each one of us, to whatever extent, by our actions influences the entire cosmos for good or ill, health maintenance is transformed from one of life's electives into a religious and social imperative. A young doctor's ambition to treat kings and merchant princes is a noble one, to the extent that it is motivated by the desire to improve the health of society by improving the health of its rulers. The king is the epitome of his kingdom, and so in a sense treatment of the king is equivalent to treatment of the entire society, because when the king is healthy, he will rule well and society will benefit in a sort of 'trickle-down' effect.

Just as a human being is a living microcosm of the universe, the universe is a living macrocosm of a human being. The Absolute Singularity is a supreme being; we might call him or her God. Every part of God's body (the universe) is as alive as every cell of our bodies is alive; neither can the parts live without the whole, nor the whole without the parts. The Absolute *exists* permanently, even when the universe resolves back into it; but it can *live*, and enjoy its life, only when it takes on a body.

The goal of the Vedic religion is to define, create and maintain a harmonious relationship between macrocosm and microcosm; the final end of the Vedic path, union with the Absolute, is achievable only after establishing right relationship with the Relative. The One exists in All, and the All defines the One; unity and duality exist simultaneously because, like the two faces of a coin, one cannot exist without the other. Absolute characteristics simply do not exist in our world of dualities; except for seers and saints, we all experience only one of the many possible states of relative truth.

Most of us view the world in polarized terms; truth must be clear and unequivocal for us to see it as true. The Semitic religions and the Greek thinkers have taught us Westerners an absolute version of duality. Even the Greek medical gods were two: Hygieia, in charge of creating health, and Asclepius, in charge of curing disease. Because of this we can easily see life as one way or another, but it is extremely difficult for us to see life as One-in-All and All-in-One simultaneously. The mechanists believe that mind had no influence whatsoever on body; even now most who do acknowledge this influence still cannot conceive of any sort of fundamental *identity* of mind and body.

India's culture sees issues not as black *or* white, but as black *and* white, and all shades of grey in between, making it easier to 'see' some of the conundrums that do not fit comfortably into the current scientific model of life. A fixed idea of the individuality of sentient beings, for example, fails to explain how a social insect like a bee or an ant can have an individual body while behaving as a mere extension of the unified consciousness that is the hive. One species of bacteria actually hunts cooperatively in teams, surrounding prey, trapping it and digesting it with enzymes. Is a single bacterium from such a colony an individual or is it one cell of a larger organism? Dilemmas like these, which include the famous conundrum of light (which is neither a particle nor a wave but behaves as either according to how one looks at it), are inherently paradoxical in our type of logic.

People who are exceptionally well adapted to life in our world are sometimes described as demonstrating 'biphasic' traits; they are, for example, both tough and gentle, serious and playful, introspective and outgoing, and so on. They intuitively understand the folly of clinging tenaciously to a single approach to life; instead they shift approaches, expressing one trait strongly and making it stand out in relief against the other, as the need arises, even though such behaviour can appear logically contradictory when viewed through our strictly dualistic spectacles. The genius of Indian thought has always been its flexibility, its ability to adapt to, and comfortably accommodate, the paradoxical. It can do so because its language is the biphasic language of paradox, not the linear language of modern science, which forces each word to conform to a specific and limited meaning.

THE UNIVERSE, EXTERNAL
AND INTERNAL

Biphasic language makes it impossible to separate the myth from the history of Ayurveda. The ancient Greeks, the forebears of Western logic, strove to clearly delineate separate human and divine realities by separating the historical from the mythic. Other cultures chose to sacrifice crisp linear historical dating in order to emphasize the inalienable bonds that link humanity and divinity. 'For the Mayans,' writes Dennis Tedlock, the translator of the Mayan story of creation, the *Popul Vuh*, 'the presence of a divine dimension in narratives of human affairs is not an imperfection but a necessity, and it is balanced by a necessary human dimension in narratives of divine affairs.' To isolate the other-worldly and the mundane aspects of reality is to ignore the all-important relationship that exists between the two. The creation myth with which the Classical Ayurvedic texts begin cannot be dismissed as a priestly insertion, for the story of the creation of the universe is also the story of Ayurveda's creation and the creation of every living being.

One of the Sanksrit words for the cosmos is *jagat*, 'the moving thing'. In the Ayurvedic model the universe is declared to be eternal and without beginning, continuously moving, periodically manifesting from a singularity and periodically resolving into unmanifestation, waxing and waning like the moon. A human being likewise begins from a zygote, a single cell containing all his or her potentialities, which explosively projects those potentialities into a physical form that, like the universe and its individual stars, grows and develops, reaches a stable plateau and then degenerates and dies.

The singularity that creates the cosmos is, like a zygote or the seed of a tree, the cause of the dualistic being it creates, which is the effect. In the words of my teacher, Vimalananda, 'Cause is effect concealed, and effect is cause revealed': the effect is concealed within the cause until the process that reveals its entirety to view is set in motion. In no way can we explain cause as separate from effect; they flow into one another because they are two time-varied states of the same thing. The principal difference is that both a zygote and its resultant human are impermanent, whereas the cause of the universe is eternal and only its effect is impermanent.

As Charaka tells it, Ayurveda appeared in our world when a number of great sages, motivated by compassion for humans whose lives were being disturbed by disease, especially those who were dwellers in towns and cities (suggesting that the dangers of urbanization were apparent even then), met and said to themselves, 'Health is the supreme foundation of virtue, prosperity, enjoyment and salvation, while diseases are the destroyers of health, of the good in life and of life itself. What is the means of remedying this great impediment to humanity's progress?' Meditating on this point, they obtained Ayurveda from the gods and translated this divine knowledge into human language, and since then human specialists have had charge of preserving and transmitting its wisdom.

Ayurveda's extraordinary seers had so developed their own awarenesses that they learned how to commune with the forces that run the universe, but they realized that very few people are capable of mustering up the stringent discipline that such communion requires, and so they thrust Ayurveda into incarnation. The eternal, divine knowledge that is Ayurveda is still available to whomever is able to locate and obtain it; for everyone else there is the seers' version, which deals specifically with the problems of embodied life on Earth. Charaka states:

This science of life is declared to be eternal, because it has no beginning, because it deals with tendencies which proceed innately from Nature, and because the nature of matter is eternal. For at no time was there a break either in the continuity of life or in the continuity of intelligence. The experience of life is perennial. . . . At no time can it be said that the science of life sprang into existence having been non-existent before, unless the dissemination of knowledge by means of receiving and imparting instruction be considered as creation of such knowledge.

The knowledge of Ayurveda is an integral part of the universal reality and manifests with each manifestation of the universe. In this sense it is eternal; but as everything that is manifested is impermanent, each manifestation of Ayurveda is impermanent, and so Ayurveda is simultaneously eternal and non-eternal.

The rishis, who are the seers of the Vedas, spent their lives contemplating the beauty of the simultaneous absoluteness and relativity of existence; in unguarded moments of exaltation their bliss escaped into verbal incarnation. These limited expressions of unlimited reality became the Vedic hymns. The seers of Ayurveda did likewise, channelling their individual experiences of the dual/non-dual nature of reality into the flow of their work. Each Ayurvedic text is a unique expression of the reality of life as expressed by a living being, which explains why all the texts do not agree on every detail. Facts are only the raw material from which life is created; a sage collects the dead, dry 'facts' of life and transmits his own life-force into them to create a living text, just as the Creator's touch sets in motion the cosmic spheres. Each sage creates and brings to life the cosmos of living knowledge that is his text.

SANSKRIT

Because the knowledge a science tries to express is moulded, consciously or unconsciously, by the language in which it is expounded, the Sanskrit language is integral to the Ayurvedic experience. English is an excellent vehicle for scientific analysis, the breaking up of larger structures into smaller ones and the description of the tiny fragments thus produced. Sanskrit, a language in which each word has many possible seemingly disparate but actually related meanings, is the definitive tongue for synthesizing and demonstrating the relationships that join tiny fragments together into larger structures. While languages like English can efficiently express specific facts, Sanskrit is unsurpassed for conveying generic truth, for which reason computer scientists study it today as part of their efforts to create artificial intelligence. Only those physicians who know Sanskrit can truly claim to know Ayurveda, no matter how much empirical knowledge they may accumulate.

Any version of Ayurveda in English is therefore bound to do it some disservice. Part of its essence will escape and dissipate, and description of that essence will have to suffice. Just as one must attempt to preserve the tone of a poem when rendering it into another tongue, retention of the 'flavour' of Ayurveda and its Sanskrit is critical when casting it into modern forms of expression. Most technical Sanskrit terms in this book have been translated into close English equivalents, but those words that express meanings that cannot be adequately or easily translated have been retained, and defined, to protect the life of the information.

CREATION

Before creation all that exists is *Purusha*, homogeneous spirit beyond time, space and causation, a single point, which, however, encompasses everything. All potentialities exist within this singularity, but none manifest until desire spontaneously arises: 'Let me manifest individuals, that they may perceive and know me.' In the moment this desire occurs, the instant of the 'Big Bang', the cosmos springs into existence by a process of evolution. We cannot speak of the cosmos separate from the *Purusha*, nor of the *Purusha* separate from the cosmos. *Purusha* is cause and cosmos is effect.

Vedic sacrifices, which are meant to establish order in both macrocosm and microcosm, take their inspiration from the great god Prajapati, the embodiment of reality's creative aspect, who at the beginning of time sacrificed himself; from his body the cosmos was created. Ritual sacrifice reconstructs Prajapati and resuscitates him, establishing divinity, and thus order, in the universe at large and on Earth in particular. A Vedic hymn called the 'Purusha Sukta' details this transformation: our sun came from the eyes of this cosmic person, our moon from his mind, fire from his mouth, wind from his breath, air from his navel, the sky from his head, the earth from his feet, and so on.

A human individual also arises from a sacrifice, on a smaller scale. When a man, the microcosmic Prajapati, sacrifices his semen into the fire that is a woman, a new microcosm springs into being. The desire that causes these two people to be overcome with the craving to unite sexually is a reflected fragment of that original desire that caused the universe to give birth to duality. The laws of thermodynamics, and especially the law of entropy, which states that systems always tend to proceed toward a state of less and less organization, discourage the development of embodied life; yet life developed, through the power of *Purusha*'s desire, which released sufficient energy to overcome the entropic tendency.

Desire is the foundation of macrocosm and microcosm. It exists in every atom of creation, because each atom is a fragment of that original person who experienced that desire to experience. In our world this desire is minimal in rocks and other 'inert' matter, and maximal in humans, but it exists everywhere, just as consciousness exists everywhere. As earthly organisms ascend the evolutionary ladder, the quality of their consciousness improves until it reaches the human, the living being that (thus far) has evolved the most sophisticated form of consciousness. Each cell in the human body partakes, to some extent, of this consciousness; each cell is aware and communicates with every other cell. To paraphrase Charaka, life is awareness. The creation of the macrocosm generated both the (relatively) unconscious physical matter and the consciousness that dwells within it, just as creation of the microcosm generates the relatively unconscious body and the conscious mind and spirit that dwell within it.

Before creation only *Purusha*, the Absolute, exists. When desire first disrupts the absoluteness of the Absolute, *prakriti*, or nature, the matrix of the manifested universe, evolves. Nature is a seamless consciousness, which differs from *Purusha* only in the conviction that it is different; its sense of separateness is the foundation of all existence. When *prakriti* becomes aware of its existence, it evolves into the state of undifferentiated transcendent intelligence or cosmic consciousness known as *mahat*. This intelligence then develops an atomized form aware of its individuality and differentiates itself into individual bundles of *ahamkara*, or ego.

Ahamkara means, literally, 'I-creator', the force that produces 'I-ness' in an organism. I-ness is itself paradoxical: the sense of individuality, separateness from all else in the cosmos, divides us from the unity of life, but without it there is no life, because only *ahamkara* can cause all the disparate parts of a being to relate to each other as part of the same separate but unified organism. The word '*aham*' is derived from *a* and *ha*, the first and the last letters of the Sanskrit alphabet, its alpha and omega. *Ahamkara* is thus the expression on an individual level of the totality of all potential manifestation; precisely how this manifestation occurs depends upon context.

Ahamkara has three *gunas*, or attributes: *sattva* (equilibrium), *rajas* (activity) and *tamas* (inertia). *Rajas*, 'I' as action, represents waves of kinetic energy, while *tamas*, 'I' as unconscious being, produces objective particles of potential energy (otherwise known as matter). The objectivity of *tamas* evolves into the five objects of the senses – sound, touch, form, taste and odour – which, in turn, produce the Five Great Elements that make up the physical universe: ether, air, fire, water and earth.

Sattva, which is 'I' as conscious being, is the subjective consciousness that perceives and manipulates matter and energy. Its subjectivity develops into the mind and the ten senses, the five senses of cognition – hearing, touch, sight, taste and smell – through which we take in information from the world, and the five senses of action, with which we express ourselves in the world: speech (which symbolizes all forms of communication), hands (which symbolize creative action), feet (locomotion), genitals (reproduction) and anus (elimination).

Embodied life is defined as the functioning as one unit in one place at one time of the Five Great Elements, the five cognitive senses with their objects plus the five active senses, the thinking mind, the ego and the intellect, and the individual soul, a fragment of the cosmic *Purusha*, which is also called *purusha*. All the principles that compose the universe thus appear in an embodied being. Embodied life refers mainly, but is not limited, to embodied human life; texts on the Ayurveda of trees, horses and elephants still exist, and may have existed for such varied animals as cows, goats, sheep, donkeys, camels and hawks.

Though consciousness is less active in lower animals and in plants, it is still present; awareness is omnipresent in the world of life. Researchers have conclusively demonstrated that plants feel fear, pain and other emotions, and it has recently been discovered that trees can warn one another of danger by releasing chemicals called pheromones into the air. The cells of your body likewise commonly think and communicate chemically; their consciousness is more automatic and less independent than is your overall consciousness, of which they form a part.

The quality of your awareness depends upon the functioning within your consciousness of *sattva*, *rajas* and *tamas*, which work by mutual suppression: whichever is strongest at any one instant expresses itself and suppresses the others. *Sattva* is 'I' as subject; *tamas*, 'I' as object; and *rajas*, 'I' as the action that connects subject with object. No ultimate distinction can be drawn between subject, object and action, as all are manifestations of *ahamkara*; they are all fundamentally identical and appear to differ only because of their relative positions. Which is subject and which object in any particular situation depends upon perspective, and can be accurately expressed only by reference to all three aspects: the figure, its background and the relationship between the two. Duality is comprehensible only with reference to how its two phases, perceiver and perceived, interact.

Because consciousness is omnipresent, there is no external permanency in the world immune to the influence of thought. As we believe, so we become, and so our world becomes as well. Our cosmos is influenced by the consciousness of all its inhabitants, the most important of whom is its creator, whose conceptualizing is stronger than the limited, hesitant imaginations of most human beings. When Jesus said that whoever has the faith of a mustard seed can move mountains, he meant that if you can conceptualize with sufficient energy, whatever you imagine will certainly come to pass. Each moment each of us regenerates our own individual realities. *Ahamkara* redefines you by disengaging from the old and embracing the new in a continual re-establishment of self. Each of your thoughts affects your organism; how strongly you hold to your past conceptions determines how long they will limit your future possibilities.

The potential for positive thoughts is unlimited, while an old fable illustrates just how dangerous negative thoughts can be. Once a man, fatigued after a long walk through the jungle, sat down under a shady tree and thought idly to himself, 'If only I had a mango right now, how happy I would be!'

Suddenly a mango dropped into his lap. He looked up at the tree and thought, 'Not only is this not mango season, this is not a mango tree. This must be the wish-fulfilling tree! This is my lucky day! Let me try it out again just to make sure!' He scrunched up his mind and thought loudly, 'Let me have a full meal laid out under this tree.' Instantly the meal appeared.

The man was so excited he was almost unable to eat, but somehow he tasted each dish and approved thoroughly of the tree's culinary skills. Then he imagined a house, a herd of cows, a beautiful wife and a million gold coins. All duly appeared, and he began to feel satiated, until suddenly he thought, 'What if a hungry tiger should come right now and eat me before I have a chance to enjoy all this?' – and there stood the tiger.

Healthy thoughts create health; dark, hopeless thoughts make your body lose hope and surrender to disease. Medicine and religion differ only in their field of activity; if your mind and spirit are at peace, your body will be too, but if your consciousness is filled with conflict and frustration, your physiology will descend into disease. Ayurveda is a good way to begin the study of spirituality; physical health makes mental and spiritual health easier to attain. Your health encourages health in your family, your community, your nation and the world, and your ill-health makes your whole environment suffer; a human is an epitome of nature. How healthy you can be depends upon your level of consciousness. A seer's mind is clear and concentrated; his mind and body communicate with one another freely, without distortion. As he visualizes himself becoming, so he causes *ahamkara* to make him become.

'Everything about the [individual] *purusha* is established in the body,' says Charaka. The spirit is the only conscious principle among all the principles that make up the universe; all consciousness in the universe is due to this *purusha* alone, and all matter evolves from it. In the context of a living being this consciousness is firmly fixed in the body, and depends on the health or ill-health of the body for the quality of its expression. The principal word for health in Sanskrit, *svastha*, means 'established in oneself'. Ayurveda, a pragmatic science, teaches living beings how to establish themselves in themselves.

THE FIVE GREAT ELEMENTS

To understand the body one must first understand the Five Great Elements. All matter in the universe is made up of earth, water, fire, air and ether. These are not elements like those in the Periodic Table; rather they are states of matter. Earth represents the solid state; water the liquid state; air, the gaseous state; fire, the power to change the state of any substance; and ether, the field that is simultaneously the source of all matter and the space in which it exists. These elements are stages in the manifestation of matter, ether being the most rarefied and earth the most solid.

Because every substance in our world is made up of these five elements, all substances can be classified according to their predominant element. Any substance that is a gas under normal conditions is said to be composed mainly of air, and anything that is usually liquid is said to be primarily made of water. Substances that are fiery are reactive; they tend to cause alteration in state in other substances. Ether predominance in a substance is shown by its rarefaction or lack of density.

Anything that is solid at room temperature, like a mountain, is said to be composed predominantly of the earth element. A mountain also possesses water, fire, air and ether, but the amounts of these elements are so much less than the amount of the earth element that the equilibrium it creates for itself is solid under normal conditions. If rock from that mountain is heated, it will liquefy, displaying its water nature, and then boil, displaying its air nature, all the while glowing brightly, radiating the heat and light of the fire element. All of these metamorphoses occur within space, the ether element.

The concept of ether resembles the modern quantum mechanical concept of the field from which all matter is created and into which all matter resolves. Ether is paradoxical: it exists and yet it does not exist. It is the source of all the other elements, the repository of the creative energy of the universe, but does not interact with the other elements. The chief quality of ether is sound, which here represents the entire spectrum of vibration: subsound, audible sound, infra-red, visible light, ultraviolet, microwave, X-rays, gamma rays and cosmic radiation. Only the slowest, lowest-frequency vibrations can travel through earth, whereas all vibrations can pass through ether.

Charaka defines a human as the assemblage of the Five Great Elements plus the 'immaterial self': 'The earth is represented in man by hardness, water by moisture, fire by heat, air by the vital breath, ether by the interstices and the self by the indwelling spirit.'

Dr Yeshe Donden, who was at one time personal physician to the Dalai Lama of Tibet, explains the functions of these elements with a vegetable analogy. Earth, he says, gives the foundation for a carrot; water is the cohesive factor that holds it together; fire enables it to ripen and mature; air makes it grow; and ether gives it the space in which to manifest and develop.

LIKE AND UNLIKE

Because life has meaning only in the context of the body, the Five Great Elements are significant to you and me only insofar as they interact with us. The microcosm exists within, and is dependent upon, the macrocosm, and yet for the duration of its life it maintains itself separate from the macrocosm, the barriers that exist between the individual and the surrounding environment selectively allowing only certain substances and other things (like thoughts) to enter or leave. Anything that does enter can exert three possible effects on the organism: it can act as food, nourishing it; it can act as medicine, balancing it; it can act as poison, disturbing it.

Depending on how the substance is employed, the five elements in it may exert one, two or all three effects. In the mental context earth can give you firmness and stability in life or it can petrify you, depending on how well you are able to make use of its innate power. Water makes your life 'juicy' or 'sticky' depending on whether your body is filled with well-digested food or with toxins. Fire gives you clarity, a sharpness of consciousness that can be used to benefit others or to manipulate them selfishly. Air may provide either vigour and exaltation or exhaustion and emaciation according to how it flows in your system. Ether gives you either the illumination of a silent mind or the ache of hollowness, depending on your condition.

The rule that governs the interaction between the environment and the organism is the Law of Like and Unlike. Charaka explains:

The like is the cause of the increase of all things at all times, and the unlike is the cause of their decrease. In the context of treatment of the body like causes increase, and unlike causes decrease, of the body's constituents. Like combines, and unlike differentiates; like is that which agrees, while unlike disagrees.

'Like increases like' is a simple principle. Your body becomes warm when you lie in warm sunlight because the warmth it takes in from the sun increases its own warmth. When you go out without a coat on a winter's night, the cold of the environment flows into you, making you feel cold. Everything you experience – food, medicine or poison – increases 'like' parts of your being and decreases those parts that are 'unlike' it.

Likewise, every thought you have changes your physiology; you become precisely what you believe yourself to be. A beneficial habit causes you to repeatedly perform an action that resonates with, and reinforces, the 'good', harmonious, altruistic aspects of your being; bad habits reinforce the unhealthy, selfish parts of you. You are what you eat, what you think and what you do; repetition and resonance create your reality for you. Knowing what is good and what is not so good for your personal self enables you to make informed choices in your life, which is Ayurveda's goal. An Ayurvedic teacher would tell his students: 'If you conduct yourself well with the gods, the sacred fire, the twice-born, the guru, the aged, the adepts and the preceptors, then the precious stones, the grains and the gods will become well-disposed towards you. If you conduct yourself otherwise, they will become unfavourable.'

Right thoughts and attitudes actually induce prosperity, and the quality of prosperity produced depends on the means employed to manifest it. Wealth that accrues as a result of natural increase (as when one's cow calves) or is acquired in the honest pursuit of one's legitimate profession (that is, by means other than thieving, cheating, lying and extorting) is 'good', healthy productive wealth, which promotes continued prosperity. Thus, although, as we have noted, a doctor's food and other possessions are ritually impure, they may still be 'well-disposed' towards him.

Wealth obtained by immoral means, such as fraud, smuggling, gambling or corrupting the innocent is polluted with strong negative emotions – outrage, greed, lust and envy. Such wealth will not promote future prosperity or remain with its possessor for long; it will be wasted on luxuries or addictions, or gambled away. Thus the admonition never to demand money from a poor person as a condition of treatment: whatever is freely offered in payment is wealth that will both endure and attract further wealth, despite its ritual impurity. By contrast, that priest who enriches himself by misguiding or impoverishing his clients will never become prosperous, no matter how ritually pure he, his victims or their food or money may be.

QUALITIES

Over millennia the Ayurvedic sages collected vast quantities of observations on how substances and activities affect living beings. A substance is the vehicle or carrier of a number of qualities. Ayurveda considers the soul, mind, time and direction (spatial orientation) to be substances, because they possess qualities that affect the life of living beings. Some of these qualities are innate to the substance and so inseparable from it, while others are added, remaining only for some time. For example, oil is oily; oiliness is one of oil's inherent qualities, which never changes as long as the oil continues to exist as oil. It can be heated or cooled, or combined with other substances, but its oiliness remains as long as it remains.

Seen from this point of view, a nervous impulse is a substance: it has a name and can be described; it has a form, albeit unstable; and it has qualities. The impulse is the progeny of the underlying matter in which it arises, and is different from that matter; its effect on the system is different from the effect of that matter on the system. All parts of the system interact with each other and with the outside world continually. When any substance, including time and space, impacts upon you, its qualities, innate and added, influence your system. Ayurveda recognizes ten important pairs of opposing qualities that influence living organisms. Each of these pairs of dualities defines a continuum of activity.

Qualities	*Continuum*
heavy and light	weight
cold and hot	temperature
oily/moist and dry	emolliency
slow/dull and intense	intensity
stable and mobile	fluidity
soft and hard	rigidity
clear and sticky	adhesion
smooth and rough	texture
subtle and gross	density
solid and liquid	viscosity

Each quality is a tendency, a movement vectored towards or away from one of the poles. The extreme ends of the continua – absolute zero and the temperatures of nuclear fusion, for example, in the case of cold and hot – are unimportant; only the relative extremes possible within the living organism are the concern of medicine. The extremes of these ten dualities are engaged in a continual tug of war, each attempting to slide the being upon whom they impact further in their own direction. The same substance that causes movement in one direction in one individual may produce an opposite effect in someone else. An inhabitant of the tropics will be chilled by autumn in a temperate climate, while a denizen of the Far North may experience the same autumn weather as balmy. The individual organism is the point of reference for everything it experiences, and, except in very special cases, the individual organism's perceptions are strongly influenced by the environment in which it exists.

A substance that is innately heavy, rough, hard, slow, stable, clear, subtle and gross is made up primarily of the earth element. One that is liquid, oily or moist, cold, slow, soft and smooth is made up primarily of the water element. A hot, intense, subtle, light, dry and clear substance is made up primarily of the fire element. A light, cold, dry, rough, clear and subtle substance is made up primarily of the air element. A substance that is soft, light, subtle and smooth is substantially composed of the ether element.

All solid, immobile body parts, such as bone and cartilage, that provide support to the organism are mainly earthy in nature. Liquid, viscid materials, including fat and vital bodily fluids like lymph, blood, semen, mucus, and sexual secretions, are predominantly watery in character. Fiery substances in the body include digestive fluids and endocrine secretions, body heat, and those materials that produce radiance in the eyes and skin, and awareness in the brain. Everything mobile or involved in movement, which especially pertains to the activities of the nervous system, is airy in nature, and all channels through which 'things' pass, be they blood and lymph vessels, pores, the organs of the gut or nerves (through which nervous impulses 'pass') are ethereal.

When earthy substances interact with an organism, they tend to augment the organism's earthy constituents, according to the principle of resonance inherent in 'like increases like', and promote plumpness, compactness, heaviness and stability in the body and mind. Watery things likewise promote moisture, unctuousness, liquefaction, union, softness and delight. Fiery items produce burning, digestion, radiance, lightness, lustre and colour; airy materials, dryness, clearness and lightness; and ethereal substances, softness, porousness and lightness.

Everything that enters a human being must be turned into a form that the human organism can utilize. Food, water, air, sunlight, touch, odours, tastes, sights and sounds and even thoughts and emotions from the outer world enter the inner world and alter it, forcing it to adapt. How well an organism responds to these challenges and adapts to new conditions, how well it 'digests' its experiences, is an expression of its innate equilibrium, its immunity to imbalance, its degree of coherence relative to the external chaos, a chaos that also is relative, composed as it is of innumerable intelligences all trying to order things to suit themselves.

Everything that enters us must be well 'digested'; whenever an experience remains 'undigested', the microcosm loses its coherence and develops a disease. Treatment is the re-establishment of this order. In jaundice, for example, the microcosm concentrates too much 'yellow' energy (bile) within it; when this excess is removed, whether by Vedic hymns or by physical medicine, there is relief. Excessive or insufficient intake of any of the elements causes imbalance and disease. Healing makes use of opposites to remove excess or remedy deficiency, thereby returning the system to equilibrium. As Charaka explains:

This much is evident to us all, namely that we treat a disease-ridden man with disease-removing measures, and the depleted man with impletion. We nourish the emaciated and the feeble, we starve the corpulent and the fatty. We treat the man afflicted by heat with cooling measures, and with hot things him who is afflicted by cold. We replenish body elements that have suffered decrease, and deplenish those that have undergone increase. By treating disorders properly with measures which are antagonistic to their causative factors we restore the patient to normal. In our hands, administered in this manner, the pharmacopeia shows itself to the best of its excellence.

THE THREE DOSHAS

The universe relies on us to preserve harmony and organization within it by maintaining harmony within ourselves. In the Vedic era people preserved harmony by means of sacrifice. Sacrificial ritual, the offering with Vedic hymns of consecrated substances into a sacred fire, aligns microcosm with macrocosm and opens a channel of communication between them, so that they can cohere harmoniously. Fire, the mediator between the two worlds, is also a deity, a divine personality; the fire altar is his body, and the sacrificial offerings, his food. In exchange for his portion of food, fire purifies the offerings and carries their fragrant essence to gratify and nourish the gods, who respond by sending timely rains of the proper amount to make the earth fertile to gratify and nourish humans. The humans feed the gods and the gods feed the humans in a symbiotic relationship. When there is harmony between the humans and the gods, the seasons come and go at their appointed time, life is fruitful and everyone is happy.

The everyday process of eating is Ayurveda's fire sacrifice, a daily offering of food into the sacred fire of digestion for the purpose of maintaining microcosmic harmony. The 'fragrance' (the chemical constituents) of these food offerings ascends to the brain, where the 'gods' (the various parts of the brain and mind) are nourished. The gods then send the 'rains' (hormones, neuropeptides and other metabolites) on to the 'earth' (the body) to make it fruitful. Sushruta's text calls a person who follows the rules for healthy eating a 'fire worshipper', and the act of eating, 'sacrificial worship'. The administration of therapy to a patient is also a sacrifice, an offering of drugs and procedures into the microcosmic sacred fire for the propitiation of one's personal 'gods' when they are afflicted by disease.

While other 'religious' references in Ayurvedic texts may be artefacts of priestly text-tinkering, this thread of thought is fundamental to Ayurvedic philosophy. Without fire to purify and digest food and to clarify and cognize thought, life could not exist. Impurity, which by preventing proper performance of a sacrificial act prevents production of the desired effect, appears as a *dosha*, a word derived from the root *dus*, which is equivalent to the English prefix 'dys': dysfunction, dystrophy, dysmenorrhoea and so on. A *dosha* is a fault, mistake, error or stain, a transgression against the cosmic rhythm, an inaccuracy which prevents success and leads to chaos. Many *doshas* can afflict a macrocosmic sacrifice, including Ancestor *Dosha*, Evil Spirit *Dosha* and Black Magic *Dosha*, all of which arise according to Malefic Planet *Dosha*, which in turn is due to Bad Karma *Dosha*.

The microcosm possesses, besides these *doshas*, three additional ones: *vata*, *pitta* and *kapha*. These *doshas* are the active, but waste-product, forms of the Five Great Elements – *vata* arising from air and ether, *pitta* from fire and water, and *kapha* from water and earth – that appear in living beings.

The Three *Doshas* are invisible forces that can be demonstrated in the body only by inference. Comparisons with the wind, bile and phlegm of Hippocratic medicine ignore their non-physical character.

Wind, bile, phlegm and other bodily constituents are merely the vehicles of the Three *Doshas*, substances that carry these forces and through which they display their qualities and perform their actions. The Three *Doshas* are 'ghosts' (spirits that possess) created by Nature in order to permit embodied life to exist. They do not really belong on the physical plane any more than ghosts do, and yet they remain here working for us; it is no surprise that they can quickly become disturbed.

Like the body's physical wastes (urine, faeces and sweat) *vata, pitta* and *kapha* keep the body healthy only so long as they continuously flow out of it and maintain their balance with each other. Urine is, in fact, an important vehicle for the removal of excess *kapha* force from the body; sweat carries away excess *pitta* force; and defecation expels excess *vata* force. Proper elimination of these wastes helps maintain healthy levels of the *doshas* within the body. It is only when *vata, pitta* and *kapha* go out of balance that they cause disease.

When an organism is healthy, its adaptability is strong and its digestion powerful, and little metabolic waste is produced; in ill health, waste prevails. Health is governed by the principle 'like increase like': those who have health tend to accumulate more of it, and those who are sick tend to get sicker, unless they change their ways.

The Three *Doshas* enable the spiritual and mental planes of existence to express themselves through the physical body. *Vata* is in charge of all motion in the body and mind. Everything that moves, from a molecule to a thought, moves because of *vata*, and every motion of any kind influences every other motion, according to the law of like and unlike. *Pitta* is in charge of all transformation in the organism. Digestion of food by the gut, of light by the eyes and of sensory data by the brain are examples of *pitta*'s activities. *Kapha* is the stabilizing influence in the living being. It lubricates, maintains and contains, and its various activities, like those of *vata* and *pitta*, are interrelated.

The smallest of the body's cells has a structure, takes in food and digests it, and expels the wastes produced. Life is inconceivable without these three activities: movement, metabolism and stability, or kinetic energy (*vata*), potential energy (*kapha*) and the force that regulates the conversion of one into the other (*pitta*). Fuel (*kapha*), something to ignite it (*pitta*) and air to support combustion (*vata*) are all essential to build a fire; if any of these is missing, no flame will be kindled.

Vata moves the food through the digestive tract; too slow or too fast a transit and digestion, assimilation and elimination will suffer. It also supports the combustion of the food by 'blowing on' various organs to induce them to secrete digestive ferments. Insufficient 'wind' means insufficient secretions; excessive 'wind' blows out the 'fire'. *Pitta* breaks down the food, preparing it for assimilation; excess or insufficiency of *pitta* interferes with the process. *Kapha* lubricates the gut and, like a cooking pot, holds the food while it is 'cooked' by the digestive fire; disturbance of *kapha* ruins the result.

In the brain *vata* is in charge of memory, the movement of thoughts from storage into present-time consciousness and back again. *Pitta* controls both cognition, the transmutation of raw sensory data into thought, and discrimination, the comparison of two thoughts that results in a conclusion. *Kapha* provides the stability necessary for the mind to function coherently. When the Three *Doshas* operate together harmoniously, so does the mind; and when they are imbalanced, the mind becomes imbalanced. Disturbance of these essential forces creates emotional disturbance: aggravated *vata* especially produces fear and anxiety; vitiated *pitta*, principally anger and envy; and disturbed *kapha*, mainly attachment and greed.

The emotions you feel directly influence your physiology, and fluctuations in your body alter your emotions. Scientists have shown that when you change your facial expression, even in jest, the new positions the muscles take alter the flow of blood to various parts of the brain, and actually change the workings of your awareness. Thus if you can make a pouting child smile even a little bit, the child will usually forget to pout. In this way all the different layers of our being continually influence and are influenced by one another.

When balanced, the Three *Doshas* cause the body's elements to cohere and function together; when unbalanced, they create chaos among all the organism's other constituents. Like all other substances, the Three *Doshas* also possess qualities, and their increase or decrease in the system depends upon the similar or antagonistic qualities of everything ingested:

vata is dry, cold, light, mobile, clear, rough and subtle;

pitta is slightly oily, hot, intense, light, fluid, sour or malodorous (a raw-meat-like smell), and mobile or liquid;

kapha is oily, cold, heavy, stable, viscid, smooth and soft.

Both *vata* and *pitta* are light, and only *kapha* is heavy; both *vata* and *kapha* are cold, and only *pitta* is hot; both *pitta* and *kapha* are moist and oily, and only *vata* is dry. Anything dry almost always increases *vata*, anything hot increases *pitta*, and anything heavy, *kapha*. Puffed rice is dry, cold, light and rough; overindulgence in puffed rice therefore is likely to increase *vata* in the overindulger. Mustard oil is oily, hot, intense, fluid, strong-smelling and liquid, and increases *pitta* in the consumer. Yoghurt, which, being creamy, cold, heavy, viscid, smooth and soft, is the very image of *kapha*, adds to the body's *kapha* when eaten. All substances and all activities increase and decrease the *doshas* according to their qualities.

All five elements, as expressed through *vata, pitta* and *kapha*, are essential to life, working together to create health or produce disease. No one *dosha* can produce or sustain life; all three must work together, each in its own way. The actions of *vata* in the body are best summarized in a passage from Charaka:

Vata in its five forms, *Prana, Udana, Samana, Vyana* and *Apana*, is the upholder of both structure and function in the organism. It is the impeller of upward and downward movements, the controller and conductor of the mind, the impeller of the senses, the conveyor of all sensory stimuli, the arranger of the body elements, the joiner of the body's parts, the inspirer of speech, the field of action of touch and hearing and the root of those two senses, the womb of laughter and exaltation, the stimulator of the gastric fire, the desiccator of morbid *doshas*, the eliminator of excrement, the divider of the gross and subtle body channels, the moulder of the fetal form, and the sustainer of the activities of life: all these are the normal functions of Vata in the organism.

Vata's abnormal functions include, but are not limited to, impairment of strength, complexion and well-being; disturbance of the mind and senses; deformation of the foetus; production of fear, grief, stupefaction, depression and delirium; and obstruction of the vital functions. Normal *pitta* causes digestion, vision, normal body temperature, body lustre, courage, intelligence, lucidity and the like, while abnormal *pitta* results in the opposite of all these. Normal *kapha* creates compactness, cohesion, firmness, plumpness, strength, virility, knowledge, understanding, forgiveness, fortitude and the like, and abnormal *kapha* produces their opposites.

No single factor can account for the production of either health or disease in living beings. When a result is produced by the concerted action of many factors or causes, the process is called *yukti*. Cloth, for example, is produced by the coming together in one place at one time with definite purpose of thread, shuttle, loom and weaver; if any of these factors is absent, no cloth results. Life exists because of *yukti*, the weaving together in one place at one time of body, mind and spirit functioning together as one unit. All sacrificial rituals, Vedic, Tantric or digestive, involve *yukti*; unless each prescribed action occurs at the proper moment the desired result is never obtained. It is no coincidence that the word 'tantra' comes from a root meaning 'to weave'.

Building a fire is a kind of *yukti*, and creating life is building a fire: a man and a woman come together at the right moment (a fertile moment) and the friction of their embrace generates the spark in the reproductive fuel that bursts into manifestation. Without the proper moment and proper conditions nothing is created, not even disease or the treatment of disease. A skilful doctor uses 'like' and 'unlike' substances to increase or decrease body elements and rekindle the organism's internal fires. With herbs and minerals as kindling, and the power of the physician as bellows, the right therapeutic fuel reawakens the flame of life when the life-force dies down, even if only embers remain.

This flame of life, called *tejas* or *agni* in Sanskrit, is different from *pitta*, which is only its more reactive form. Likewise, *vata* is the unstable form of prana, or *vayu*; and *kapha* the inert, 'dead' form of *ojas*, or *soma*. Prana, *tejas* and *ojas* are the essences of the air, fire and water elements as applied to embodied life. Prana is grosser than *vata*, says Dr Donden; he compares prana to electricity, and *vata* to the light that electricity can produce when it is directed into a bulb.

TABLE OF ESSENCES

Essence	Element	Reactive Form	Physical Vehicle
prana	air	*vata*	nerve impulses, etc.
tejas	fire	*pitta*	bile, enzymes, etc.
ojas	water	*kapha*	phlegm, synovial fluid, etc.

According to an ancient analogy, prana is the life-force that strings body, mind and spirit together like beads on a strand of breath. Prana is not air, though oxygen is one of its vehicles; prana is the force that causes the physical *yukti* necessary to keep living beings alive. *Tejas* burns windows into the barriers that exist between the body, mind and spirit, permitting them to communicate and influence one another in spite of their differing planes of existence. *Ojas* is the subtle glue that cements the body, mind and spirit together, integrating them into a functioning individual.

When an organism functions at peak efficiency, the Three *Doshas* are produced in quantities just sufficient to meet physical needs. In systemic imbalance the *doshas* are overproduced or underproduced at the expense of the body's vitality, adaptability and immunity. When digestion is strong, the prana contained in the food is efficiently taken into the system, and only a little *vata* is produced; when digestion is weak, only a little prana can be assimilated and much *vata* is generated. A person who suffers from aggravated *vata* often seems to be a bundle of energy, but on closer inspection he or she proves to be merely a bundle of nerves. All the healthy prana that should be invigorating each cell has instead evolved into nervous energy, which is useless for most bodily functions and must be burned away. Likewise, a superabundance of fire guarantees inflammation of body or mind because of *pitta*, and plentiful 'juice' loads the system with sticky toxins due to *kapha*, if *tejas* and *ojas* are not adequate.

Vedic medicine did not need the Three *Doshas*; it dealt with life at the level of prana, *tejas* and *ojas*. Ayurveda, a medical system for the masses, makes use of the *doshas* because its principal field of activity is the physical body, where the *doshas* hold sway.

3

ANATOMY

EARTH AND SKY

Humans, whose consciousness is tethered to physical bodies, live on the gross Earth plane; the gods, who are personifications of cosmic forces, are non-physical beings who inhabit the subtle sky plane. The humans and the gods need one another, and both are dependent upon the cosmic rhythm that created them. Because the gods exist both within and without the individual they can be propitiated by internal as well as external sacrificial rites. Since the keys that unlock the secret esoteric significance of the Vedic hymns have been lost, esotericism is now the property of the tantras, which developed from the magic of the Atharva-Veda and which, like the Vedas, personify the forces of the universe to facilitate subjective communication and interaction. When much of Vedic ritual became fossilized after its priests forgot its inner significance, iconoclasts who insisted on the primacy of personal experience over dead dogma rebelled against the system and established virile but often misunderstood new rituals.

Tantric personifications are mentioned in the later Ayurvedic literature, just as the Vedic gods are mentioned in the earliest works, and probably for similar reasons: to remind the average student not to ignore non-physical reality even when attending to the mundane, and to introduce esoteric medicine to the exceptional student. Because Ayurveda is mostly exoteric, mainly concerned with the physical plane, its esoteric aspects are only hinted at in the Ayurvedic literature, finding full expression in the tantras. Tantra is a system of internal sacrificial rites that uses the inner environment to influence the outer environment. Many people mistakenly believe Tantra to be a religion of sexual excess, when, in fact, sexual rituals form only one of the methods of Tantric worship. Tantra, which neither shuns physical existence nor embraces it indiscriminately, teaches that because consciousness is established in the body, the body should be one's temple or fire altar; everything one does with that body should be an act of worship.

Internal worship resembles external worship in essence and differs in detail, much as the microcosm is both identical to and different from the macrocosm. At an external sacrifice the celebrants first invoke the Earth to establish stability for the sacrificial setting and then invoke the gods of the skies, inviting them to come to the place of worship to be fêted. The ritual sacrificial stake or post, which symbolizes this aligning of Earth and Sky, is a paradox, at once part of both worlds but belonging to neither. The maypole, which was once central to Nature worship and fertility festivities, is one representation of this axis; others in India include the Flag of Indra (the king of the gods) and, more commonly, the Shiva Linga, the phallus of the god Shiva, which rests in a base formed of the vagina of his wife, Parvati, an icon that may have antedated even the Vedas.

Yet another form, familiar to anyone who has ever visited a doctor's office, is the caduceus, the winged staff with twin snakes twined around it, which is a representation of the spinal column, the internal sacrificial post that connects the 'earth' polarity at the perineum with the 'sky' polarity in the brain. The tantras and the Vedas use this inner stake for their internal rituals. A dividing cell produces two poles within itself, and then polarizes its being into two parts, which accumulate at the two poles. Two poles also develop during human manifestation, centred at what become the head and the base of the spine. These are the microcosmic representatives of the two macrocosmic poles of our existence: the limited Earth, which holds us to her that we might live, and the unlimited Sky, the vast universe. Earth represents for us all that is individual and particular in existence, and Sky stands for all that is cosmic and general. Mother Earth stands for the contraction of energy into matter, and Sky-Father for the expansion of matter into energy.

A developing foetus extends itself from the ethereal world into the physical world along this spinal axis. A fully formed human is a bipolar beast, containing both Earth and Sky. At the base of the spine resides the cosmic energy that has projected into flesh, and which, as long as it remains there, identifies with the body. In Ayurveda we call it *ahamkara*, the I-creator; the tantras call it the *kundalini shakti*. In the average embodied being *kundalini* lies 'sleeping' at the base of the spine, totally identified with the body. The spinal cord provides humans with a mechanism by which to vary their state of consciousness. The lower into the body your consciousness drops, the more it will plug into the physical world; the higher it rises, the more it will tune into the ethereal.

THE FIVE SHEATHS

Like an onion, a human being is composed of concentric layers, or sheaths. These sheaths are generated as consciousness descends into denser and denser matter, providing platforms for the expression of that consciousness. The subtler sheaths act as patterns or templates for the grosser, each level of organization building on the previous level. Consciousness remains unitary, but because it is expressed under different conditions on each level there is a limited individual consciousness in each sheath.

Five sheaths are recognized by esoteric anatomy: food, prana, mind, special wisdom and bliss. We will concern ourselves only with the first three. The physical body is the Sheath of Food; it is nourished, imbalanced and healed through the juices extracted from our food. The Sheath of Prana, which connects the Sheaths of Food and Mind and permits them to operate together, is nourished, imbalanced and healed through prana. There are actually two methods of nutrition for the body's prana: 'instant', in which the lungs during breathing absorb the prana found in the air, and 'delayed', in which the colon absorbs the prana found in well-digested food. This mutuality of function explains why the lungs and the large intestine are so closely connected in Ayurvedic physiology, and helps to explain, for example, how a few minutes of slow, deep breathing can reduce hunger. The Sheath of Mind is the astral body, composed of mind-stuff and nourished, imbalanced and healed through words, images and emotions.

Consciousness is a very complex phenomenon, whose quality depends upon how and and where it is manifested in the organism. Human awareness is the product of millions of years of evolution of a physical form that encourages the expression of consciousness, and 'self-awareness' in most people is a composite of the projection of consciousness through these three sheaths. For example, awareness of your hand is a composite of awareness of its physicality (bones, muscles, skin, nails, etc.), its ability to act (to grasp, clench, extend and so on), its ability to sense (temperature, pressure, pain and like sensations), and your own personal positive or negative 'image' of it as useful or useless, shapely or misshapen, and so on. This awareness, or lack thereof, extends to each limb of your body. The quality of your consciousness is the aggregate of all these individual limb-awarenesses plus that integrating-awareness that makes you *you*. How much you are aware of the various aspects of your existence determines the state of your overall awareness.

The job of the Sheath of Food, in which *tamas* predominates, is to stabilize your consciousness. If you become too attentive to the physical body, your consciousness will become clogged with *tamas*, making you too fixed in your ways to change easily; if you are not enough 'in your body' you will be too changeable, unable to be stable. The Sheath of Prana, in which *rajas* predominates, makes you either sufficiently active, too active or inactive, depending upon how much of your attention it takes up. If *ahamkara* fixes your awareness in the Sheath of Mind after carefully training and disciplining your mind, then *sattva* will predominate in your consciousness and your system will tend to remain in equilibrium; otherwise you will remain a prisoner of your mind's storms of *rajas* and curtains of *tamas*. *Tamas* and *rajas* form a duality of stability versus change, of bodily and mental orthodoxy versus somatic and psychological innovation, which can be mediated only by *sattva*, whose task it is to preserve balance.

The purpose of the Vedic sciences, including Ayurveda, is to assist individuals to learn enough about themselves to know how much and what kind of awareness they require, and to teach them methods to develop this awareness. Tantra is called a religion of the body because it teaches that only by first cultivating the Sheaths of Food and Prana can mind be made sufficiently stable to function under its possessor's control. Hatha yoga is one of the methods by which the Sheath of Prana is trained, while Ayurveda's main interest is with the Sheath of Food.

The Sheath of Prana

The Sheath of Prana is mentioned only infrequently in the Ayurvedic texts. Sharngadhara, who was strongly influenced by Tantra, invokes subtle anatomy when he describes the vessels that arise from the navel and spread throughout the body, constantly supplying prana to the tissues. He describes how the prana near the navel moves up to the heart and emerges from the throat to drink 'the Nectar of the Feet of the Preserver'. Having partaken of this nectar, it moves inside quickly to enliven the entire body and enkindle the digestive fire. These vessels are the ethereal nerves (*nadis*), and the navel is the site of one of their plexuses (*chakra*). Through these structures, which make up the Sheath of Prana and are extremely important in Tantric practice, moves the life-force. Despite the insistence of some modern Ayurvedic authorities that the nectar Sharngadhara mentions is oxygen, it is clearly prana, the life-force, which is carried both in the food we eat and in the air we breathe.

The central staff of the caduceus represents the most important *nadi* in the body, which is also the least used by the average individual. This *nadi*, called *sushumna*, flows within the central sulcus of the spinal cord, the six most important *chakras* arranged along it like flowers on a garland. The two snakes represent the body's next two most important *nadis*, which flow in conjunction with the two nostrils. Most of us breathe through only one nostril at a time, shifting unconsciously from one to the other in cycles lasting two to three hours. The left nostril (or, rather, its *nadi*) cools and calms the organism, while the right heats and excites it. Heat expands, and cold contracts; in the body of a living being heat generally dilates the channels, and cold constricts them. The two great *nadis* that terminate in the two nostrils govern and maintain the rhythmic contraction and expansion of the body and its physiology, and this duality of heat and cold, in turn, fuels the circulation of *vata* in the body, very much as it fuels the circulation of atmospheric air.

Scientists now know what the Vedics have long known, that

Earth's atmosphere is modulated by what happens on its surface; our lives literally change the life of our Earth, and it, in turn, alters us in response to our activities. Likewise, each of our activities affects and is affected by the circulation of our internal 'atmosphere', our 'inner wind', which exerts its effects by stimulating the physical nerves that flow in synchrony with its nadis. Those nerves there stimulate the endocrine glands, which translate their impulses into physical form. An entire science of breath called *svarodaya* details the proper functioning of the *nadis* and their use in diagnosis and treatment.

Some argue that since neither *nadis* nor *chakras* can be demonstrated in a dissected corpse, subtle anatomy must be entirely imaginary; but as these structures (a word we must use advisedly) reside in a layer of existence far more subtle than the physical, more subtle than even the *doshas*, at most it is their effects that can be detected in the physical body. Other people compare human anatomical charts with Tantric *chakra* and *nadi* maps and make a great deal of unwarranted one-to-one correlation of the six most important *chakras* with nearby physical glands and plexuses, ignoring the fact that these *chakras*, which exist within the centralmost *nadi*, function only when their *nadi* is open and freely functioning.

Various traditions disagree over the number and precise location of the *chakras* because their practices 'awaken' only certain ones. Unless energy is actually flowing through a *chakra*, it remains in an inactive, potential form, like a sperm or ovum before they unite, and cannot really be said to exist. In all but the most spiritually advanced individuals the 'energy vortices', 'spinning patterns' and other concentrations of power that have been detected by sensitives are flows that, though generated ultimately by the *chakras*, actually overlay the *chakras*, existing near them in more superficial layers of the organism.

Light in our world comes from the sun. The light that we see on Earth changes in quality according to changes in our atmospheric conditions. While our atmosphere possesses a dramatic power to affect those of us who live beneath it, it exerts only an infinitesimal effect on the sun itself. Similarly, conditions in the more superficial layers of the average human being have a nearly negligible effect on the *chakras* themselves, even though they may affect the consciousness dramatically. The *chakras* affect us, but we are hard-pressed to affect them.

The six principal *chakras* are knots in the energy axis that connects the ethereal to the physical world. They come into existence in order to bind down *ahamkara* into self-identification with the elements that make up the universe so that the physical body can be assembled from those elements. Each of these *chakras* forms the joint, the point of interaction, between *ahamkara* and an element; each plugs *ahamkara* into the frequency of that element. *Ahamkara* can continue to recognize and manipulate that element within the body only so long as this connection remains intact, for the *chakra* in effect broadcasts its element into the organism. The element associated with the *chakra* tends to predominate in that region of the body nearest the *chakra*, and, accordingly, the organs that evolved near those *chakras* predominate in that element.

The base of the spinal cord at the lowest part of the torso contains the incarnated cosmic energy, which 'sleeps peacefully' in the *Muladhara Chakra*, the seat of the body's earth element, the element that provides our bodies with solidity and stability. Above it is the *Svadhishthana Chakra*, the centre for the water element, near which is the predominantly watery genito-urinary system. Next is the *Manipura Chakra*, which occupies that region of the subtle body near the physical navel. The *Manipura Chakra* permits *ahamkara* to relate to the fire element, and so the fiery digestive organs are clustered in this area.

The station for communication with the air element is the *Anahata Chakra*, between the shoulder blades at the level of the chest, close to the ever-moving (and so air-predominant) heart and lungs. Speech, a function of the ether element (which has sound as its special quality), manifests at the throat, where lies the *Vishuddha Chakra*, the home of the body's ether element. At the brow is the *Ajna Chakra*, where *ahamkara* and mind mate, producing (indirectly) the structures of the brain that serve the mind, especially the pineal gland, the seat of *ojas*.

Marmas

The details of subtle anatomy are important to those Vedic and Tantric practitioners whose consciousness is sufficiently subtle to perceive them. Today only a few Ayurvedic practitioners have even been exposed to *svarodaya*, and while many learn the doctrine of *marma* while in college, few make use of it in practice. A *marma* is a point on the body beneath which vital structures, which may be physical, subtle or both, intersect. Some of these points are identical with acupuncture points, and others are nearly identical. Damage to *marmas* by trauma from without or by metabolic imbalance within has severe and potentially fatal consequences.

Marmas apparently have been known since Vedic times. Warriors targeted *marmas* on their enemies to inflict maximum damage, and surgeons employed the knowledge of *marmas* in their treatment of such injuries. Sushruta classified 107 *marmas* on the basis of the structure involved (muscles, blood vessels, ligaments, nerves, bones, joints) and regional location, dimension and consequences of injury (swift death, death after some delay, death as soon as any foreign body is extracted from the wound, disability, or simply pain). Though the practical application of the knowledge of body *marmas* has disappeared from most of India, it persists in the southern state of Kerala among the practitioners of the martial art known as *kalarippayattu*.

In its current form, dating from approximately the twelfth century AD, *kalarippayattu* is, in the words of Professor Phillip Zarrilli, 'similar to the practice of hatha yoga in that a set of preliminary physical exercises leads not only to extraordinary physical control, but ultimately is thought to lead inward to the discovery of more subtle aspects of practice'. *Kalarippayattu* is thus linked to Dhanur Veda (the science of war), Ayurveda and meditational practice. The masters of *kalarippayattu* recognize 160 to 220 *marmas* in martial practice, and use the 107 marmas of Sushruta in therapy. *Kalarippayattu* views the human being as three intricately interwoven bodies: the changeable body of fluids, including the tissues and wastes; the relatively less changeable body of muscles, bones and *marma* points; and the subtle body with its *nadis* and *chakras*.

These 'bodies' are not discrete, absolute structures, but, because of their specialized functions within the unified structure, they are treated as such. There is no contradiction between this classification and that of the Five Sheaths; they are simply different ways of looking at the same reality, because of the different purposes to which each classification is put.

According to *kalarippayattu*, injury to a *marma* blocks or cuts the associated *nadi* at that point, interrupting both the flow of prana, the life-force, and the flow of *vata*, prana's waste product and servant, in that area. Profound damage occurs only if there is a penetration of at least one *angula* (about one inch) into the tissues beneath the spot – a mere slap will not damage it. Immediate first aid for such an injury is a firm stroke or slap to the similar *marma* on the opposite side of the body, to get prana moving again to get the victim out of danger. Such a counter-application must be given within a certain time in order for it to work, and must be followed by treatment for the imbalance of the *doshas* caused by the injury.

Like a *chakra*, a *marma* is not even really a structure in that it does not exist at all times. Professor Zarrilli emphasizes that *marma* exists only insofar as there is prana in the body – that is, a dead body has no *marma* – and that any *marma* is activated fully only when prana is actually moving in it; the death or damage predicted as a result of injury to a *marma* occurs only when such a *marma* is attacked. Prana's movement through, and concentration in, the body's *marmas* is controlled by the lunar day; in this the doctrine of *marma* is strikingly similar to that of Indian sexology, which details the specific areas of a woman's body that are awake to erotic excitement on particular lunar days because of the movement of prana therein.

The Sheath of Food

Even in Ayurveda's study of the physical body the idea of structure never quite becomes concrete, because knowing how the body's constituents interact is more meaningful than knowing their gross anatomy. While the texts do name each bone and most of the organs, Ayurvedic anatomy is more concerned with the overall organization of the system than with its many parts. Aristotle taught that the body's tissues exist to serve its organs, while Ayurveda teaches that the organs exist to serve the production and nutrition of the tissues.

The Ayurvedic idea of organ includes, but is not necessarily limited to, that which modern science calls an organ. Ayurveda sees the 'heart' as the centre of circulation of blood and *vata* and the seat of the mind, intellect and consciousness, while the head, known as 'the best of the limbs of the body', is regarded mainly as the residence of the sense organs. Heart disease is not limited to disease of the pumping muscle, but also includes disorders of the forces and substances of the chest region that may involve the heart only secondarily; abdominal disorders, such as distention of the colon with gas, which can disturb the heart by exerting pressure on it through the diaphragm; and even heartache and heartbreak. Another possible interpretation is that if the seat of consciousness is the heart, wherever consciousness is situated in the system is at that moment the organism's heart, the centre in which *ahamkara* holds prana's reins. Damage to that 'heart' could prove fatal even if it were not a generally accepted vital organ.

Concern with organ structure is replaced in Ayurveda with attention to *dosha* location, movement and function. The Three *Doshas* pervade the body, working in every cell of every tissue every moment of the day, but concentrate themselves in those tissues in which they are particularly required. *Vata* accumulates below the navel to help counteract the force of gravity by pumping blood, lymph and wastes from the lower parts of the body back into the torso; *kapha* accumulates above the diaphragm to keep *vata* from moving upward too strongly, and to ensure lubrication for those organs that most need it (the heart, lungs and alimentary canal); and *pitta*, the mediator and fulcrum between *vata* and *kapha*, occupies the region between the diaphragm and the navel, near the body's centre of gravity.

Concentrations of each of the *doshas* are normally stored in certain body organs:

vata in the brain and nervous system, heart, colon, bones, lungs, bladder, pelvis, thighs, ears, skin;

pitta in the brain, liver, spleen, small intestine, endocrine glands, skin, eyes, blood, sweat;

kapha in the brain, joints, mouth, head and neck, stomach, lymph, thorax (especially lungs, heart and oesophagus), fat.

There is actually only one *vata*, one *pitta* and one *kapha*, but, according to the specific duties they perform, each is divided into five aspects. The five *kaphas* manifest in specialized body lubricants: stomach mucus, pleural and pericardial fluid, saliva, synovial fluid and cerebrospinal fluid. The five *pittas* appear in transformative substances: digestive juices, haemoglobin, melanin, rhodopsin and various neurotransmitters.

The five *vatas* divide the body into spheres of influence. The field of activity of *prana vata*, the 'forward-moving air', extends from the diaphragm to the throat; it is in charge of taking things, like food, water and air, into the system. All five *vatas* are derived from prana, but since this *vata* is particularly involved with the intake of the life-force, it has been given the same name.

The field of *udana vata*, the 'upward-moving air', extends from the throat to the top of the head, and controls self-expression: speech, endeavour, enthusiasm, memory, vitality, complexion (one of the body's means of expressing its innate state of health) and the like.

The field of *samana vata*, the 'equalizing air', extends from the diaphragm to the navel. It is in charge of digestion and assimilation, and helps keep prana and *apana* in balance.

Vyana vata, the 'pervasive air', pervades the entire body from its seat in the heart, distributing nourishment by causing blood and other fluids to circulate, and producing locomotion, extension and contraction, perspiration and other such actions.

Apana vata, the 'downward-moving air', operates from the navel to the anus. It expels matter from the body: urine, faeces, gas, semen, menstrual blood and the foetus.

As we have seen (p. 53), the *doshas* must be produced and excreted in the right amounts, and remain in balance with each other, for the body to be healthy. Excess *kapha* causes mucus and other lubricants to be overproduced and to accumulate within, creating obstructive conditions like indigestion, lethargy, cough and nausea. Insufficient *kapha* leads to other problems, like weakness, dryness of skin and mouth, body ache, palpitations and insomnia. Even the proper amount of *kapha* may cause disease if some obstruction prevents its expedient excretion.

The same holds true for *pitta* and *vata*. Overproduction of *pitta* creates such conditions as anger, acidity, increased body heat, burning sensations, yellowness of body and mind, diminished sleep, and excessive hunger and thirst. Obstructed *pitta* may also cause these and other problems, and insufficient *pitta* can cause coldness,

lack of vigour and joy, stiffness, loss of lustre and weakened digestion.

Excess *vata* promotes weakness, emaciation, dryness, flatulence,
constipation, various sorts of pains, insomnia, tremors and tics,
giddiness, and impairment of sensory and motor functions, while
decreased *vata* reduces all bodily activities, disturbs the digestion,
induces aches and pains, and encourages nausea, loss of taste and
depression.

The tissues and the wastes

Vata, *pitta* and *kapha* display their abilities by acting through the
tissues and waste products that make up the body. In one sense it is
the *doshas* that make up the body, because the tissues are arranged
and nourished, and the wastes sequestered and excreted, by the
doshas. A human being is a factory in which raw materials are
operated upon by the *doshas* to produce products and by-products,
an organism that exists by constantly exchanging matter and energy
with its environment. While the factory building, machines and raw
materials are all essential to production of the product, without the
workers (the *doshas*) nothing gets produced.

The products of digestion are the seven tissues, or *dhatus*, which
anchor mind and spirit firmly in the physical body (the word *dhatu*
comes from a root meaning 'to support'). The grosser body tissues
act as raw materials for the subtler, and the nutrients are progressively concentrated by this processing chain as they proceed deeper
into the body until *ojas*, the ultimate product of metabolism, results.
At each stage are also produced *upadhatus*, or secondary tissues,
which undergo no further transformation, and wastes, each of
which has its own job to do as it is expelled from the body. Faeces,
for example, provide temporary strength to the colon; urine maintains body-fluid balance; and sweat lubricates the skin, controls heat
and fluid balance, and promotes growth of body hair.

Nutrition of the body begins when the first 'juice' is extracted
from the food; this juice is acted on by a special form of fire, which
converts it into *rasa*, another untranslatable concept. *Rasa* (its root
means 'to move') means, according to context, liquid, potion,
nectar, essence, semen, sap, aesthetic appreciation, artistic delight,

melodious sound, the element mercury or the other minerals used with it in alchemy, the expressed juice of fruit, leaves or other plant parts, an extract of meat (usually its soup), and emotion. In sum, *rasa* represents every juice that makes life possible and worth living.

In the physical body *rasa* is chyle or plasma, the body's 'sap', the nutrient liquid that moves ceaselessly throughout the body bathing each cell in its fertilizing flow. Nourishment of body and mind, and the exaltation that ensues therefrom, is its task. The same sort of bliss you feel after a truly satisfying meal is felt by all the little cells of your body when they are immersed in fresh *rasa*. When the complexion is ruddy, the flesh and fat well-formed, the bones solid, the nervous system strong, and the skin and eyes full of lustre, one may safely conclude that the tissues are well-nourished and full of 'sap'. *Rasa*, which is mainly composed of the water element, has the greatest affinity for *kapha* among the Three *Doshas*, and *kapha* is the waste produced during its production.

Breast milk and menstrual blood are *rasa*'s secondary tissues. *Rasa* nourishes blood by providing it with plasma, which nourishes those things, particularly the red blood cells, that make blood red. Its secondary tissues are blood vessels and tendons, and its function is invigoration, the vitalizing of body and mind, a function associated with the colour red. *Pitta*, blood's associated waste, is carried mainly by blood; in both the fire element predominates. Sushruta, aware of the surpassing importance of blood to a surgeon, went so far as to call blood the fourth *dosha*. Blood is the red essence of a being, and healthy blood is described as the colour of such things as the red lotus and heated gold.

Blood nourishes flesh, which is composed predominantly of earth and is in charge of 'plastering' the skeleton to contain and protect everything within. Its secondary tissues are ligaments (or perhaps certain muscle bodies, the translation is unclear), and the six or seven layers of skin. Flesh is *kapha*-like in nature, and its wastes are the so-called 'space wastes' (in Sanskrit, *kha mala*), the wastes that fill body cavities, such as ear wax, navel lint, nasal mucus and smegma.

Flesh nourishes fat which is also predominantly earthy and *kapha*-like. Fat's job is *snehana*, a word that means both lubrication and love, suggesting that the lovelorn may overeat fat because it provides them with a chemical substitute for love, just as chocolate provides the same chemical that is generated internally by romance. Fat's secondary tissue is said to be the subcutaneous fat (some sources say the sinews), and its waste is sweat, especially that grease that forms part of sweat.

Fat's essence goes to nourish bone, the only tissue in which *vata* predominates. Bone is composed mainly of the air element, being filled with spaces, and supports the body, providing the personality with 'backbone'. The teeth form its secondary tissue, while body and head hair, beard and nails are its wastes (some say head hair is also a secondary tissue).

Bone's essence nourishes marrow, the tissue that 'fills' the bones. Since anything encased within bone qualifies as marrow, this tissue includes the brain and spinal cord as well as the red and yellow varieties of bone marrow. *Kapha* predominates in marrow, which is unctuous, and its waste is that fatty material that collects in the corners of the eyes (some say instead it is that basic oiliness of flesh and skin, which, even if washed, will not disappear).

Marrow's essence goes to create *shukra*, the reproductive fluids of both male and female. *Shukra* has no secondary tissue (unless one counts the foetus it creates), and no waste. The action of a very subtle form of fire on *shukra* generates *ojas*, the glandular secretion that cements body, mind and spirit together. A male's *shukra*, his White Essence, is mainly composed of the water element, while a female's Red Essence, called *artava*, is fiery in nature (female *shukra*, which is ejaculated by some women during orgasm, more closely resembles male *shukra*).

Each Ayurvedic author amended this scheme to suit his purposes. These classification systems explain what their authors require them to explain; differences arise because of the point from which the system is viewed.

Charaka states that *shukra* is produced in the marrow and, oozing through the porosities in the bones 'like water filled in a new pot', spreads throughout the entire body. Ayurveda knows well the functions of the testicles. The *shukra* that oozes through the holes in the bones is neither the sticky white semen that a man ejaculates nor the fluids that ooze from an excited woman; it is, rather, that force produced by the combined action of electrical, magnetic, mechanical, glandular, nervous and mental energy that governs and makes possible sexual activity. The Taoists of China speak of a similar phenomenon when they talk of filling the bones with *chi*, the life-force, and circulating that *chi* throughout the body. Recent discoveries that bone is a natural rectifier, a transducer (which converts force into electricity and vice versa), and a light-emitting diode in the infra-red band supports the view of bone as an integral part of the body's energy system.

When the mind becomes filled with the desire for sex, it begins to identify strongly with the sex organs, drawing the consciousness down to that part of the body along with the blood and other nutrients needed to successfully perform the sex act. Charaka speaks of *shukra* being melted from the places it is stored in the body because of 'the exhilaration of sexual desire born of love' (or lust), and then flowing like water from a higher to a lower region. Here height and lowness refer to the location of the organism's awareness along the spinal cord rather than to the location of the physical *shukra*. The process, which culminates in ejaculation, begins with a disturbance in *ojas* that makes it move downwards, thereby impelling the downward movement of *shukra*.

The texts say it takes from seven to thirty days for ingested food to proceed through the tissues to nourish *shukra*, and thus *ojas*, since *shukra* is the raw material from which *ojas* is produced, though milk, honey, onions and alchemically prepared mercury are some of the substances reported to replenish the body's *shukra* almost instantaneously. *Ojas* is the finest refinement of 'sap' the body produces, and when *ojas* is firm and 'plump', mind and body are also firm and 'plump'. Excessive loss of sex juices robs mind and body of their firmness by desiccating *ojas* and *shukra*, thereby weakening immunity and digestive capacity. Unrestricted sexual activity is therefore regarded as one of the acts most detrimental to health, not because sex itself is bad but because by straining the nerves and exhausting the bodily juices, it increases *vata*, the only dry *dosha*, and decreases *ojas*, the essence of the body's water element.

Lustre and aura

Rasa is the foundation and *ojas* the apex of the body's nutrition pyramid. *Ojas* permits *tejas* to project from the subtle body into the physical body, where it appears as the digestive fire. *Ojas* is therefore both the cause and the effect of good digestion, and its conservation is essential to good health because it controls the immune system and generates the body's aura, the lustrous halo that projects the essence of one's being out into the world to act as a subtle shield against the entry of dangerous ethereal forces. 'There is no man without aura and lustre,' says Charaka. 'The shadow which is seen in water or a mirror or against the sun, and which is the exact replica of the original, is the reflected shadow. The "other shadow" (the aura) is dependent on the body's color and radiance.' The aura overshadows the body lustre, while the lustre enhances the body colour. The aura is sensed only from close quarters, while the body lustre shines from afar.

Body lustre originates from the fire element and is of seven types: red, yellow, white, dark brown, green, pale white and black. That lustre that is expansive, glossy and broad is auspicious, while a dry, soiled or contracted lustre is inauspicious and betokens disease. The colour of the aura reflects the predominant element in the individual. That aura due to the ether element is pure, blue, glossy and lustrous; that due to air is dry, dark reddish-brown and devoid of lustre; fire's aura is clear red, fiery and delightful to the eye; that of water is clear like pure water and very glossy; and earth's is stable, glossy, dense, smooth and dark or white. The air aura, which manifests when prana is imbalanced, portends death or great suffering, while the others indicate health and happiness. It is said that Gautama Buddha's aura extended to a distance of fifty miles from his body, and that everyone who came within this circle of influence automatically became a little more peaceful.

CHANNELS OF FLOW

The *doshas* when balanced support the body by irrigating the tissues with nutrients like water irrigates a field. Like field crops, the tissues require a canal system through which the nutrient juices can flow to reach them. A *srotas* is such a canal, a bodily channel in which nutrients, tissues or wastes move. Such channels exist on every layer of existence except the subtlest; a *nadi*, for example, is a *srotas*. The body's form emerges from the channels, which guide food to the tissues and mould them during their nutritional metamorphoses.

Many channels, like the digestive tract, look like pipes even to the naked eye, while the flow of others that are more subtle is not confined by the walls of a fleshy tube. The digestive tract is the most important of all the bodily channels, since it takes in the elements necessary to replenish body tissues and maintain the system's continuity. When all flows well in the various channels, the organism is healthy and happy. Disturbed flow, due usually to disturbed *vata*, creates disease and consequent misery.

There are four possible disturbances to flow in a channel: increase, decrease, a 'knotted' condition (obstruction) and deviation. Taking the alimentary canal as an example, diarrhoea is a condition of excess flow, and constipation a condition of insufficient flow. Tumours and twistings of the intestine, such as volvulus and intussusception, are varieties of obstruction, and the release of the canal's contents into the peritoneal cavity (as after perforation of a peptic ulcer or rupture of the appendix) is a deviation of flow.

One important cause of such disturbances is the restraint of the thirteen urges that must never be restrained, the urges to: expel urine, faeces and flatus; vomit, sneeze, belch and yawn; eat when hungry, drink when thirsty, cry when sad, sleep when sleepy, pant after exertion and ejaculate semen when irresistibly aroused. Restraint of these urges causes *vata* to move in an abnormal direction in these channels. Because *vata* is the force that transports materials through the body, improper direction or velocity of *vata* vitiates first the channel involved and then the entire system. Many other urges, which are not physical reflexes, including especially the negative mental urges like greed, sorrow, fear, anger, envy, pride, shame, disgust and the like, ought always to be restrained, though not suppressed.

Physical reflex urges may disturb the body even when they are not restrained. For example, one is advised to always clench the teeth tightly while urinating or defecating to prevent the strongly downward-moving force of *apana vata* from loosening them. The implications for health of the movements of *vata* are often difficult to comprehend. While all animals yawn – even fish and reptiles –

psychotics rarely do, nor do the severely ill, in whom yawning is often a sign that they are beginning to recover. Though we cannot yet say exactly what yawning does for living beings, we know that it should not be suppressed.

Given that, as Charaka noted, 'there is as much functional diversity in the systems of circulation in the human body as there is elemental diversity in the structural composition of the body', the body's channels are effectively innumerable. Ayurveda therefore singles out the most prominent of these and describes them so that, in Charaka's words, 'the ordinary practitioner will know enough to practice successfully and the intelligent physician will be able to infer the nature of those which remain unmentioned'. Of the sixteen major channels, fourteen are common to both sexes and two appear only in the female. These fourteen channels fit into four main groups: those that deal with the intake of nutrients, the nutrition of the tissues, the expulsion of wastes, and the mind.

Channels concerned with intake of nutrients

The Prana Channel is composed of the respiratory system and the heart. This 'heart' probably refers both to the physical pumping station in the chest as well as the portion of the brain that controls its function. Both are 'hearts', central essentials, of the system; both act as seats of life and of *ojas*, the functions attributed to the heart in Ayurveda. In the context of the physical body the Prana Channel mainly governs respiration.

The Water Channel, which governs the balance of the liquid element in the body, extends from the palate to the *kloman* (which apparently is the pancreas).

The Food Channel extends from the region of the oesophagus and stomach to the large intestine.

Channels concerned with nutrition of the tissues

While the *Rasa* Channel is described as consisting of the 'heart and the Ten Great Vessels', it also includes those other structures, such as lymph and blood vessels, that transport *rasa* from the gut to the heart. The two channels peculiar to the female, namely the Milk

Channel and the Menstrual Channel, are both secondary to the *Rasa* Channel. The Milk Channel includes the breasts and nipples, and the Menstrual Channel the uterus, cervix and vagina. Their functions are the production of milk and the expulsion of menstrual blood respectively. That the two are related is evident from the fact that ordinarily a woman does not menstruate while she breast-feeds.

The Blood Channel is based in the liver and spleen. This agrees in principle with the tenets of biomedicine, which assigns to the liver the role of king of the reticulo-endothelial (blood-forming) system and to the spleen the task of destroying old red blood cells.

The Flesh Channel consists of the muscles and skin.

The Fat Channel includes the kidneys and *vapavahana* (which may be the omentum).

The Bone Channel consists of the fat and the hips (the 'hinder parts').

The Marrow Channel consists of the bones and the joints and everything encased in bone, namely the red and yellow bone marrow and the brain and spinal cord.

The *Shukra* Channel consists of the testes and penis in the male, and their corresponding structures (the ovaries, vagina and clitoris) in the female. This channel in a woman is called the *Artava* Channel, the word *artava* being derived from *rtu*, or season, which implies, among other things, that even a healthy woman is fertile only 'in season', during that part of each month when she ovulates.

Channels concerned with the elimination of wastes

The Urine Channel consists of the bladder and kidneys; the Faeces Channel, the colon and rectum; and the Sweat Channel, the fat and hair follicles.

The fourteenth channel, the Channel of Mind, pervades the entire body. The body is, in a sense, the mind's special channel. There is nowhere in the body that mind cannot and does not go.

CONSTITUTION

One definition of life is: 'The link between the future existence and the past one'. This refers to both reincarnation and the present incarnation. Despite the ceaseless change of taking in things from the environment and releasing other things into the environment, an impermanent organism projects an illusion of permanence by maintaining a stable form. Molecules come and go, atoms enter and leave the body, but the body goes on. I was not the same person yesterday that I am today, and tomorrow I will be yet a different person, but the physical and metabolic patterns of my body and the principal elements of my personality remain the same. Who I am today depends on who I was yesterday, and who I will become tomorrow depends on what progress I make today.

The stability that permits me to remember who I am also discourages me from changing my ways. Some mental and physical patterns, like handedness, are so deeply embedded in the organism that it is almost impossible to eliminate them. It is very difficult to change from being right-handed to being left-handed, or vice versa, a difficulty that is associated with the very real differences that exist between right-handed and left-handed people. There is more than a little truth in the observation that lefties have a greater affinity for the arts while righties are more comfortable with the linear logic of letter and number. These are inherent, innate tendencies, which resist alteration.

As we favour hands and brain hemispheres, so we favour other organs. Each of us favours particular glands, hormones and even thoughts and images; we *favour* them, preferring them to other tissues and concepts in the organization of our lives. Modern medicine does consider variations in susceptibility to certain illnesses – for example, proposing that so-called Type A people are more likely than the general population to suffer from peptic ulcer and hypertension – but Ayurveda has synthesized metabolic tendencies and character traits into a system. It is not a clean, quantifiable system that can plot your existence with clinical precision, because such straight-line graphs cannot accurately represent human systems; humans are better represented as complex waves generated by the force of ego's gravity trying to keep the individual functioning as a well-integrated unit.

Ayurveda calls a person's characteristic physical and mental constitution *prakriti*, to be distinguished from *vikriti*, the condition or current state of a person's health, which differs from moment to moment. The sages used the word *prakriti*, which also means the manifested universe as a whole, because an individual's *prakriti* is a systematized expression of that individual's personal universe. *Prakriti* is both the first creation, which occurs when a human is created, and the first reaction of that individual's body and mind to stress. Knowledge of *prakriti* allows you to select appropriate habits and lifestyles to enhance health maintenance.

Prakriti is fixed at the moment of conception, determined by conditions in the parents' bodies and minds at the time of coitus. If, for example, the force of *vata* was increased in the father and *pitta* predominated in the mother, the child will always be, all through its life, constitutionally prone to overactivity of both *vata* and *pitta*. Other sorts of disease may come and go, and severe conditions may make consideration of the underlying constitution irrelevant, but that underlying pattern is etched permanently into the genetic material and changes during life only if the genes and chromosomes change. The parents' heredity, the diet and activity of the mother during pregnancy, and conditions in the womb during pregnancy and in the birth canal during delivery also influence the child's health and happiness, but these are all secondary to constitution.

Your constitution shows where you fall on the scales of biphasic traits, the most important of which is heat–cold. *Pitta*, the hot *dosha*, tends to create extra heat in the internal environment, and *vata* and *kapha* tend to produce more cold, *vata* causing a dry cold and *kapha*, a wet cold. A *pitta* person often feels 'hot under the collar'; usually such a person hates hot climates and loves colder realms, while a *vata* person hates to be cold and generally loves heat. *Kapha* people most enjoy the changes of the seasons, which stimulate their systems. The 'climate' of your microcosm affects you in ways similar to the climate of your homeland, and its influences are much more difficult to shut out. The three basic microcosmic constitutional types are fundamentally identical with the three basic macrocosmic types of climate: arid, torrid and humid.

The similarities between climate and constitution suggest that certain races of people should share certain constitutional characteristics, which is, in fact, the case. Natives of the tropics tend to be leaner and longer-limbed than natives of colder climes, who are stockier with shorter extremities. The former have higher surface-to-volume ratio, which more efficiently radiates heat; the latter have less surface area and so conserve heat better. Metabolic rate and blood flow are also highest in residents of a cold climate and lowest in those who live in heat. Skin colour helps regulate the amount of the body's vitamin D, which is produced by the action of sunlight on oils in the skin. In a sunny climate a dark skin helps protect against the accumulation of excess vitamin D, which can cause kidney disease; and in the northerly latitudes, where the sun is weak, a light skin helps the body absorb more sunlight to help prevent rickets, which is caused by lack of that vitamin.

Other racial differences include those between muscle fibres (which help to determine if you can be a sprinter or a long-distance runner), apocrine sweat glands and ear wax. Differences in eye colour mean that different colours are preferentially absorbed into the system, causing differences in endocrine balance and other metabolic values. There are plenty of differences between the sexes as well, and all these influences affect one's heredity.

Analysis of constitutional type is basically analysis of how the organism utilizes its matter and energy. *Pitta* people are hot because all their channels tend toward dilation. *Kapha* people tend to have congested channels, and *vata* people usually have constricted channels, though the channels in a *vata* person tend to fluctuate between dilation and contraction more readily than do those of other types. Generally *vata* people have little ability to retain either matter or energy and *kapha* people have too great a tendency to retain both. Only *pitta* people have an innate knack for managing both well, and too often they overmanage. *Vata* makes people erratic, *pitta* makes them intense, and *kapha* relaxes or over-relaxes them.

Vata, composed of the air and ether elements, is changeable, being the ever-moving wind. Because motion is what it knows, it always tries to move to the maximum – further and faster. This refers to both the organism's external activities and its internal metabolic processes. *Pitta*, the fiery *dosha*, which heats the organism and cooks its food, maximizes by becoming hotter and more intense. *Kapha*, composed of the heavy water and earth elements, stabilizes by nature; it maximizes its expression by maximizing immobility, especially by accumulation.

How you feel inside depends upon how these *doshas* work within your system. In the winter everyone's extremities become cold because of exposure to external cold, but many *vata* people have cold hands and feet all the time, because their extremities suffer from exposure to internal cold, a cold created by excessive expenditure of energy. *Pitta* people feel hunger more easily than do other types because their digestive fire is always hot, anxious for something to digest. This may manifest as hunger for physical food or as the hunger of ambition; both are due to the system's inherent fieriness. *Kapha* types gain weight more easily and lose it with more difficulty than do other constitutions because their systems are engineered to store matter and energy, and do so whenever the opportunity arises.

Constitution affects all layers of consciousness. *Kapha* people tend to accumulate money more easily than do *vata* people, who are the archetypical impulse-buyers. When *vata* obtains energy, whether it be physical energy or the energy of money, there is an innate tendency to make use of it, just as the *kapha* person experiences an innate tendency to try to save it. The *pitta* person is better at managing all sorts of energy, including money. *Vata* people are naturally good at original thought, and naturally poor at putting it into action. *Pitta* people are born engineers, knowing in their bones how to apply theory to practical situations, but they are often too demanding and irritable to be good managers. *Kapha* people often lack the incisive minds that characterize the other types, but are naturals at managing organizations.

Everyone has inherent strengths and weaknesses. If you know yours, and know how your constitution causes them, you can adjust for them and make your life happier and healthier. When you evaluate your constitution, you must see yourself as you are, not as you would like to be. Because constitution is fixed at the moment of conception, look at the tendencies that have persisted in you from childhood. Whenever you cannot decide, or it seems that you shift between characteristics, score yourself as *vata*. The most reliable characteristics are generally those that are most physical, as they are easiest to observe and most difficult to ignore. For example, the less compact and more disproportionate you are (unusually short or tall, unusually long or short legs compared to your torso), the more the influence of *vata*.

Moderation being central to Ayurveda, proportion is important to *prakriti* and the height of your body should equal the span of your outstretched arms from middle fingertip to middle fingertip. Ayurveda's individuality extends even to body measurements, which are made in units derived from the body of the person being measured, like the *angula*, which is related to the size of the finger, and the *anjali*, the volume of the two hands cupped together. A small person's *anjali* will differ from a larger person's, making each measurement proportional to the size of the person measured, not statistically standardized according to means and medians.

TABLE OF CONSTITUTIONS

Characteristic	Vata	Pitta	Kapha
Body frame	thin, irregular	medium, usually proportionate	broad, heavy, well-proportioned
Weight	easy to lose, hard to gain	easy to lose, easy to gain	hard to lose, easy to gain
Skin	dark or tans deeply, often cold to touch	light, sunburns easily, warm to touch	medium shade, tans easily, cool to touch
Sweat	scanty, even in heat	profuse in heat	moderate, consistent
Hair	dry, coarse, curly, often dark	fine, often straight, light colour, may be oily, tends to go grey or bald early	oily, lustrous, thick, usually brown
Eye colour	grey, violet, slate-blue	hazel, green, light or electric blue	brown, occasionally blue
Appetite	variable	intense	regular
Evacuation	erratic, often constipated	usually regular, sometimes loose	regular, slow
Climate	prefers warm	prefers cool	enjoys changes of season
Stamina	poor, tends to overexert	medium, over-exerts when competing	good, tends to underexert

Characteristic	Vata	Pitta	Kapha
Sex drive	variable	often intense	steady
Fertility	poor	medium	good
Sleep	Variable, often poor, deep when tired	sleeps easily, rises easily	sleeps easily, rises with difficulty
Speech	talkative, may ramble	speaks purposefully	slow, cautious
Emotion	fear often primary	often afflicted with anger	likes to avoid confrontation
Thinking	usually verbal	lots of visual imagery	frequent use of feelings, emotions
Memory	learns quickly, forgets quickly	learns quickly forgets slowly	learns slowly, forgets slowly

Vata people do things quickly: they are quick to learn and to forget, quick to become enthused and to lose that enthusiasm. They walk, talk and change their minds and moods quickly. Even their bodies change quickly: some days their digestion is good while on others it is poor; some nights they sleep well while on others they remain sleepless. Like their bodies, their minds tend to inconstancy and unsteadiness, and both body and mind tend to restlessness. Their energy comes in bursts. When energy levels are high they chat, worry, think, run or do whatever else they may be addicted to until that energy is exhausted; then they must hibernate for some time to accumulate a new store of energy, which they then go out and spend. *Vata* energy is like the capitalist business cycle: periods of boom followed inexorably by periods of bust.

Vata people often have trouble making decisions, and suffer frequently from gas, constipation and cold extremities. *Vata*'s dryness makes their bodies dry (their skins tend to crack and their joints to make noise) and often rough. Being 'cold-blooded', they tend to dislike cold weather and to love light and heat. Fear or anxiety, generated from within by the anxiety their cells feel at the erratic supply of nutrients, is their predominant negative emotion, which often arises when they miss a meal. They gain weight with difficulty and lose it easily, have imaginative minds and irregular habits, are exciting and excitable, and can be extroverted and introverted by turn. The *vata* constitution is, because of its spend-thrift ways with matter and energy, the most difficult constitution to keep healthy.

Pitta people are efficient, precise and orderly, mentally and physically. They tend to hate heat, preferring cool climates and cooling foods unless they have developed an addiction to stimulation. Their skin tends to be warm and soft, and to sprout moles, freckles, pimples, rashes and wrinkles easily, and their hair greys and falls early. They are strong-minded and forceful, and often unconsciously try to impose their will on their neighbours. They love to eat and to compete. Being easily irritable, they tend to be intolerant of disagreement and of hunger, and impatient with those who are less quick and efficient than they. They value regularity and tend to perfection-ism, which can manifest as criticism of self and others. They are determined and efficient, and tend to be so one-pointed at whatever it is they do well that they may sacrifice everything else for success. When well-disciplined, their natural heat creates courage; otherwise it produces anger, especially when they are hungry. Heat, physical and mental, creates most of their diseases.

Kapha people like the slow, relaxed life. They tend to gain weight easily and lose it with difficulty. Their body tissues are usually firm, well-nourished and healthy. They sleep deeply, and are usually slow to get going in the morning. They usually eat, walk and talk slowly, and their digestion is slow. They learn slowly, but, like elephants, rarely forget. They dislike damp cold and are prone to congestion of the sinuses and other parts of the body, but their stamina is superior to the other types and they can skip meals without physical discomfort. Skipping meals may, however, create mental discomfort in them, because underneath their placid, calm exteriors they are very emotional, often introverted, beings. They effortlessly attract prosperity to themselves and may enjoy collecting wealth.

One's *gati*, or gait, is characteristic of one's *prakriti*. Every animal possesses a characteristic gait: frogs jump, crows hop, dogs trot, and elephants and rhinos lumber. A human's gait, like an animal's, reflects his or her internal energy equation. A *kapha* person's physical gait, like his or her pulse's gait, is often described as being that of a swan, an animal that swims regally through life. Of all constitutional types the *kapha* type is easiest to maintain in a state of health.

There are eight principal *prakriti* types: *vata*, *pitta* and *kapha* each predominating alone; *vata–pitta* or *pitta–vata*, *pitta–kapha* or *kapha–pitta*, and *vata–kapha* or *kapha–vata* predominating together; all three *doshas*, tending to imbalance; and that rarest of constitutions in which all three *doshas* always tend to remain in balance. Most people have double predominance, but when one considers the various possible proportions of all these *doshas* to one another, the number of constitutional types becomes infinite, which is as it should be, since everyone is an individual. *Prakriti*-typing is neither a way to reinforce limitations nor a source of convenient labels for pigeon-holing people. It is instead a tool for self-examination and self-development, for use in locating and settling into one's own niche in the cosmos.

The above is only an outline of the process and implications of constitutional analysis; for further information please consult *Prakruti: Your Ayurvedic Constitution*.

4

ROUTINE

A LIFE WELL LIVED

This life is the only life you, as yourself, will ever have, and you owe it to yourself and to the world to make the best of yourself. The practical Charaka condenses the four Vedic aims of life – right livelihood, pursuit of wealth, enjoyment of desire and realization of the transitory nature of existence – into three pursuits: the pursuit of life, the pursuit of wealth and the pursuit of the afterlife. Most important of these three is the pursuit of life, which implies the pursuit of health, for without health one cannot enjoy life or achieve one's aims. As health is impossible without right relationship, affluence, satisfaction and at least a certain degree of non-attachment, one must simultaneously guard both one's health and one's direction in life.

From the Ayurvedic perspective, bodily health is the paramount objective. Charaka writes:

An intelligent man should therefore specially devote himself to those endeavors which assure the body's well-being. The body is truly the support of one's well-being, since humans are established in the body. Leaving everything else, one should take care of the body, for in the absence of the body there is the total extinction of all that characterizes embodied beings.

This is no Epicurean atheism; Ayurveda clearly proposes the primacy and ultimacy of spirit, but worldly success requires practicality. Once a healthy life is secured, a householder should pursue wealth; Charaka says, 'Surely there is no wretchedness more wretched than that of a man possessed of long life but lacking the appurtenances that make life worth living.' With the help of health and wealth one can live a long and dignified life according to one's own right livelihood, during which one can, by performing appropriate spiritual practices, prepare comfortably for the afterlife.

Ayurveda proposes three stages in the quest for good health: routine daily and seasonal activities to prevent illness, purificatory and palliative therapy for disease, and rejuvenation of the system to enhance health and quality of life. Ayurvedic preventive medicine is called *svasthavrtta*, 'establishing oneself in good habits', and its salient principle is that one must reject excess in everything. Harmony and health are possible only when everything in life is enjoyed at the proper moment in the proper amount.

LAND AND SPACE

As soon as sperm and ovum unite, the being thus formed becomes limited by our universe's time, space and laws of cause and effect. Health requires keeping our internal spaces and time cycles in harmony with the external spaces and time rhythms of the outer jungle, the world of wildness that is our external environment. If we fail to maintain ourselves within ourselves, bacteria, viruses and other vermin can swarm in and take us over. Civilization is the order humans impose upon Nature's wildness, and the ancient Aryans enlisted the land itself in the civilizing process by imprinting it with temporal and spatial order.

A house is a closed space whose structure, like a mould, shapes the lives of those who inhabit it; an orderly house makes for orderly residents. Villages and towns are collections of ordered spaces that structure the civilization of the community they comprise. The human mind is a space in which civilizing education creates an inner ordering of consciousness; a text is an ordered space that moulds that knowledge poured into it. A human being is a space that is by nature unstable, perpetually prone to fall into disorder.

A righteous ruler effortlessly imbues his or her kingdom and subjects with order by offering them a noble image they can accept and identify with. In a country where ruler and ruled think together and work together, the seasons, proceeding in their proper order, fill both the land and its inhabitants with the 'juiciness' needed for a happy life. And, as the disease consumption exemplifies, an unrighteous ruler disturbs the order of space and time and opens the door to wildness, epidemic disease and the breakdown of civilization.

Francis Zimmermann, in his excellent book *The Jungle and the Aroma of Meats: An Ecological Theme in Hindu Medicine*, shows how the Aryans polarized the space of India, and how this polarization affected and was affected by Ayurveda. They classified the land they found as arid ('having scanty rainfall and vegetation, swept by high winds, and enjoying abundant sunshine'), humid ('having abundant rainfall and luxuriant vegetation, few high winds and little sunshine') and balanced, and preferred for colonization the arid regions, in which *vata* and *pitta* predominate, to the humid ones, in which *vata* and *kapha* predominate. A dry climate is inherently healthier than a wet climate because it is easier for *rasa* to stagnate in the body in a wet climate. Stagnation encourages obstruction of the channels, which permits the breeding of parasites. Parasites, barbarian organisms that in or out of the body breed in stagnant water, disturb order; a well-ordered system is easier to maintain in the absence of stagnation.

Water is essential for life, but too much water ruins health. The substances found in a humid climate tend to be full of humidity themselves, and so are 'heavy' for digestion; they contribute too much water to the system, making it difficult for the digestive fire to remain hot enough to function efficiently. Substances from arid climes are arid themselves, and so 'light' for digestion. Anyone who has ever tried to build a fire from wet wood knows the antipathy that exists between fire and water. Dry fuel lights quickly and burns cleanly, and that is what we need to keep our own digestive fires well-stoked. Just as it is easier to irrigate a parched field than it is to dry out one that is waterlogged, it is easier to add *rasa* to a body living in an arid climate than it is to remove it from one living in a humid climate.

RASAS

Be a climate arid or humid, everything in its landscape (plants, animals, soil) is permeated by a particular flavour, a particular mix of juices that affects us even if we are not sensitive enough to perceive it. The sun 'cooks' water and soil nutrients into plants, whose sap becomes *rasa* in the bodies of the animals who eat them. When these plant and animal juices are eaten by a human, their qualities are taken up by the *rasa* tissue; as you eat, so you become. A *kapha*-type individual who lives in a humid, *kapha*-type climate, which encourages accumulation of wetness in the body, will find it much more difficult to stay well than a similar individual who lives in an arid climate, which tends to remove wetness from the body. A *pitta* person will find a torrid climate a very difficult place to live in comfortably, and a *vata* person will always suffer more than other types in an arid climate, because of the effects of the climate itself and of the 'juices' in the climate that are consumed as food.

The characteristics of the environment in which *rasa*, the tissue that nourishes all the other tissues, is formed impregnate it and generate its 'flavour'. Your personal experience of life, the flavour of your life, is generated from this 'sap', which pervades your existence and your consciousness, making your personality sour or salty, your existence bitter or sweet. This flavour is your reality, the reality in which you live your life, which makes your life blissful or miserable according to its quality. Saints and other self-controlled people find all the bliss they need within themselves. Those of us who cannot do so, must extract the flavours we require from our environments, making ourselves into cooking pots, processing what we take in to obtain a tasty 'soup' to satisfy our souls.

How you experience your life is determined by the flavours of your being. The most commonly used of the several systems of Ayurvedic flavour classification is that of the six tastes. These tastes apply to each sense organ, but they are called tastes (*rasas*) because their most important influence is on the make-up of the *rasa* tissue in our bodies.

Sweet Appearing mainly in substances in which earth and water predominate, sweet is cold, oily and heavy, and increases *kapha* while reducing *vata* and *pitta*.

Sour Earth and fire are the predominant elements in substances with this taste. Sour is hot, oily and light, increases *kapha* and *pitta*, and relieves *vata*.

Salty Because water and fire predominate, the saline taste is hot, oily and heavy, and, like sour, it increases *kapha* and *pitta*, and relieves *vata*.

Pungent (or spicy) The combination of air and fire make pungent hot, dry and light. It increases *vata* and *pitta*, and relieves *kapha*.

Bitter Here air and ether cooperate to make the bitter taste cold, dry and light. It increases *vata*, and relieves *pitta* and *kapha*.

Astringent Air and earth predominate in the astringent taste; it is cold, dry and heavy, increases *vata*, and reduces both *pitta* and *kapha*.

The tastes are six possible combinations of the three pairs of polarities that predominate in the *doshas*. The tastes and the *doshas* are two different subjective expressions of the system's direction of movement, the tastes being six directions in which the organism can shift when influenced by sense objects like food, and the *doshas* being three directions in which the system can skew in conditions of imbalance. Like the *doshas*, the tastes of the food and drink you eat modify your feelings and emotions, which, in turn, produce their associated tastes in your *rasa*. Sweet is associated with desire and its gratification, sour with envy, salty with greed, bitter with grief and frustration, pungent with anger, and astringent with fear.

Quality, taste and emotion are the expressions on three different levels (body, body–mind interface, and mind) of the same principle, whose manifestation differs because the perspective from which the organism perceives it differs. The same sort of pathological changes that occur in the lungs of asthma patients, which are often caused or worsened by fear or anxiety, also occur in the lungs of people who are exposed to extreme cold. Cold and fear, and the astringent taste (which causes extreme constriction), are all equivalent from your organism's point of view. Which you experience most depends on which you are exposed to first and how your system reacts to that exposure.

If your aim is to achieve happiness in this life, you must consciously select appropriate tastes in the food, drink, medicine, activity, climate, seasons and other 'substances' that you take into yourself to ensure that the *rasa* that results after digestion is sweet. When your internal space is filled with sweet *rasa*, it attracts external sweetness to it, according to the principle of 'like increases like', and harmony in life multiplies.

TIME CYCLES

Ayurveda calls space a substance because, in our world at least, space possesses qualities, like cold and wetness, that materially affect our lives. Climate is one quality of that space; another is orientation, which is governed by the Earth's magnetic field. More than two dozen animals, including the dolphin, tuna, salmon, salamander, pigeon, honeybee and the human have small amounts of iron embedded in a bone in their forehead. This iron, which is affected by magnets, is an internal compass, which sensitive individuals can actually use to locate north in a dark room. Magnetic fields, both natural (generated by the Earth, the sun and the moon) and artificial (human-generated), also affect our brain waves, pineal secretions and other physical and mental functions.

The gravity of the sun and the moon also affects us, as do their heat and cold, their light and darkness, and the seasons that all these influences together generate. The seasons control Earth's *rasa*, from which we derive our *rasa*. 'Time is change,' says Charaka, while Vagbhata declares, 'Time is, in fact, God.' Change in the relative cold or heat, wetness or dryness, and heaviness or lightness of the external world changes the balance of the body's *doshas* by constricting or dilating its channels. Change being ceaseless in our world, our efforts to adapt to it must be equally ceaseless. Plants and animals have no conscious time sense; their instincts keep them in synchrony with the seasons. We humans, who have traded most of our instincts for conscious senses, must create synchronous rhythms if we wish to live well.

Rhythm is essential to life, moment by moment. The lungs and heart work rhythmically, the intestines produce peristaltic waves and the brain generates brainwaves, all of which are intricately interrelated with one another and with the external environment. *Rtam*, the rhythm of the universe, appears in our little world as *rtu*, or season, a 'time to every purpose under heaven'. Like the Mayans, the Vedics created the image of cosmic *rtam* on Earth by establishing a system of days, months and seasons that 'calendrifies' or (in Dennis Tedlock's pun) 'day-ifies' the gods. The Vedics and later seers carefully signposted the seasons with festivals to help people keep themselves synchronous. By re-creating the seasons, such festivals reinforce the cosmic rhythm.

Ayurveda recognizes four main seasonal cycles: day and night, the seasons of the year, age and digestion.

Day and night

The day–night cycle is one of warming and cooling. Overall, *pitta* is predominant during the day, which is warmer than the night, during which *kapha* predominates. *Vata* predominates at dawn and dusk, the junctions of day and night. Within this larger cycle occurs another smaller cycle: from dawn to mid-morning the force of *kapha*, inertia, predominates, as sunlight stimulates the system to expel its excess water and become more active. Mid-morning to mid-afternoon is the time of *pitta*, when heat is maximal in the system. Mid-afternoon to dusk, as the dried organism cools, is ruled by *vata*. Likewise for night: *kapha* predominates from dusk for slightly more than one-third of the night, *pitta* predominates during the midnight hours, and the pre-dawn hours are ruled by *vata*. Chinese medicine's scheme of which organs work at what time of day and night corresponds fairly closely to this.

The seasons of the year

Charaka divides India's three seasons – winter, summer and the rains – into six two-month seasons to integrate the lunar calendar with the solar year. There are actually two slightly different sets of seasons. The first contrasts the three intense seasons – cold, hot and wet – with the three milder 'shoulder' seasons that separate them. The other emphasizes the natural progression in *rasa* in the environment, which develops as a result of the cold, heat and wetness of the seasons.

The sun is said to capture *rasa* from our planet, and the moon to release it again to us. During the six months from the winter to the summer solstice, as the sun, the lord of the fire element, grows stronger daily, it progressively withdraws 'juice' from the world, drying it out. From the summer to the winter solstice, the sun's power grows daily weaker, releasing that 'juice' again to us. This half of the year is ruled by the moon, which is the lord of the water element. The terrestrial environment and its denizens must perpetually adjust to this cyclical withdrawal and release of 'juice'.

Each season has its own taste, which pervades everything in the environment, altering its own innate, climatic 'constitutional' flavour. The permutation of these flavours and the effects of the variations between hot and cold and dry and wet weather, which affect the 'heaviness' and 'lightness' of the *rasa* in the environment, generate a pattern of *dosha* increase and decrease. Charaka provides detailed instructions for the proper regimen to be followed during each season to guard against the *dosha* imbalance caused by these fluctuations; for example, eating jaggery (sugar-cane juice boiled until it solidifies) mixed with ginger powder during the rainy season and jaggery with sesame during winter.

The seasons of temperate countries are different from those in India, but in most of them *kapha* accumulates in winter and becomes aggravated in spring; the *pitta* accumulated during spring becomes vitiated in summer, when *kapha* is calmed; and the *vata* that accumulates during summer predominates in autumn, when *pitta* calms down. *Vata* then calms itself during winter (unless the climate is inordinately cold).

Women have an extra season, the menstrual (monthly) cycle. Most women are more sexually interested and active during the full moon. Ideally, a woman ovulates with the full moon, the astronomical moment when the moon is pouring abundant *rasa* on to the Earth, and menstruates with the new moon, when the sun is drawing that *rasa* away again. In a healthy woman *kapha* predominates after the menstrual flow ends until ovulation, *pitta* predominates from ovulation until the flow begins, and *vata* predominates during the flow.

Age

Life follows a trajectory, rather like a boomerang, into and then back out of manifestation in the world of *rasa*. *Kapha* predominates strongly until age sixteen while 'juice' is being taken into the system; its domination persists until about age thirty while integration of body and mind progresses. Because of this predominance teenagers are more susceptible to colds (usually a *kapha* condition) than people over fifty. *Pitta* predominates during middle age, when a person has attained metabolic balance and mental maturity, and *vata* predominates after sixty, as body and mind gradually disintegrate. Age involves loss of life's 'juice'; people shrink with age, and the aged also feel cold more acutely than the young as *vata* desiccates their insulating body fat.

Digestion

Immediately after eating, the large inert mass of ingested food causes *kapha* to predominate and *pitta* to increase. During the digestive process *pitta* predominates, *kapha* becomes calm, and *vata* accumulates. After digestion and during assimilation and excretion of wastes *pitta* cools off and *vata* (which circulates the 'juices' in the body) predominates.

MIND AND BODY

The nostrils switch on and off every few hours, the *nadi* connected with the left nostril tending to cool and calm body and mind, and the *nadi* connected with the right nostril tending to heat up and agitate the system. Tantric hygiene requires the functioning of the nostrils to be synchronized with the lunar day and month, and advises the use of specific nostrils for particular activities; for example, the right nostril should be working when one eats, and the left when one is listening to a lecture.

Establishing a rhythm in each cycle is to physical health what satisfaction is to mental health. Only when the body's metabolic processes function with the proper frequency and intensity is physical happiness and health possible, and the mind remains in balance only when it is pleased. Daily and seasonal routines try to ensure that the body's needs are satisfied no matter where the mind may roam, since most people are unwilling or unable to develop the perception necessary to know what is happening within their bodies. Neither activity nor rest should be excessive; the body requires moderation in all things. A healthy routine establishes moderation and order in both body and mind, helping you to flow in the direction most appropriate for you.

Like Aristotle, Ayurveda teaches that one should always seek the golden mean; those who are naturally timid must learn courage, and vice versa. While there is no one 'good' that is good for everyone, certain values, such as honesty, are generally regarded as being beneficial for everyone, as others, such as dishonesty, are seen to be generally detrimental to long-term happiness. Charaka fills an entire chapter with advice on how best to 'discipline' the senses, including information on personal hygiene, moral elevation and religious observation ('remind yourself constantly of the vanity of things', 'do not be a slave to your sense-appetites or pander to the fickle mind'), followed by a list of practices to eschew, a catalogue of moral imperatives that is especially striking when compared with its total lack in much of modern medical training.

We are told that one should always cultivate the company of those who, because they have conquered passion and ignorance, never speak untruth. Saints impregnate their surroundings with saintly vibrations; mean, cruel, envious, fickle-minded scandal-mongers radiate selfishness and negativity in all directions. Since we become impregnated with the 'flavour' of our environment, communion with the low lowers our consciousness as surely as the companionship of the noble elevates us. Noble beings, including saints, experts and teachers, truly deserve reverence, a bowing down of the ego in humility to Providence appearing to us in the form of the guardians of tradition.

Learned people, says Charaka, are of two types: those who think of others and are happy and satisfied, and those who are selfish, unhappy and dissatisfied. Whom you choose to learn from determines the quality of what you learn, and that knowledge, which is a sort of nourishment, influences the quality of your mind and consciousness. Like the student of Ayurveda, who is expected to test his guru before beginning to study with him, everyone must test their teachers before daring to accept uncritically any of their pontifications.

SEASONAL ROUTINES

Ayurveda tells us that 'diseases are generated at the junctions of the seasons', the moments when one season changes into another. Every adaptation to changed circumstances that a system must make increases the likelihood of disease. Ovulation and menstruation are the joints of the menstrual cycle, dawn and dusk are the 'joints' of day and night, and adolescence and menopause are the junctions of life. Regular seasonal purifications help protect against potential ailments at the seasonal joints. Many such seasonal practices have been institutionalized into holiday rituals to make their observance by the general public more automatic.

Seasonal routines must account for constitutional differences in their practitioners. For example, at the junction of winter and spring *kapha* becomes predominant. A person of *kapha* constitution will require a more strenuous purification, such as therapeutic vomiting, than will a person of *pitta* constitution, who may be best purified with mild purgation. It is often best for a *vata* person to gradually eliminate *kapha* from the system with medicines rather than with active purification, which may increase *vata*. Between spring and summer both *pitta* and *kapha* people may profit from purgation, which may or may not be appropriate for *vata* people, according to their specific conditions. *Vata* people do respond well to medicated enemas at the joint between autumn and winter, though their enemas must be more unctuous than that prescribed for the autumnal purification of *pitta* and *kapha* people.

A healthy, well-balanced person ordinarily tries, by adjustment of food and activities, to control *kapha* during late winter and spring, *pitta* during summer, and *vata* during autumn and early winter, while a strongly *vata*, *pitta* or *kapha* person will often need to control their predominant *dosha* all year long. A *vata–pitta* or *pitta–vata* individual will usually aim to control *vata* in autumn and winter and *pitta* in spring and summer; a *pitta–kapha* or *kapha–pitta* individual, to balance *pitta* in spring and summer and *kapha* in autumn and winter; and a *vata–kapha* or *kapha–vata* type will be concerned with allaying *vata* in autumn and early winter and *kapha* in late winter and spring, summer being generally beneficial to them.

A *kapha* person must be careful not to impede digestion by sleeping or otherwise becoming inert immediately after eating, lest *kapha* increase. *Pitta* people must concentrate on avoiding heat-producing mental or physical activity during the period when digestion is in full swing, lest *pitta* become irritated. *Vata* people must remain calm and decrease their activity during the food's assimilation, or *vata*'s increase then will inhibit proper nutrition of *rasa*.

Age can be analysed in like manner: the increase in *pitta* during middle age and of *vata* during old age may prove beneficial to a *kapha* person. *Vata* people must begin preparing early for their senior years, which, when they arrive, will compound *vata*'s power and predispose to imbalance. Everyone tends to fall prey to *pitta*-type diseases (such as ulcers and gallstones) more readily during middle age, but *pitta* people are even more susceptible than are other types and must guard their health more carefully then. Every cycle requires attention if health is to be preserved.

DAILY ROUTINES

Comparing the body to a city or a chariot, which needs regular maintenance and careful attention, Charaka explains at great length the importance of using perfumes and wearing clean clothes, flower garlands, jewels and ornaments; used apparel, except from one's guru, should never be worn. This practice of regular adornment attracts, by the 'like increases like' law, more jewels and other such crystallizations of prosperity to you.

Seasonal purification routines help to prevent disease by removing from the body wastes that would otherwise clog the channels. The daily routine has the same purpose: physical and mental purity are essential prerequisites for eating, the daily sacrificial ritual that replenishes the bodily field and exhilarates the gods of the microcosm. Arising before dawn in order to enter the new diurnal cycle awake and alert, one eliminates urine and faeces, mobilizes metabolic wastes and expels sweat through massage and exercise, removes external wastes, gross and subtle, by bathing, purifies the sense organs by 'purging' the head; and eliminates mental wastes by meditation.

Purification drains excess 'juice' from the bodily field and must be followed by oiling, to prevent *vata*'s dryness from emaciating the individual. Mineral oil and other inedible oils must never be applied to the skin, which is a digestive organ; whatever is applied to it eventually enters the system. Charaka avers that all sensory response is referable ultimately to the sense of touch. Daily oil massage strengthens the skin, improves its colour and texture, and makes it soft and unctuous. The oil reduces *vata*'s dry, light and rough qualities, and the rhythmic movement relieves *vata*'s erratic nature and alleviates stiffness.

Massage increases the circulation to remove wastes from the tissues while improving their nutrition by keeping the lymph (*rasa*) freemoving and pure. Massage alleviates old age and fatigue, improves the vision and the sleep, and strengthens resistance to stress and injury. The type of oil to be used for massage depends upon the season; a cool oil (olive, coconut, sunflower) for summer, a warmer oil (mustard, almond, sesame, safflower, peanut) for winter. Massage should not be done when the body is suffering from an excess of *kapha* or an acute disease, especially a fever, because it would increase toxins.

The heart, navel, genitals, joints, anus and all hairy areas (the armpits, pubes, chest and head), all seats of *vata*, must always be well oiled, working in the direction in which the hairs grow, which is the direction of *vata*'s flow. Massaging to move the body's energy downward facilitates the action of *apana vata*, while moving the energy upward provides a more meditative quality. Oiling of the navel improves the flow of prana in the many *nadis* centred around it. One Ayurvedic ailment for which there is no modern equivalent is 'dislocation of the navel,' a condition in which the navel is displaced from the centre line of the body. This is said to disrupt the movement of *vata* in the intestines, resulting in constipation and/or diarrhoea, distention and the like. Manipulation of the navel is necessary to return it to its original position.

Massage of the head strengthens and calms the sense organs. The most important part of the head to be oiled, say the Vedics, is the *agnishikha*, the whorl of hair at its back. The *agnishikha*, which means 'crest of fire', is hooked up to certain important *nadis* through which the life-force must flow freely if consciousness is to be clear.

A true Vedic always keeps a long tuft of hair growing at this whorl, which he twists at oiling time in the direction in which it grows. Different races have different directions of whorl; in most Europeans it is counter-clockwise; in most Japanese, clockwise.

Massage has always held an important place in Indian culture, and even today people often trade foot and leg massages. Traditionally, children are massaged daily during their first years of life, and weekly thereafter. A ceremonial massage is administered before marriage, and the treatises on sexology advise regular sensual massage with aphrodisiac oils. Pregnant women are often massaged gently during their pregnancy and more strenuously during the first forty days or so after they deliver. Some 'modern' doctors in India now tell new mothers not to oil babies because this produces colds and bronchitis; besides the clear physical benefits of regular massage, however, the simple act of holding and caressing a child stimulates its immune system. Human and animal infants can die if they are not regularly cuddled and fondled, and since rocking has been shown to stimulate the development of the cerebellum, baby massage is truly essential to a baby's development.

Adult massage, which is passive exercise, must be complemented by active exercise, which enables more prana to reach the tissues by cleaning and clearing all channels, promoting circulation and the excretion of wastes, improving lung efficiency, destroying fat and increasing stamina and resistance to disease. Stress interferes with immune activity; exercise improves it. There are three types of strength: natural (inherited strength of body and mind), periodic (dependent on season and age) and acquired (accruing from diet and exercise). Because we have practical control only over the third variety, proper diet and exercise are profoundly important to health.

Excessive exercise can cause physical injury, and evidence suggests that people may be genetically programmed to burn a set amount of calories before they die. A higher-than-programmed metabolic rate, which can result from over-exercising, might actually shorten the life-span; you *can* get too much of a good thing. Exercise is food for those people whom it helps increase their muscle mass, medicine to the obese, and poison to those who become addicted to it for the endorphin thrills it delivers (such addiction is common among *vata*-type people).

Exercise is best performed in the early morning to balance *kapha*, which predominates then. At no time should you expend more than half your available energy on exercise; if, for example, you become exhausted after running for an hour, never run for more than half an hour at a time. Exercising until sweat appears on the forehead is sufficient to strengthen the circulation. Only *kapha*-type people should exercise very vigorously; everyone else, especially *vata* types, should be more moderate. Exercise is contraindicated in *vata* diseases such as chronic respiratory complaints, in pitta conditions such as blood disorders and severe inflammations, in severe indigestion, and for very young and very old people.

Soap is not meant for use on the body except when one is truly grimy, and even then, as modern medicine agrees, it should never be used on mucous membranes. This aspect of Ayurveda has been forgotten in all parts of India except Kerala, and almost every Indian today, including those who must bathe on the street, soaps up vigorously. Bathing is prohibited within an hour after eating, and when one is suffering from diarrhoea, abdominal distention, chronic cold, indigestion and most acute illnesses. The yogis always advise cold water for bathing, while Ayurveda suggests hot water, except on the head, where only warm should be used lest it weaken the sense organs. Because bathing with water cleans only the outer body, the subtler bodies must be cleansed by other means, such as by chanting mantras or singing devotional songs while bathing, which makes the bath or shower water into a vehicle for those vibrations and transports their purifying power into the deepest levels of being.

Purification of the body 'space' should also be accompanied by purification of the 'space' of the house in which one lives. In Vedic rituals the sun, fire and fumigation were used to destroy parasites and other malignant organisms, and Sushruta prescribed fumigation to purify operating theatres, hospital wards and the like. Plants like apamarga (*Achyranthes aspera*), cedar, mustard and calamus have been shown to actually kill airborne bacteria when they are used to fumigate.

After all these purifications the organism is ready for its daily activities. Just as the quantum of exercise determines whether it is beneficial or non-beneficial to an organism, it is the amount and intensity of these daily activities that determines whether they enhance or weaken health. Of all life's activities three are most essential, and most in need of quantity control. Charaka calls them life's main supports, its Three Pillars: eating, sleeping and sexual activity. Eating will be discussed in the next chapter.

Sleeping

Sleep is the world's upholder and nurse. Normal sleep, which is due to disengagement of the mind from the outward-pointed senses, is necessary only for the mind; it is good for the body, but the body could gain the same benefit from simple deep rest. Sleep is necessary to prevent mental indigestion, to permit the mind to digest everything it took in during the day. Sleeping during the day for longer than a brief nap is permissible only in certain cases of weakness and exhaustion, or in very hot weather; otherwise it increases *kapha* and clogs all the channels. Staying up all night does the opposite, increasing *vata* and decreasing *kapha*.

Sleeping on the left side makes the right nostril and its *nadi* more active, and is good for digestion and to activate the body, but may aggravate *pitta*. Sleeping on the right side makes the left nostril and its *nadi* work harder, cooling and calming the system to encourage more relaxing sleep, but sometimes aggravating *kapha*. Sleeping on the back does not encourage free movement of either *nadi* and so increases *vata*, while sleeping on the stomach aggravates all three *doshas*. If you sleep with your head pointing to the north, the Earth's magnetic field reduces your peripheral blood flow and increases restlessness, irritation and confusion in your thinking. This orientation is, however, said to be good for promoting out-of-body experiences by weakening the ties that bind the astral and the physical bodies. Sleeping with your head to the east promotes meditative sleep; to the south, deep, physically restful sleep; and to the west, overactive or violent dreams.

Dreaming is an integral part of mental digestion, for in a dream the mind can do all those things it is unable or forbidden to do in waking consciousness. Dreams can also be prophetic, and sometimes accurately presage changes in health. Everyone without right-brain damage dreams at night; in fact, apparently all animals but the spiny anteater dream. Cows sleeping in barns dream twice as much as those sleeping in meadows; perhaps their minds roam further to make up for the relative inactivity of their bodies. Modern research shows that children dream more than adults do, and foetuses seem to dream all the time, which agrees with the Ayurvedic concept of pregnancy as a time when the newly reincarnating soul is reviewing and reliving its past life, ruminating over plans for its life to come.

Sexual activity

Consciousness exists in both egg and sperm. A woman is born with all the eggs she will ever have, eggs that developed by the end of the fourth month after she was conceived, so you were influenced in the womb by the conditions of your maternal grandmother's pregnancy; your mother and maternal grandmother were directly affected by your maternal great-grandmother's pregnancy; and so on. In addition, your genetic material preserves the flavour of its previous users; this connection is strong enough that your consciousness is affected by the seven generations of ancestors. The seers long ago became aware of the importance of heredity and of maintaining good relationships with your family members, with whom you share your genes.

How a child is conceived makes an immense difference to its development in the womb and its birth experiences, and colours its whole life after birth. It is trapped in its constitutional pattern, which is fixed at the moment of conception. A child conceived in fear and lust in the back seat of a car begins its life with several strikes against it. A child conceived during a blissful sexual experience unconsciously remembers some of that ecstasy. That whiff of joy becomes a firm foundation for a happy and healthy life – 'well begun is half done'. According to Sushruta, the ideal setting for a tryst provides a feast for each sense organ: a full-moon night in a bower of flowers, soft silk garments, sweet intoxicating perfumes, light and nourishing food, sweet music. When each sense has been fully fed, the satisfaction permeates the consciousness and the ensuing orgasmic sacrifice of the male's *shukra* into the female's fire satiates both partners; sex is, as Vimalananda used to say, 'eating with the lower mouth'.

101

After touch, smell is the most important sense to be fed during sex; one Sanskrit verb meaning 'to kiss' also means 'to smell'. The cells that set puberty in motion originate in the nose and only later migrate to the brain, and many people with smell disorders lose interest in sex. The creative use of fragrances can improve the timbre and flavour of sexual enjoyment. Women have a better sense of smell than do men; they detect musk, Ayurveda's premier perfume and heart stimulant, better than any other odour, and detect it 100 to 100,000 times better during ovulation and menstruation. Pheromones, the hormone odours contained in the sweat of both sexes, also seem to affect women more than men. Male pheromones help to regularize a woman's menstrual cycle, and women who live together usually develop synchronized menstrual periods through the effect of their own pheromones on each other.

The ancient authorities knew another fact that scientists today are only now accepting: a woman's sexual experience is far superior to a man's. The female brain is wired to deliver a better orgasm than is the male brain; a male orgasm is more of a reflex, like the orgasm of lower mammals. A woman is a man's teacher in the realm of sex, and so Charaka is faulted by some modern sexologists who feel he is over-concerned with the male's excitation. They offer in comparison texts such as Vatsyayana's *Kama Sutra*, which extensively addresses the question of a woman's excitation. There is some truth in such accusations, though in Charaka's defence we may observe that he was concerned mainly with his clients, most of whom were men, and he was more concerned with procreation than with pleasure. In his discussion on virility even Charaka clearly states that the best aphrodisiac for a man is a woman who loves him: 'All the delectable objects of the senses are found together in combination only in the person of the woman, nowhere else. . . . In her also are established righteousness, wealth, auspiciousness and the two worlds, this and the other.' A man must, therefore, honour his partner as the embodiment of the goddess of wealth and prosperity. When he offers his libation of seed into her, he worships the fire she embodies, and from this sacrifice prosperity manifests through her. This is an internal sacrificial rite.

The Tantric religion, a religion of the body, respects sexual intercourse as a sacred act, which can, if properly performed, become an act of worship. Just as today's Ayurveda owes much to Tantra, ancient India's sexology reflects the secularizing of Tantra's researches into human sexual response. A glance at the table of contents of Kalyana Malla's *Ananga Ranga* discloses discussions on which lunar day prana causes passion to reside in which female limb, and how to awaken that passion; sexual compatibility by size and qualities of genitals, by personality, by homeland, and by astrology, palmistry and physiognomy; the varieties of enjoyment, including kissing, use of the nails, yoga postures used as sexual positions, and so on; alchemical aphrodisiacs, rejuvenatives and remedies; and charms and spells for both men and women to attract the opposite sex.

In the Tantric religion the two sexes are absolutely equal. After this sexual knowledge was secularized, however, a subtle sexism crept in. Men stopped seeing sex as a sacrament, and began to view it as a pleasure to be indulged in. It is easy to become addicted to indulgences, and through the eyes of addiction many men came to view women as objects of indulgence. Recovered 'sexoholics', in turn, saw women as temptresses who had taught them to indulge. The average Indian male's ambivalent attitude towards women dates back at least to Manu, India's best-known lawgiver, who in his *Manu Smruti* wrote both 'Where women are not honored, no sacred rite can yield rewards' and 'Her father protects her in childhood, her husband protects her in youth and her sons protect her in old age; a woman is never fit for independence', because of her supposedly insatiable sexual appetite. Sudhir Kakar quotes a Punjabi proverb in his book *Intimate Relations*: 'A woman who shows more love for you than your mother is a slut.'

Religious law states that a man should never refuse a woman who requests him to unite sexually with her, but the texts provide sufficient ritual prohibitions to invoke that he may protect himself almost all month long from this fiery partner, who would, by devouring his *shukra*, dry out his 'juices' and his *ojas*. One must certainly protect one's *ojas*, and so Ayurveda advises orgasmic sexual activity a maximum of two to three times a week in the healthiest season of the year, and not more than twice a month in climatic extremity.

Orgasm, a sudden discharge of tremendous nervous energy, can disturb *vata*, so after orgasm, one should urinate (to regulate the activity of *apana*), wash the face, brush the teeth, clean the armpits, legpits and ears (to free the passage of *vata* and prana on the surface of the body), and do stretching or mild exercises. Sex should be avoided immediately after meals and during acute disease or convalescence. Indiscriminate sexual activity and a multitude of partners increases the likelihood of disease, including, but not limited to, venereal diseases. Any kind of proximity causes an exchange of all sorts of 'things', such as pathogens, emotions and even thought forms, between people; sleeping near someone, kissing and sexually uniting progressively increase the opportunity for 'things' to be exchanged.

The priests who demanded all-or-nothing attitudes to life took these health-oriented restrictions to sexual activity and made of them a ritual-based dogma that utterly separated sex from spirituality. Women then became the gateway to hell, both physically and mentally, and men in India started to see women either as sluts or saints, and nothing in between. Though Sanskrit literature contains enough examples of tender, devoted love between man and woman to suggest that some men continued to regard their wives as goddesses incarnate, anti-sensual attitudes have persisted. Ayurveda teaches that a healthy, emotionally satisfying sex life is a critical factor in a woman's health; when it is missing she falls prey to imbalances, which are then transmitted to her children, the next generation. Men who search for ways to improve society and civilization need look no further than their own sexual attitudes and practices.

PREGNANCY AND CHILDBIRTH

Chapter Three of Charaka's section on the body contains a debate between his teacher, Atreya, and the seer Bharadvaja over how a foetus is formed. Atreya maintains that embryos can be said to be born from the mother, the father, the spirit, the *yukti* of time and place, and from nourishment, all connected together by mind. After some verbal sparring, Bharadvaja inquires how all these factors know how to integrate themselves together, and Atreya responds, 'When the embryo-forming elements find themselves in the human mould they emerge in human form.' When, inspired by the desire-mind, the sperm, ovum and nutrients mix together in the crucible of the womb at the right moment under the right conditions, a sort of ethereal species template or mould, which in Sanskrit is also called a womb, shapes that new life into a human form. All the humans who have gone before have contributed to some degree to this pattern of humanness, and the child who is created from this pattern will contribute to it as well.

This morphogenetic pattern (to use the modern term) is one of the fundamental factors that shape the final form of the being to be born, others being the parents' racial templates, the family patterns of the mother and father, and the patterns resulting from the previous incarnations of the incarnating child. All these influences are then acted upon by the minds of the mother and father before, during and after conception, and the result appears nine months later. A couple ought to want the strongest, most attractive, healthiest, highest-minded, highest-souled child who has ever popped out of the human mould, and should organize their lives to actualize this aim. Requesting the gods, elements, adepts and all other influential beings in the universe to assist them in this endeavour, they should proceed elatedly and determinedly. After extensively purifying and rejuvenating their bodies, they should unite their seeds with joy and exaltation on an auspicious night at an auspicious moment, to germinate a healthy embryo.

Then, says Charaka, their physician should make the parents consider which qualities they want in their child, and should, to replace any existing negative patterns of life with positive patterns, have the woman imitate in 'diet, recreation, care and paraphernalia' the people of that culture that most closely resemble the image they have visualized. The woman does not simply sit and imagine her child developing in a certain way; she pours herself into the appropriate mould, and reinforces her thoughts with her actions, reinforced themselves by the cultural and racial mould of the people she imitates. Although the child's sex is fixed at the moment of conception, sons have been preferred to daughters since the early days of the Aryan race, because sons marry and remain with the family while daughters are given away in marriage to other families. Ayurveda therefore also offers couples a ritual that can shift the sex of an unborn female child to male.

The foetus is aware inside the womb. One hero of the *Mahabharata* learned a military manoeuvre while yet unborn by listening to his father describe it to his mother. Today tiny babies seem to be able to recognize the theme songs from the soap operas their mothers watched during pregnancy. A child who is carried for nine months by a mother who does not want it or by a mother whose spouse does not want it will grow up feeling unwanted, no matter how much attention is lavished upon it thereafter. Wilful abortion of a foetus is not good, especially, they say, after the foetal heart begins to beat, but physical abortion's effects are often preferable to the permanent scarring of such mental abortion.

Everything a pregnant woman eats and does, as well as her milieu, should therefore be 'soft, palatable, cooling, pleasant and delicate'; in a word, 'wholesome', to reassure and strengthen the child and to interfere as little as possible with its self-expression. 'Like a pot brimful of oil,' says Charaka, 'a pregnant woman should be handled without being upset in any way.' Sudden fear, injury, very hot food and drinks and the use of alcohol are a few of the activities and mental attitudes that can cause miscarriage. Potential causes of damage to the foetus include the mechanical (such as travelling over a bumpy road), the physiological (addiction to bitter foods, which aggravates *vata* and yields weak or emaciated offspring) and the psychological (intolerance in the mother, which creates a fierce, deceitful or envious offspring). Charaka emphasizes that all such prohibitions apply both to male and female up to the moment of conception, and that the psychological prohibitions apply to both parents indefinitely.

Some of the peculiar cravings a pregnant woman feels are due to physical imbalance or deficiency because of donation of much of her *rasa* to the foetus, and because of the foetal wastes, which strain her own waste-management systems. The stereotypical craving for pickles and ice cream reflects the system's craving for more sweet, heavy, milky juice for nourishment, and for the sour and spicy tastes needed to help digest it. Most of these desires, though, reflect the preferences and aversions of the foetus, which are carried over from previous existences and transmitted to the mother through the channels that connect them, influencing her feelings and perceptions.

After conception, the soul awaiting birth hovers near the womb. When the foetal heart begins to beat, the latent mind of the soul becomes activated into the consciousness of its new existence, and in this 'two-hearted' state mother and child function as a psychological unit. Strange maternal cravings must be satisfied to ensure the child's future mental and phsyical well-being unless the mother might be harmed thereby. If she insists that her desire is overwhelming, she can be permitted to indulge herself, but only with an antidote, something that will prevent that indulgence from disturbing the *doshas*.

A variety of tonics and supplements can be given to an expectant mother, including the medicated ghee (clarified butter) called *Phala Sarpis*, decoction of the root of *bala* (*Sida* spp.), and Ayurvedically prepared iron. The soul finally enters the child irrevocably in the eighth lunar month, a critical moment for both mother and child, as *ojas* is transferred between the two. About one month before delivery, the expectant Ayurvedic mother during the classical era was ushered with ritual and music into a light, airy maternity room in the southwest corner of the house, facing east. She remained there, living quietly and meditating on her soon-to-be-born child, until going into labour, while the father-to-be busied himself before, during and after delivery with the performance of protective rituals. About two weeks after the birth, when the period of ritual impurity ended, the emergence of mother and child from the lying-in room would occasion a big feast. Such lying-in rooms are rare in modern India.

During labour the physician might use decoctions and medicated enemas to encourage the free, strong downward motion of *apana vata*, and might give herbs such as saffron, calamus and *ashvagandha* (*Withania somnifera*) to promote delivery. Sushruta advises that *Gloriosa superba* root be tied to the woman's limbs for an easy birth. Eight abnormal presentations (including breech and shoulder presentations) are mentioned in the texts, and forceps delivery is described. Surgeons were also taught to extract any foetus that had died in the womb.

Immediately after delivery the mother is given herbal decoctions to reduce her aches and pains and strengthen her nerves; in some parts of India she is later fed sweets made of gum arabic to help her body regain its strength. She may also require treatment for general malaise, fever due to exertion, tremors, thirst, heaviness of the limbs, oedema, colic or diarrhoea. The mother's body, which was until recently filled with child, has now been suddenly emptied. In order to control *vata*, which tends to accumulate in any empty space, she must be regularly massaged after she delivers, and her well-oiled abdomen should be bound tightly with a cloth to support her internal organs and encourage her uterus to involute. Uterine tonics such as betel-nut jam may also be prescribed.

The new-born child is often given honey mixed with fresh butter or with aloe vera juice to purify its digestive tract and hasten the expulsion of meconium. Sometimes a baby's first food is a mixture of honey and ghee into which a bit of pure gold has been rubbed, so that the baby's first taste of its new world is one of auspicious substances of auspicious colour, that its whole life may be auspicious. The child is also regularly massaged, and to its skin are applied pastes of such substances as turmeric, mung beans and grated coconut. If at all possible, the child should live exclusively on breast-milk for at least six months. Should it become ill, its remedies are administered to its mother so that their active principles emerge, made milder, in her milk. A few herbs are also given directly to infants, such as dill water for colic, and calamus root, which is given daily in tiny amounts during the first several months of life to strengthen the immune system.

Diseases of the breast and its milk, including especially those abnormal qualities of breast-milk that develop when a mother indulges in inappropriate food and activities, and can cause such common conditions as eye irritation, respiratory congestion, eczema and nappy rash, require special attention. It is particularly bad for a child to drink the milk of a mother who has become pregnant again, because of the increased wastes that circulate in her blood. The mother is not, of course, the sole source of all the baby's ailments, but adequate treatment of the mother and her milk can prevent or cure many of baby's illnesses.

Nursing is an occasion of joy for mother as well as baby. Sushruta observes that:

just as semen comes out of the body of its own accord by the sight, remembrance, hearing or touch of the woman loved, sheer pleasure being the cause of its discharge, so it is with breast milk. It flows freely by the touch, sight, remembrance and fondling of the child, and the cause of continuous lactation is the love of the mother toward the child.

The let-down reflex, which causes milk to flow, closely resembles the male orgasmic reflex; that is, the release of milk provides a woman with the same sort of joy and satisfaction that release of semen does for a man. The nipple, like the penis, becomes erect during sex, and the breast itself, like the penis, becomes tumescent, enlarging during sexual excitation. Semen and milk are both cool, sticky, white essences subject to the same sorts of disorder. Women, therefore, are twice-blessed, with the bliss of both orgasm and nursing.

Children in India are sources of joy for everyone in a home, and young children are the centres of attention in most Indian households, everyone nurturing and indulging them ceaselessly. Ayurveda strictly directs that pregnant women, the sick and the young always be served first, and that harsh words never be used to the aged, the sick or children. Nor may one beat children, though mild spanking is permissible, nor should the child be awakened suddenly, snatched or thrown into the air, or otherwise irritated. Parents are forbidden to use the 'bogey man' (in the form of ghosts, goblins or ferocious animals) to make the child eat or otherwise obey them.

Charaka's text also contains detailed instructions on the care of the young child, including when it should be encouraged to sit up; the size, shape, texture, colour and safety of toys; and the variety of amulets it should wear. A child must be protected and kept happy at all times at all costs, as this is crucial for its healthy psychological development. Sudhir Kakar observes that 'with compassion and tenderness for the young, Ayurveda strives to develop the adult caretaker's capacity to comprehend the needs and emotions of the child — needs that are apt to be overlooked since they are articulated in voices that are frail and words that are indistinct.'

This capacity has taken such deep root in the Indian psyche that tens of millions of Indian devotees have learned to worship God as a child, taking for themselves the attitude of God's parents. Their natural love, compassion and tenderness for all children transfer easily and naturally from a human baby to a baby Krishna or baby Rama.

SAMSKARAS

The increase in desirable qualities, reduction in negative qualities, and introduction of previously absent qualities into a substance is the process of *samskara*. *Samskara*, the 'lending of other properties to a substance', literally means 'doing well', as in the proverb 'Anything worth doing is worth doing well.' Herbs, animal products and minerals undergo *samskaras* when they are processed into medicines; in a 'cold' thing there is always a little heat that can be enhanced, and a 'hot' thing can always be cooled. The study of medicine is itself the study of how to create new realities, new character traits and tendencies, in living beings by means of *samskara*. The various daily and seasonal rituals are *samskaras*, regularly repeated activities meant to maintain order in the individual and in society; neglect of such routines carries with it the ever-present risk of a retreat into individual or cultural chaos.

Such training must begin early in life, because it is often too late to learn images of healthy living if you wait until severe disease strikes. The first *samskara* in the Vedic tradition occurs when a child is ritually introduced to, and inducted into the family by its naming, usually within the first month of life. At the age of three or four months it is taken outside for the first time to look at the sun and the moon, a ritual introduction to its universe. Between six months and one year comes its first meal of solid food, usually cooked rice, an introduction to eating, which marks the onset of weaning. Around the sixth month its ears are pierced, a practice that was originally a sort of permanent acupuncture treatment. In most communities a boy has had his first haircut by the age of three; his head is often fully shaven as part of a death-and-rebirth ritual.

Education traditionally began between five and seven years and was followed between eight and twelve by investiture with the sacred thread, which, with its death and rebirth symbolism, transforms the child into a young man. There is a proverb: 'Treat a son like a king for the first five years, like a slave for the next ten and like a friend thereafter.' Even today Indian children are spoiled by their families until they go to school, and then worked mercilessly at their studies until they graduate.

Though these *samskaras* were, and are mainly, performed for upper and middle caste boys, and only rarely for girls or lower caste boys, they still affect all strata of society; for example, most of what the Indian populace knows of Ayurveda is the legacy of the training in preventive medicine that all students of the Vedas were taught as a *samskara*, training that diffused over the centuries into every part of society. And no matter how limited their implementation may have been they compare favourably with the attitudes towards children that have been present in the West since antiquity. A father had absolute control over his children under Roman law, and could kill or sell them into slavery at his whim. Infanticide, torture, sexual abuse and abandonment were common until the end of the Middle Ages, and declined only slowly thereafter. Today's decadent Western culture shows signs of again retreating into brutality, for decadence is not far removed from barbarism, and both are distant from civilization.

Only a life cultured by *samskara* can be truly satisfying and happy. The stability and health of your family and society originate with you, so you must be patriotic – or better yet, 'matriotic' – to be truly healthy, in the sense that you must both love your homeland unconditionally and strive to remove its flaws. Every substance you contact, including your country and your food, is a 'being in transition' with which you form a relation. The result of creating many orderly, healthy relationships is sweetness.

At the end of the chapter on routine in *Ashtanga Hrdaya* there is a verse that captures the essence of self-improvement. It defies simple translation, but in essence it advises you to pass your nights and days in reflection on the transitory nature of existence, examining what is wholesome and what is not for yourself, your family, your country and the world. By taking only those courses of action that are beneficial to all concerned and appropriate to your capacity to act (your age, strength, state of health and so on), you ensure for yourself a life of sweetness without tasting misery until your dying day.

5

FOOD

_____

The life of all living beings is food, and all the world seeks food. Complexion, clarity, good voice, long life, understanding, happiness, satisfaction, growth, strength and intelligence are all established in food. Whatever is beneficial for worldly happiness, whatever pertains to the Vedic sacrifices, and whatever action leads to spiritual salvation is said to be established in food.

CHARAKA

The most important of all *samskaras* is proper eating, a human's daily fire sacrifice. While the Vedas class substances according to their utility as sacrificial material for the external sacred fire, Ayurveda classifies them according to their use as food offerings to one's internal fire. You can no more make a silk purse from a sow's ear than you can construct healthy tissues from unhealthy food, unless you have become a Tantric adept. Ideally your food should be grown in your own field or garden so that you have full control over what physical and mental inputs it imbibes, but since this is impossible for most of us nowadays, the role of the food preparer becomes paramount.

Many of India's cooks and doctors are Brahmans, because these professions, like that of a Vedic priest officiating at a sacrifice, involve the selecting, mixing and offering of substances to a fire. The cook in a traditional Indian household is, in many ways, its sacrificial priest, preparing live food for the sacrifice of communal eating, which 'cooks' individuals together into a family. Like an alchemist, the cook extracts the essence from the raw materials and feeds it into human fires for the production of sweet *rasa* and *ojas*. A good cook personalizes food, projecting love and nourishment into it, killing it and then bringing it back to life. Every thought

thought by the cook affects the food and, after ingestion, the eater. Only one who loves you and is ready to devote the effort needed to transmit that love into the food should cook for you. Menstruating women are not allowed to cook in India because menstruation is a time of purification during which it is difficult to harness the mind adequately to concentrate on this exceedingly important work.

Though a good cook can improve the qualities of almost any food, the effect of the food on the system finally rests with the digestive capacity of the eater. Yoghurt, for example, is forbidden to the *kapha* person, and to everyone during *kapha* season, climate or disease, because under those conditions it is more likely to remain undigested and thus to act more like a poison than a food.

Food goes through three stages during its digestion: the 'raw' stage in the stomach, governed by *kapha*, in which sweet is the predominant taste; the 'cooking' stage in the small intestine, governed by *pitta*, in which sour predominates; and the 'cooked' stage in the colon, with pungency predominant, governed by *vata*. As long as the food remains raw in relation to the eater, it is impure, and potentially poisonous; once it has been thoroughly 'cooked' by the digestive fire, it becomes pure, fit to be assimilated into the body.

Taste is the effect of the food on the body after ingestion and before digestion. *Virya*, or potency, is the effect it exerts during digestion and *vipaka*, or post-digestive effect, is the expression of a food in the system after it has been digested and assimilated. Charaka says, 'Every action is the result of potency.' Although there are four pairs of strong potencies, including heavy and light, the most important is hot and cold. Hot food enhances the fire available to the body, while cold food reduces it. Generally sour, salty and pungent substances are hot, and sweet, bitter and astringent substances are cold.

There are three types of post-digestive effect: sweet, which tends to increase the tissues, cause *kapha* and build up the body; sour, which causes *pitta* and may burn away the tissues; and pungent, which increases *vata* and dries out the tissues. Generally, substances that are sweet and salty in taste have sweet *vipaka*, sour substances have sour, and bitter, pungent and astringent substances have pungent *vipaka*. Since sweet, sour and pungent are the tastes produced during the three stages of digestion, *vipaka* is a measure of both the natural qualities of the food ingested and the strength of the digestive process.

Your choice of food is determined principally by its taste. Everyone craves for the taste they are missing in themselves. Because no one food is fit for everyone at all times in all places, you should always consciously select those tastes and other qualities that will help you balance your *doshas*. Body and mind may both crave a certain taste, but because most people are not trained to examine the tastes of their food, their minds' emotions and conditioned preferences will crave for specific foods of that taste, while their bodies crave any food of that taste so long as that food's other qualities (soft or hard, light or heavy, oily or dry, etc.) provide the chemical context the body needs to help it remain in balance. It is always best to know exactly what you need and to select your food accordingly instead of permitting your mind to convince you that the things it likes are good for your body.

Children love the sweet taste, and need it to feed their growing bodies. But when they try to get this sweetness from candy and other sugar-filled, nutritionally disastrous treats, the excess sugar increases their blood levels of adrenalin (the chemical that causes us to prepare for either fight or flight), producing uneasiness, the precise opposite of the satisfaction that wholesome sweet food should produce. Sweets are also associated with endorphin release, which increases pain tolerance, so sweets are a joy to the poor, and chronic pain patients sometimes eat sweets alone, with eventual side-effects like hypoglycaemia and diabetes.

Selection of food items to ensure good effects on the eater depends mainly on eight aspects: its natural quality, preparation, combination, amount, the climate, the season (internal as well as external), the rules of eating, and the eater.

NATURAL QUALITIES

These qualities are innate to the foodstuff. Black gram, beef, pork, and milk are innately heavy for digestion, while mung beans, venison and rice are innately light. Heavy food should form at most one-third to one-half of your meal, while you can eat your fill of food that is light. In general, raw food is heavier than cooked, and preserved food is heavier than fresh, but aged wine and grains are lighter than new wine and grains. The flesh from the lower part of a male animal or the upper part of a female is lighter than the rest; the flesh from animals native to water or wetlands or that eat heavy foods are heavy, as is the flesh of any pregnant animal; and flesh is heavier than blood, fat than flesh, and marrow than fat. Semen is heaviest of all.

Some substances have unique natural qualities that make them unusually useful in the diet. Fish is generally hot and sweet, so it can help strengthen the body without much danger of aggravating *kapha*, as most sweet foods do. The amalaki fruit is cold though sour, and it can improve digestion without aggravating *pitta*. Rock salt is not very hot though it is salt, and so aggravates *pitta* less than ordinary salt. Natural quality must be amended for those of us who live in an unnatural world. Although fresh rain-water is said to be the best water to drink, in areas where acid rain falls, rain-water will not be pure. Nor is food grown with chemical fertilizers and pesticides pure, but when it comes to a choice between an organic, non-chemicalized food that you know you cannot digest and a food grown with agricultural chemicals that you know you can, your choice should always be that which is digestible.

PREPARATION

The qualities of a food can be altered by *samskara*. Rice, which is naturally light, is made even lighter when puffed by roasting or baking, and the flour of puffed rice can be made heavy by being made into balls and fried. Milk becomes lighter when heated with spices such as saffron, and rice becomes heavier when cooked with milk. Honey, which is hot, should never be baked or otherwise heated, which increases its heat; likewise peacock meat, which is hot, should not be roasted on a spit of castor wood, which is also hot.

The basis of Indian cuisine is the prevention of possible food side-effects by appropriate *samskaras*. Fish is often cooked with fennel or with coconut milk or is served with lemon to cool it and make it less likely to aggravate *pitta*. Turmeric is always added when beans or lentils are cooked, to prevent them from making blood 'impure'. Legumes are ordinarily also cooked with oil, with something sour, like tamarind, and with spices such as ginger, garlic and asafoetida to prevent *vata* disturbance. Sometimes antidotes to a food are found on the same plant: the astringent strawberry leaf is an antidote to the sour berry, just as the cold, bitter inner seed kernel of the mango is an antidote to the hot, sweet fruit. The seeds of the lemon and lime are negative antidotes to the otherwise ambrosial effects of those fruits.

All food should be 'alive' so that it can give life to its eater. Overcooked, undercooked, burnt, bad tasting, unripe or overripe, putrified, stale or otherwise revolting food should never be consumed. Spices should, optimally, be ground fresh for each use. Refrigerated food gets heavier, as does food preserved by other methods. Left-overs should be heated up or, better yet, avoided, and cold food and ice-water are generally forbidden. Even the container in which food is stored must be sagaciously selected; for example, when water is stored in a copper pot, as is common in many parts of India, within four to six hours almost all bacterial contamination is eliminated; the same is true of a silver pot. Food should not be cooked or stored in aluminium vessels.

Raw food is more 'alive' than cooked food – its prana is more intact – but it is also more difficult to digest and can occasionally cause imbalances in the system. For example, many of the members of the brassica family, including turnips, cabbage, swedes and soybeans, contain chemicals called progoitrins, which, when overeaten in raw form, can produce a disease called cabbage goitre, a condition that is prevented when they are eaten cooked. Only those people whose digestive fires are exceptionally strong can make raw food their sole diet.

COMBINATION

Certain combinations of qualities disturb the *doshas* and should be avoided. Raw and cooked food should not be mixed at the same meal, unless the amount of one is small, like a small amount of raw chutney, nor should fresh food and left-overs be consumed together. Both fish and milk are sweet in taste, but milk is cold and fish is hot, so they cannot be combined, raw or cooked. One of my fellow Ayurvedic students found she could safely enjoy fish by itself and milk by itself, but would develop a skin rash whenever she ate both foods on the same day, even at different meals. Honey is hot and ghee cold, but they may be taken together as long as they are not equal in amount. Excess of a quality is also forbidden: because alcohol, yoghurt and honey are heating, other hot food should not be consumed with them.

Many otherwise incompatible combinations are permissible if the eater is *satmya*, or habituated, to them, or if the incompatibility is slight, or if the eater has a strong digestive fire, or is young or is strong from exercise. Combination for providing an antidote can also change these rules. Although the texts specifically prohibit the consumption of milk and radish together, because milk is cold and radish hot, when they are consumed in the proper proportion they provide an antidote to each other, each helping the other get digested. Cooking foods together also often makes their product more digestible because their incompatibilities are neutralized in the cooking process, the qualities of the result often differing from the qualities of its raw ingredients.

AMOUNT

'Stomach capacity' in Ayurveda refers not to the volume of the stomach but to the strength of the digestive fire. An acute digestive fire (characteristic of *pitta*) can cope with all dietary 'indiscretions', while a dull fire (characteristic of *kapha*) cannot. *Kapha* fire is, however, regular (it is impaired by indiscretion but normal otherwise), while *vata* fire, being irregular, often becomes impaired for no apparent reason. The idea of *matra*, or measure, is all-pervasive in Ayurveda. You can safely eat only that amount of food that will be promptly digested without any impairment of health; to take less or more than this is to invite disease. At any one meal you should ordinarily fill your stomach one-third full of solid food and one-third full of liquid food, leaving the last third empty to permit free movement of the *doshas*.

CLIMATE AND SEASON

It is generally best to eat food that is opposite in qualities to the climate and season in which one lives. Eating cold, wet things in a humid climate is generally incompatible, as is eating such foods in winter unless the person is habituated to such food. However, the mango, which is a hot fruit, appears in the hot season, and so everyone in India attempts to become habituated to mangoes in order to fully enjoy them then. Consuming too many mangoes at once tends to cause skin rashes or diarrhoea, but if you begin with just a slice and slowly increase your dose it may be possible to build up your capacity to several mangoes a day, even if you have a tendency to high *pitta*.

Some foods exert different effects on the body according to season or climate. For example, yoghurt, being sour, increases *pitta* when taken in the hot season, and so exerts a 'hot' effect on the system, whereas in the cold season its qualities of heaviness and stickiness increase *kapha*, thus exerting a congesting effect on the system, which is effectively 'cold' even though yoghurt is itself 'hot'.

RULES OF EATING

Charaka writes, 'Even food, which is the life of living creatures, if taken in an improper manner destroys life, while poison, which by nature is destructive of life, if taken in the proper manner acts as an elixir.' His fundamental rules for healthy eating include:

Eat heated food, to stimulate digestion.

Eat unctuous food, which excites the digestive fire and nourishes the body.

Eat properly combined food in due measure after digestion of the previous meal, so that there is a free passage for all substances.

Eat in a congenial, quiet place with all necessary 'accessories' (clean tablecloth, flowers, etc.), either alone or with affectionate people so that the mind is not depressed (eating, excreting, sex and meditation should always be performed in private).

Eat neither hurriedly nor leisurely, so you may appreciate the good or bad qualities of the food you are eating, and so that the 'gait' of the food as it moves through the digestive tract will be proper.

Eat without laughing or talking, with concentration, considering your constitution and what is good and not good for you as you eat it.

Other rules include:

Do not eat when you are not hungry, and do not fail to eat when you are hungry. Do not eat when you are angry, depressed, or otherwise emotionally distraught, or immediately after exertion.

Keep as large a gap as possible between meals.

Sit to eat, whenever possible facing east.

When possible, ensure that your right nostril is functioning.

Pray, thanking the Creator for the food you are offering into your digestive fire. Reverence for everything in the universe is the healthiest of all attitudes to life, and food is the universe sacrificing itself to you.

Never cook for yourself alone; the gift of food is the best gift of all. In India it was once common to make a five-fold offering of food before eating: to the home fire, a cow, a crow, a dog and a stranger.

Feed all five senses: look at the food and appreciate its appearance and aroma before you begin; listen to the sounds it makes, especially while cooking; eat with your hands so that you can enjoy its texture; chew each morsel repeatedly, to thoroughly extract its flavour. Feel reverence and love for it because it is soon to become a part of you, and the emotional charge that you apply to it will be carried by it deep into your tissues.

Stroll about a hundred steps after a meal, to assist the digestive process, but do not exercise, enjoy sex, study or sleep within an hour of eating. You may, however, relax, lying on your left side to encourage the functioning of the right nostril, which will encourage good digestion.

Do not eat heavy or *kapha*-producing food like yoghurt and sesame after sunset, and nothing at night within two hours of going to bed.

Never waste food.

THE EATER

Eating is a religious observance; in the words of the Taittireya Upanishad, 'Brahman (the Absolute) is food; only they eat who know they eat their God.' Even those people who have neither the time nor the inclination to worship God in any other way could revolutionize their lives if they only took the time to become conscious of what, how and why they eat, and to thank the universe for providing them with food. The simple act of gaining control over your diet provides you with the discipline to control many more aspects of your behaviour, because you are what you eat; your food contributes to your consciousness.

Many people use food as an addiction, a crutch, a substitute for love, almost anything except what it should be. Occasional fasting helps control food addictions, purifies the body, rests the digestive organs, returns the taste sense in the mouth to normal and heightens it, and encourages a more reverential approach to the act of eating. It is traditional in India for people to fast twice a month, or sometimes once a week, living on a single food or beverage for a day, living on water alone or even doing without water. Longer fasts for purification of the body, as are popular in some circles in the West, are generally frowned upon in Ayurveda, though they are sometimes used as spiritual penances, because they cause degeneration of the body's tissues and loss of cohesion between body and mind. During certain seasons, especially the rainy season, which is generally the least healthy time of year, many people in India restrict their diets for an entire month, for religious purposes. Sharngadhara also describes an astrologically inauspicious fortnight at the junction of autumn and winter called 'the Fangs of Death' during which one can be healthy only if one consumes small amounts of food.

When you become habituated to a food, your system learns how to cope with its negative effects, knowing that you will be eating it regularly. The negative effects are still experienced, but in a less acute way; they accumulate in the body and wait for an opportunity to express themselves. Anyone who smokes tobacco or drinks alcohol probably remembers a strong reaction to that first-ever smoke or drink, a reaction that subsided after a day or two when the body realized that these substances were to become regular visitors. To cope with such drugs the body reorganizes itself, creating a new metabolic balance based on their regular ingestion, sweeping their poisons into storage, where they can cause chronic diseases, and feeling acute discomfort only when these poisons do not enter the system regularly.

Alcohol and tobacco are two dramatic examples of what happens to everyone who becomes habituated or addicted to anything. Food itself is an addiction, a necessary dependence on substances from outside to perpetuate embodied life. To maintain your health you should become habituated only to healthy things, keeping the poisons aside for occasional or medicinal use. If you become habituated to unctuous food, such as milk, ghee, oil and meat soup, and to all six tastes, you will be strong, able to resist disease and long-lived, says Charaka. If, however, you become habituated to dry things or to only one taste, your vitality will be low, you will lack resistance and you will be short-lived. A baby is given butter and honey as its first food, even before its mother's milk, so that it will have a head start on obtaining that inherent oiliness of face and skin, which cannot be washed off, that shows healthiness of marrow, and so *shukra* and *ojas*.

This is true up to a point, say the yogis, but every addiction should be eliminated. They teach that one should progressively reduce the amount and heaviness of one's physical food, replacing it with breathing exercises and other methods to extract prana from the environment. If you know how, you can imbibe prana through your eyes, or even directly through your mind, as well as through your nose and mouth. Such well-digested prana can produce strong *ojas* without having to clog up the body with greasy substances.

Some modern scientists suggest that human life can be extended by lowering the body's temperature, as yogis learn to do, and by living on an absolute minimum of food. Other people counter by saying that even if you did not live forever on such a regimen, it would seem like forever, because you would be denying yourself and your tissues the satisfaction of consuming and digesting delicious food. Both approaches to life are valid, depending upon one's goals, but unless the body is carefully induced to learn to live happily on a minimum of food, the organism as a whole will never truly be healthy because its cells will remain unsatisfied.

Those of us who are still addicted to eating owe it to ourselves to become habituated to healthy foods. The best foods to which one can become habituated include ginger, buttermilk, rice, wheat, barley, the white daikon radish, grapes, mung beans, amalaki fruit, pomegranates, fresh pure water, onion, garlic, rock salt, wild game or the flesh of animals from arid regions, goat's meat and milk, cow's milk, cow's ghee, and honey. Foods one should consume only occasionally and never become habituated to include yoghurt, dried meat, fish, beef, pork, mutton, frog's flesh, sheep's milk and ghee, safflower oil, dried vegetables, molasses, cheese and heavy legumes such as black gram. Although salt is regarded as the best substance in the world for improving the taste of a food, the excessive use of common salt is 'especially forbidden', as it causes flabbiness and debility in body and mind, premature baldness or greying of the hair, premature wrinkling of the skin and impotence.

Charaka lists sugar as a food to which one can afford to become habituated, but sugar is now so overused that its beneficial effects are rarely seen any longer, having been supplanted by its negative qualities. Overuse, misuse and abuse of foods tend to make people sensitive or allergic to them. The foods listed above that one may become habituated to, with the addition of a few other common foods such as lamb, sweet potatoes, pears and green beans, generally do not cause adverse reactions, whereas overuse of the forbidden foods and citrus fruits, eggs, nuts, shrimp, tomatoes, wheat, bananas, chicken, chocolate, coconut, coffee, mushrooms, plums, potatoes, soy products, spinach and sugar are often implicated today in sensitivity or allergic reactions.

Habituation to unhealthy foods should be eliminated gradually, to permit the system to adjust to the changed conditions in which it finds itself when a familiar food is withdrawn. The texts speak of reducing the amount of the offending food by fourths; that is, on the first day eating one-fourth less of the food than normal, on the second and third days eating one-half less, and on the fourth to sixth days eating only one-fourth as much as one was habituated to eating, so that by the seventh day one is free of the addiction. Today people are more intensely addicted to more substances, since food is available to us in greater abundance and variety than ever before, and so the modern body often needs more than a week to adjust, but the principle of gradual removal is, when feasible, far better for the system than the sudden, 'cold turkey' method.

QUALITIES OF SPECIFIC FOODS

The chief article of diet for the average person should be grain. A typical Indian meal, like a typical meal from many other traditional cultures, consists of a large quantity of grain served with a smaller quantity of legumes, with meat, vegetables, greens and all other foods added as optional condiments to enhance the tastes and qualities of the main grain.

Grains

Barley

Dry, cool, sweet and not heavy, barley increases *vata* unless prepared soupy, increases faeces, stabilizes the body, is astringent but promotes strength and cures *kapha* increase. Barley is a primary food for all *pitta* afflictions and for respiratory and assimilation disorders. Barley gruel is much used in convalescence. Barley's alkali, extracted from its ash, is used in treating urinary stone and retention of urine, especially with coconut water, and is used in treating colic and respiratory diseases and as a substitute for salt.

Corn

Dry and hot, corn tends to increase *vata* if not prepared with unctuous substances. It is eaten particularly in North India in winter with mustard greens to promote heat in the body. Corn-silk tea is diuretic.

Rice

India's principal food grain, rice is sweet and cooling, sweet in post-digestive effect and light. Rice forms condensed stools, cures *pitta* and may be slightly *vata*-stimulating. As a gruel it is the primary diet in illness, especially fevers and intestinal inflammations, and in convalescence. Rice cooked with flesh, vegetables, fat, oil, ghee, marrow, fruit, black gram, mung beans, milk or sesame is strengthening, nourishing and cordial ('hearty'). It is used in the preparation of various medicines and is itself a medicine (for example, it is repeatedly washed and the wash water given in excessive menstrual bleeding).

Wheat

Wheat is sweet, cool, heavy and unctuous. It helps the tissues adhere together, cures *vata* and *pitta*, and is vitalizing, aphrodisiac and stabilizing. Wheat-eating North Indians sometimes deride rice-eating South Indians for their relatively shorter, slighter stature, and South Indians often retort that while wheat creates brawn, rice creates brain, an estimation possibly derived from Ayurveda.

Legumes

Black gram (*Phaseolus radiatus*)

This looks exactly like the mung bean but is black rather than green. It is astringent and sweet in taste, hot in potency and sweet in post-digestive effect. Being heavy, oily and strengthening, it cures *vata*, and 'quickly imparts virility'. It increases the quantity of faeces and is beneficial for nervous diseases and for cough and fever due to weakness. A medicated oil in which it and goat's flesh are the primary ingredients is used for treating muscular and nervous weakness and paralysis.

Chick-pea, lentil and the common pea

These are astringent and sweet in taste, cool, light and pungent after digestion. They are beneficial for *pitta* and *kapha*, as they strongly dry the body, for which reason they are not good for *vata*, the lentil being particularly dehydrating.

Kulattha (*Dolichos biflorus*)

This small, light-brown legume is used more as a medicine than as a food. Its decoction is used in treating urinary tract disease, leucorrhoea and menstrual disorders, and in the purification of metals and minerals.

Mung bean

The best of all legumes, the mung bean is astringent and sweet, cool, and pungent in post-digestive effect. Being dry, light and purifying, it cures *kapha* and *pitta*. Its soup is ideal in illness and convalescence. *Khechari* or *khichadi* (split mung cooked with rice) is a purifying and nourishing dish that can be safely fed to almost anyone in almost any state of health; it purifies the body of toxins. Mung is also said to strengthen the eyes.

Yellow lentil (*Cajanu cajan*)

This is probably the most popular legume cooked in India today. It aggravates *pitta* when taken in excess. Its seed and leaf paste are sometimes applied over a woman's breasts to stop the secretion of milk.

Sesame

Charaka includes sesame among the pulses. It was the only oil-seed used in the Vedic era by the Aryans, and a lump of sesame was found at Harappa. It is sweet, bitter, astringent and hot, and exerts a sweet effect after digestion. Being oily and heavy, it promotes *pitta* and *kapha* while it relieves *vata*. It is especially good as a tonic for the skin and hair. The seeds, which have been used to produce abortion, can be crushed and made into a poultice for ulcers, and the black seeds are rejuvenators for hair and bones. Sesame oil is used as the base for most Ayurvedic medicated oils.

Meat

In the *Sutra Sthana* Charaka says, 'For those who are wasted, convalescing, emaciated, deficient in semen, and desirous of increased strength and complexion, meat juice is to be regarded as nectar itself.' Of all meats, that of the rooster is most strengthening to the body. As noted above, however, except for venison and perhaps goat and chicken, one should never become habituated to meat; its daily use should be limited to 'those who exercise constantly and indulge in women and wine, to prevent them from becoming weak or falling ill'. Even in these cases meat is still essentially a condiment, better consumed as a broth or soup rather than as a steak or chop.

Beef

Beef is used to calm an unusually intense digestive fire and to counteract atrophy of the flesh. It is generally used to treat only those diseases that are caused by *vata* alone.

Fish

Sweet, heavy, oily, hot, aphrodisiac and strengthening, fish cures *vata*. River fish are said to derange *pitta* and blood and cause bulky stool, whereas fish from a pond are more palatable and control *pitta*.

Goat

Goat's flesh is not as heavy or greasy as other meat, and does not disturb the *doshas*; it is good for rebuilding the body.

Pork

Pork is heavy, aphrodisiac and strengthening. It promotes fat, builds the body, cures *vata*.

All meat is heavy, but some meats, such as those derived mainly from animals living in arid areas, are relatively lighter than others, such as those from humid areas. In addition, one must avoid the meat of emaciated, very fat, very old or very young (like veal) animals, or from an animal that was not slain while 'roaming at will in its natural habitat'. This last caveat eliminates from consideration most of the meat available to us today, which comes from animals who are pumped full of hormones and antibiotics, and live in unnatural surroundings where they can do nothing but stand around in their own waste all day long, stuffing their metabolic wastes deep into their tissues. When to these poisons are added the chemicals produced by the terror the animals feel as they are about to be slaughtered, the meat is clearly unfit for consumption. Unsurprisingly, red meat has been implicated as a causative factor in diseases such as cancer of the colon.

Other disadvantages of meat include the following facts: the production of one pound of meat protein consumes about ten times the natural resources needed for the production of one pound of vegetable protein; animals also possess consciousness and have as much right to life as we do; and food collected with violence tends to create violence in the consciousness of the eater. Even when appropriate for the physical body, meat remains inappropriate for the mind, in which it promotes both overactivity and rigidity. In the context of individual life-preservation Ayurveda prescribes the eating of meat, because 'in all circumstances one must safeguard one's life'; but when there are other means than meat of safeguarding one's life, and the purpose of violence against animals is merely to fatten oneself, such violence is wrong.

Vegetables

Most of the vegetables that existed in Charaka's day have been supplanted in the popular diet by the tomato and potato, both imports from the New World. Notable exceptions include the cucumber, which is sweet, heavy, drying, cooling, slows the movement of food through the intestines, and is diuretic. It helps reduce the intoxication due to alcohol and is applied to the skin as an astringent. Karavellaka (*Momordica charantia*) is a very bitter cucumber-like vegetable, which is widely eaten by diabetics to keep their blood sugar down. The pumpkin strengthens the system. The aubergine has two main varieties, one with large fruits (the kind usually available in the West), which is cooling, hard to digest, laxative, diuretic and provokes *kapha* while it alleviates *pitta* and *vata*; and another with small fruits, which is bitter, pungent, light for digestion, strengthens the digestive fire and tends to increase *pitta*. Some varieties of loofa, which, when dried, are sold as a bath sponge, are also vegetables, while others are emetic and purgative.

The qualities of the vegetables that are common today must be determined by their users. In general roots (beetroots, carrots, parsnips, radishes, swedes, turnips), being heavy and earthy, tend to be good for *vata* and not so good for *kapha* or *pitta*, while leaves (spinach, lettuce, the cabbage family, and so on) and squashes tend to be good for *kapha* and *pitta* and not so good for *vata*. 'Hot', pungent vegetables, such as the radish, are better for *vata* and *kapha*, while cool ones, such as the cucumber, are better for *pitta*. When tender, the radish rebalances the *doshas*, but when overdeveloped, it imbalances them. Sweet potatoes are better for *vata* and *pitta* than they are for *kapha*. Okra, which is a species of hibiscus, is high in protein and is diuretic, and its mucilage is soothing in dysentery. The seeds when massaged on the teeth whiten and strengthen them. Turnip is astringent, intense, good for *vata, kapha*, piles and to help the body heat up; it is not good for *pitta*.

Asparagus is perhaps the best of our vegetables, and tomato the worst. While tomato soup is sometimes good for weak people and during convalescence, it is not for daily use, as it aggravates both *kapha* and *pitta*. Raw tomatoes disturb *vata* as well. Strict Ayurvedic tradition holds that most vegetables should be avoided while undergoing therapy, as most of them are astringent and so cause the channels to close up just when they need to be free-flowing. Three vegetables, however, come in for special praise because of their amazing utility: garlic, ginger and onion.

Garlic

The writings of the ancient Egyptians, Babylonians, Romans, Greeks and Chinese have all mentioned garlic as a wonderful remedy for a wide variety of disorders. In the Sanskrit texts it is known variously as 'The Disgusting', 'The Supreme Medicine', '*Vata*'s Enemy', 'Beloved of the Greeks' (or 'Heretics') and 'Lacking-One-Taste', this last because garlic possesses five of the six tastes, lacking only sour. *Bhavaprakasha* says that the root is pungent; the leaf, bitter; the stalk, astringent; the tip of the stalk, salty; and the seed, sweet.

Garlic is called 'Rahu's Residue' because the demon Rahu, who had happened to sneak a sip of the nectar of immortality illicitly, had his head severed from his body by the discus of Lord Vishnu, the Preserver of the Universe, and garlic sprang up from a drop of Rahu's blood that fell to earth. It thus possesses both ambrosial and infernal properties; it is an elixir for the body but it makes the mind intolerant and increases *tamas*. Islamic myth agrees with this assessment, stating that garlic sprouted from where Satan's left foot touched the earth.

Garlic relieves both *vata* and *kapha*, and increases *pitta*. It is heavy and aphrodisiac, assists parents in obtaining an intelligent child, promotes strength and memory, sweetens the throat, purifies the vision and improves the complexion, digestion and tissue nutrition. It is useful in healing fractured bones and in treating dry skin diseases, *vata* diseases, worms, haemorrhoids, colic, cough, heart disease, chronic fevers, asthma, *kapha* diseases and indigestion.

Garlic juice, which has been shown to kill harmful bacteria without destroying useful ones, was diluted with water and used on sterile bandages by the British during the First World War to prevent wounds from becoming infected. Garlic has been used to cure or improve cases of typhoid, diphtheria, whooping cough, pneumonia, bronchitis, bronchiectasis, influenza and tuberculosis, to reduce cholesterol and to scavenge heavy metals from the tissues. It improves the appetite and the circulation, and decreases high blood pressure and body and joint pain. One cause of garlic's effectiveness is its ability (which it shares with such substances as fenugreek and honey, and many poisons) to penetrate to all parts of the body very quickly. When you rub garlic on the bottom of your feet, as some people do to treat the common cold, or take an enema of decoction of garlic, its odour will come on your breath within a few moments. It is this property that makes a dog who is fed garlic an unpleasant host for fleas, since its sweat will be redolent of garlic.

Garlic is administered as juice, powder, paste, decoction, poultice, collyrium, medicated milk, oil and ghee, medicated wine and jam, and as an ash, and it appears as an ingredient in many Ayurvedic pills. Some people prefer to use the milder garlic sprouts or grass rather than the bulbs, and strict Brahmans never eat it (beloved as it is of heretics), though they are permitted to consume the milk or milk products of a cow fed garlic.

Ginger

There is a pill made from ginger alone known as the 'Universal Remedy', and indeed ginger comes close to being just that. Dried ginger, which is mainly used in medicine, is pungent and sweet, hot, and sweet after digestion; it controls and balances the three *doshas* (though in excess it may increase *pitta*). Fresh ginger, which is used mainly in cookery, has a stronger pitta-increasing property and is forbidden when *pitta* is high, such as in bleeding disorders, skin disease, fever and the summer season.

The ancient texts call ginger 'satisfaction killer' for its property of inflaming the appetite. *Bhavaprakasha* suggests that one should always eat a little fresh ginger and rock salt before a meal, to intensify the digestive fire, increase appetite and clean the tongue and throat. As part of the powder known as *Hingvashtaka Churna*, ginger relieves bloating and abdominal distention due to gas. Powdered ginger, as research in Britain has proved, can prevent motion sickness, and it is given with rock salt and cumin with water after meals to treat chronic diarrhoea. With lime juice and sugar or salt it is a popular Indian first-aid remedy for sunstroke. Ginger is Ayurveda's supreme toxin-digester, used, for example, as a strong tea with castor oil in treating rheumatism and rheumatoid arthritis.

Ginger promotes circulation, especially when applied to the body. Ginger baths promote warmth and help relieve musculo-skeletal aches and pains. Paste of powdered ginger on the forehead relieves some kinds of headache, juice of fresh ginger alleviates certain kinds of earache, and burnt ginger and salt is beneficial for the gums and teeth. Consumed with turmeric in hot milk, dry ginger loosens and liquefies thick respiratory congestion; for productive cough, it is given with honey, either alone or mixed with black pepper and long pepper (*Piper longum*; see p. 234). For dry cough, pharyngitis, bronchitis, nausea and vomiting, fresh ginger juice is used with mint juice, lemon juice and honey. Fresh ginger juice is often given with fenugreek decoction and honey to people suffering from influenza. Dry ginger and solidified sugar-cane juice make urine and faeces flow more freely, and sweetened ginger tea helps some cases of disturbed or absent menses.

Onion

Charaka maintains that the onion promotes *kapha* and cures *vata* but not *pitta*. The *Harita Samhita* disagrees, stating that onion reduces both *vata* and *kapha*, and other authorities aver that onion reduces both *pitta* and *kapha*. Which of these effects an onion will produce depends upon its variety (red onions are generally hotter and therefore more *pitta*-producing than either yellow or white onions) and its condition (cooked onions lose most of their pungency and are more *kapha*-promoting).

Everyone agrees, however, that the onion is strengthening, heavy and appetizing. Onions are sweet and pungent (raw) or sweet (cooked) in taste, hot in potency, and sweet in post-digestive effect. They stimulate the heart, promote bile production, reduce blood sugar and relieve intestinal gas and colic. Fresh onion juice is moderately bactericidal and makes a good heart tonic when given with honey or aged (more than seven years) jaggery. The onion is a reputed aphrodisiac, especially when mixed with honey, ginger juice and ghee; it is one of those substances, like honey and ghee, that are said to immediately increase semen when eaten. One of its Sanskrit names, *kandarpa*, is also a name for Kamadeva, the Indian Eros.

Innumerable popular recipes make onion a trusted home remedy. Its juice is instilled into the eyes (with honey, for pain and cataract), nose (for runny nose and nosebleeds, and for loss of consciousness) and ears (for earache). A paste of onion on the soles of the feet is said to cure headache, as is the smelling of a crushed onion, which is also prescribed for nausea and vomiting. Used in food, it is said to protect one's teeth, and in various combinations it has been employed to treat alopecia, asthma, laryngitis, diarrhoea, dysentery, urinary stone, retention of urine, haemorrhoids, amenorrhoea, mammary abscess, heat stroke and rheumatism.

Fruits

Apple

Satyananda Stokes was an American who moved to India and, adopting it as his own country, became the Indian Johnny Appleseed, planting apple trees in many parts of the Himalaya. Thanks to him, apples are now freely available all over the country. The whole fruit cures constipation, while the pulp or juice controls diarrhoea. Being astringent and sweet in taste, cold in action and pungent after digestion, raw apples tend to increase *vata*. Apple bark and root are used in folk medicine.

Banana

Named in Ayurveda after the celestial dancing damsel, Rambha, the banana is reputed to promote fertility and so is used to decorate marriage halls. Many people in the west and south of India use the fresh leaves as plates for their meals, and the flowers are used to treat dysentery and excessive menstrual bleeding. The fruit is said to be aphrodisiac, while the juice of the stem is reported to be anti-aphrodisiac and to calm mental agitation and hysteria. The fruit can be used to treat either diarrhoea or constipation.

Coconut

Sweet, oily and cool, the coconut strengthens and builds up the body. It is called 'auspicious fruit' in Sanskrit, as it is used in almost every religious ritual. The inner water of tender coconuts flushes out the kidneys and cools the system; as the coconut gets older and drier, this water gets hotter. Coconut oil is especially nourishing for the hair, and extracts of coconut are sometimes used to treat tuberculosis and yeast infections.

Related to the coconut palm is the toddy palm, whose sap, fruit and root are cooling and relieve gastritis. The sap, which, like the water of tender coconuts, flushes the urinary tract, ferments soon after collection. The resulting alcoholic beverage, toddy, is a pleasant laxative, and is also used in poultices with rice flour on inflamed body parts.

Date

The date is sweet, aphrodisiac, heavy and cool, and builds body. Dates help reduce alcohol intoxication and are used in diseases of *vata* and *pitta*. One use for the seed kernels is as a tonic for racing bullocks.

Fig

Sweet, nourishing, strengthening, heavy, delayed in digestion, laxative, cool, controls *vata* and *pitta*.

Grape

This fruit is sweet, cooling, strengthening, aphrodisiac and unctuous. It cures thirst, burning sensations, fever, shortness of breath, 'heat in the blood', wasting of the body due to *vata* or *pitta*, indigestion, alcoholism, bitter taste in the mouth and cough. The leaves are used in treating diarrhoea; and the sap of young branches, in skin diseases. Kept in the mouth, raisins allay thirst, heat, cough and hoarseness. They are also soaked overnight and chewed the next morning for all the above benefits, and are good for anyone, even pregnant women.

Guava

Eaten without the rind, the guava causes constipation. The unripe fruit is used to control diarrhoea, as is a decoction of the bark. Decoction of the leaves is gargled to relieve swollen gums and mouth ulcers, and the leaves are made into poultices and used to treat anal prolapse in children.

Jambu (*Eugenia jambolana*)

India resides on the continent known as Jambudvipa, the Rose Apple Island. *Jambu*, the rose apple, is said to be the god of clouds incarnated in fruit form, as it supposedly is the colour of the sky as a thunderstorm approaches (it is actually much darker). Rose apple is astringent and sweet, cooling, and pungent after digestion. Though heavy, the fruit balances the Three *Doshas*, while the seed decreases *pitta* and *kapha* and can, in excess, increase *vata*. The fruit helps blood carry prana to the tissues and is used in treating diabetes, enlarged liver, diarrhoea and bleeding piles. The vinegar or medicinal wine made from the ripe fruit is diuretic and stomachic. The seed has a stronger anti-diabetic effect than does the fruit, and is good for treating diarrhoea and dysentery, as are the bark and the leaf juice. The latter is purifying and invigorating and is used externally to cure chronic sores. It is said that an infusion of the fresh tender leaves helps to correct sterility and the tendency to miscarriage.

Lime

The Indian lemon or lime (*Citrus acida* or *C. medica* var. *acida*) is sour, bitter, astringent and cooling, and sweet post-digestively. Though it does not aggravate normal *pitta*, it must be used with caution once *pitta* is elevated. Its juice is applied externally on mosquito and other bites, on skin eruptions and on the scalp to remove dandruff. It is used in treating all sorts of digestive disorders, including diarrhoea and dysentery, and it is added to food to improve both digestion and appetite. It has also been used in treating fevers, constipation, diabetes, diseases of the liver and spleen, poisoning, gout, rheumatoid arthritis and even cataract (the brave put drops of it into their eyes). Some authorities claim that there is no disease that this fruit, properly prepared, cannot cure.

Mango

The most important fruit tree of India, the mango is known as the King of Fruit, and its juice as Rasaraja, the King of Juices. The largest mango tree in the world is reported to yield more than fifteen tons of fruit yearly, appropriate for a fruit that symbolizes fertility and abundance. Myth has it that the mango flower is Cupid's arrow, and the fruit, which is shaped like a woman's breast, provides a juice that is nectarean and aphrodisiac. The tree is used in marriage, birth and death rituals, and strings of mango leaves festoon auspicious sites.

The ripe fruit is laxative, diuretic and cools the blood. It subdues *vata* and increases flesh, semen and strength. In the hot season I have often lived happily on mangoes and milk alone. The unripe fruit can be used to prepare a cooling drink during the hot season, and the kernel inside the seed can cure the diarrhoea caused by overindulgence in the fruit. The bark is used in treating uterine haemorrhage, haemoptysis (the vomiting of blood) and diarrhoea.

Orange

This fruit is sweet, slightly sour, cordial and heavy. It promotes relish for food, is difficult to digest and cures *vata*.

Peach

Not very hot, the peach is heavy, sweet and tasty. It is strengthening, quickly digested and wholesome.

Pear

The wild Indian variety is hard and astringent and increases *vata*, while the commercial variety controls all three *doshas*. Both are heavy and cool.

Pomegranate

This fruit is sacred to the Zoroastrians and is used in their rituals. It is said that Muhammad advised his followers to eat pomegranates to help them purge envy from themselves. The fruit rind and root bark are astringent and bitter, while the fruit is sweet, sour, astringent, cooling, and sweet, after digestion. The sweet variety of pomegranate is digestive, stimulant, unctuous and cordial. It controls all three *doshas* and cures *vata* and *pitta*, while the sour variety aggravates *pitta* and *vata*. The juice of the sweet variety is rejuvenative, and is prescribed by the sagacious juice sellers of Bombay for diarrhoea and cases of 'bad stomach'. The seeds are made into a digestive powder, the root bark is given for worms, and the flower or fruit rind is given to treat diarrhoea and dysentery, used as a douche for leucorrhoea, and applied as a paste for ulcers and piles.

Tamarind

Its name means 'Date of India'. It is sour both before and after digestion and it is hot. Unripe, it decreases *vata* and increases *pitta* and *kapha*, while ripened, it decreases both *vata* and *kapha*, and if sweet will decrease *pitta* as well. Tamarind is used in the diet to increase appetite and digestion, and has a laxative effect. When boiled in water and sweetened, it is given to cool the body in fevers and, with other ingredients, to relieve the effects of alcoholism. Tamarind pulp is a popular snack among schoolchildren, and is used to polish brass. Its seed can be made into flour, and is applied as a paste on scorpion stings and styes. The seeds are also taken internally, after soaking and removing their shells, for leucorrhoea and backache.

Nuts

Most nuts, including almond, walnut, pine nut, pistachio and cashew, are sweet, heavy, hot, oily, aphrodisiac and strengthening. They build up the body, cure *vata*, and increase *pitta* and *kapha*. Of these, almond is regarded as superior, being rejuvenative.

Dairy

The Aryans were apparently nomads for centuries before they and their lyre-horned cows moved to India. Though Ayurveda prescribes beef, and though bulls apparently were once employed in India as sacrificial animals and the Vedas appear to have permitted the consumption of sanctified beef on certain occasions, Ayurveda also prescribes, in the context of preservation of society, the worship of cows. The cow has been sacred in India for ages, partly because she is the foundation of the Vedic way of life. Cows produce milk and butter for food, dung for fuel, urine for medicine, and when they die, their hides go to make leather. Before the advent of tractors, the bullock was the principal beast of burden in the subcontinent. To slaughter a cow was as much an economic as a religious sin, and part of the reason cows were made sacrosanct was to prevent peasants from consuming their bovine wealth and impoverishing both themselves and their country.

Milk

Milk is regarded by Charaka as the best of those substances that make you feel alive. 'Milk is the semen of the god of fire,' says the *Shatapatha Brahmana*. Ayurveda respects it because it is the pure essence of the *rasa* of plants, concentrated into White Essence by the animal's organism. It is also the only common food in the world that can be collected with no violence whatsoever; in fact, a contented cow loves to give milk. Milk is good for infants, for people with a strong digestive fire, and for those who are emaciated, old, sexually active or sleepless. It is not good at night, cold or mixed with other foods (notably fruit, leafy vegetables, fish, sour things or salt). Warm milk straight from the cow is like ambrosia; homogenized milk is not. The Tibetans like to use skimmed milk to treat recurrent common colds, and to cause a moving sickness to settle in one place, from where it can then be removed with medicine. Though the many races who cannot digest cow's milk denigrate dairy products, the Aryans and the Masai, whose diet is almost entirely cow's milk, continue to enjoy it.

Cow's milk is sweet, cool, unctuous, thick, glossy, viscid, heavy, slow to digest and clear. Because it shares these qualities with *ojas*, it nourishes *ojas*. Fresh cow's milk is foremost among vitalizers and rejuvenators. Milk of the water buffalo, which is most commonly available in India today, is heavier, fattier and more cooling than cow's milk. The water buffalo represents the embodiment of *tamas*, and its milk is good for insomnia and to calm an intense digestive fire. Goat's milk increases human milk production and removes emaciation and cough, while donkey's milk is a popular remedy for whooping cough. Human milk is vitalizing and is used as nose drops in nosebleeds and as an eye application in eye disorders. Other milks include those of the camel, mare, ewe and elephant.

Yoghurt

Yoghurt is an appetizer and a digestive stimulant. It is nourishing, increases unctuousness and strength, and is aphrodisiac. Being sweet and sour, hot, and sour after digestion, yoghurt cures *vata* and increases *pitta* and *kapha*. It is good for treating diarrhoea, certain fevers, loss of appetite, urinary problems and emaciation, but should not be used in hot seasons, *kapha* conditions or *pitta* illness. Because it is *abhisyhandi* (causes stagnation of the water element in the tissues), Charaka emphasizes that yoghurt lovers must not eat it cold, at night or without mixing it first with ghee and sugar, mung-bean soup, honey or the powder of *Emblica officinalis* (the *amalaki* fruit; see p. 220).

Colostrum (the first milk a cow gives after delivery) and cream cheeses are heavy, nourishing, aphrodisiac and cure *vata*.

Butter

Butter in India is usually made by first fermenting whole milk into yoghurt and then churning the yoghurt. It is commonly then clarified into ghee. The whey or buttermilk that remains after churning cures *vata* and *kapha* and cleans the channels. A text comments, 'After food drink buttermilk; after sex drink hot spiced milk.' Buttermilk is regarded as a sovereign remedy for piles, assimilation disorders, diarrhoea and dysentery, and is also commonly used in treating some varieties of oedema, suppression of urine, loss of appetite, indigestion, anaemia and many other diseases. When fresh buttermilk is unavailable, non-fat yoghurt diluted with an equal amount of water and liquefied can be substituted.

Ghee, says Charaka, the best of all unctuous substances, is the best substance to cure both *vata* and *pitta*. Cow's ghee, which is sweet both before and after digestion and is cool, promotes memory, intelligence, the digestive fire, semen, *ojas* and fat. It removes toxicity from the system and cures insanity, consumption, chronic fever and lack of prosperity. Properly prepared, its potency increases a thousandfold and it becomes efficacious in a thousand ways. Aged ghee is used to treat alcoholism, epilepsy, fainting, consumption, insanity, toxic states, fevers and pain in the vagina, ear or head. Hundred-Times-Washed Ghee is used externally only, for wound healing and to calm *pitta*. The ghees of other milks have the qualities of those milks.

Fats and Oils

Oil does not have quite the positive association for the Aryans that ghee does. Charaka writes, 'By the use of oil, in olden days, the kings of the demons became unaging, free from disease and fatigue, and endowed with great strength in battle.' Like garlic, vegetable oils produce more *raja* and *tamas* in their consumer than does ghee, which usually creates *sattva*. Moreover, oil, if consumed regularly, is said to cause skin and eye diseases. Oils are mainly used externally in Ayurveda, though now that ghee is so expensive, the average Indian cooks with oil.

Sesame oil, the best of all oils, is good for the skin, hair, intelligence and digestive fire, strengthens the system and is one of the best remedies for *vata*. It is sweet with an astringent after-taste, hot and diffusive, and increases *pitta* but does not much increase *kapha*. Safflower, the worst of all oils, is hot, pungent after digestion, heavy, irritant and provokes all the *doshas*. Mustard oil is not held in high regard by the texts either, though North Indians swear by it.

Other oils have qualities according to the foods they are derived from, as do animal marrows and fats. Oil, animal body fat, bone marrow and ghee are in order increasingly better for *pitta* and decreasingly useful for *vata* and *kapha*.

Sweets

Sugar cane promotes the production and free flow of urine. The juice you obtain by chewing and sucking it is aphrodisiac, cooling, laxative and nourishing, while machine-pressed juice is irritating. Jaggery, which is created by boiling the juice, gets heavier as it concentrates; it increases marrow, blood, fat, flesh, and worms. The purer the sugar produced from the juice, the cooler it is.

Being drying and astringent, honey is good to apply to burns and wounds. It is aphrodisiac and strengthening, and because, like poison, it quickly moves to the deepest tissues, it is the best of medications, but indigestion due to honey is reported to be very difficult to treat. Honey must be used raw, never cooked.

Spices

Spices are medicinal herbs used to alter the qualities of food items to make them more digestible and to reduce possible negative effects.

Bay leaf

The Indian version is *Cinnamomum tamala*, a cousin of cinnamon (*C. zeylanica*). It is pungent and sweet, hot, and pungent after digestion. It reduces both *vata* and *kapha* and increases *pitta*, and is given mixed with cinnamon and cardamom for respiratory congestion. Its bark is sometimes used as an adulterant for cinnamon.

Black pepper

Black pepper is the unripened fruit of *Piper nigrum* dried in the sun; white pepper is the same fully ripened (in Kerala the seeds of *Moringa oleifera* are used for white pepper). Both varieties of *P. nigrum* are pungent, and hot and pungent after digestion. They decrease *kapha* and *vata*, and increase *pitta* only slightly, because their drying quality counteracts *pitta*'s oily quality. The unripened, undried green version of this spice is heavy, has a sweet post-digestive effect, is not too hot and is pickled in western India for use as a condiment.

Black pepper powder is sprinkled on cold food such as cucumbers, melons and bananas to counteract their coldness. It burns toxins from the body, and its mixture with ginger and long pepper into *Trikatu* (the Three Pungents) is used to inflame the digestive fire, treat cold fevers and relieve respiratory congestion. Because black pepper dries secretions, it can irritate mucous membranes if over-used or misused and so it is made into a medicated ghee for nasal applications to relieve sinus congestion and headache.

Caraway

While *Carum carvi*, the true caraway, grows wild in the northern Himalaya, and other species of *Carum* are found in India, it is cara-way's cousin *C. copticum*, known as *ajowan*, which is mainly used in Ayurveda. *Ajowan* and caraway have similar properties, being pungent and bitter, hot, and pungent in post-digestive effect. They control *vata* and *kapha* and tend to increase *pitta*. *Ajowan* is used main-ly for the digestive tract, especially as a decoction for gas and colic, and the seeds are chewed to improve the digestive fire.

Similar in activity to *ajowan* are anise (*Pimpinella anisum*) and *ajamoda* (*Apium graveolens*), which is an ingredient in the famous digestive recipe *Hingvashtaka Churna*.

Cardamom

Although cardamom is sweet and pungent in taste and hot in potency, it does not increase *pitta*; instead it increases *tejas* and *ojas*, the essential, pure forms of the fire element. Cardamom reduces all three *doshas* and, being sweet after digestion, it rejuvenates the system. Popular as a spice and chewed after meals as a digestive, it is especially useful despite its heat for reducing improper or waste heat in body and mind. It can remedy indigestion, abdominal distention, piles, urinary complaints, weakness of the heart and body, cough, asthma and consumption. Because it relieves acidity, Middle Eastern-ers add it to their coffee. It appears in many compounds, including *Sitopaladi Churna*, which is used for respiratory congestion. A related species, 'Great Cardamom', whose pods are black and are larger than those of the usual cardamom, is used mainly in cookery.

Chillies

Being pungent, hot and pungent post-digestively, chillies reduce *kapha* and increase *pitta*. At first their heat helps to control *vata*, but their pungency increases *vata* after long-term use. Though chillies are not native to India, they have been enthusiastically adopted into its cuisine. Eating hot chillies in a hot climate helps to keep the body cool by inducing sweat production, but regular use eventually overheats the system. Chilli powder is applied by villagers to dog and other animal bites, as it is believed to kill pathogens, including the rabies virus. It is also used internally as first aid in acute diarrhoea and cholera and for intestinal and uterine bleeding. Repeated use for these purposes will aggravate the problem it is trying to solve.

Cinnamon

Its Sanskrit name means 'bark', the part of this tree that is most useful. It is pungent, sweet and bitter in taste and hot in potency, but is sweet in post-digestive effect and therefore controls both *vata* and *kapha* without aggravating *pitta*, unless it is consumed in excess. It is less likely to aggravate *pitta* than is ginger, but still eliminates *kapha*. It is an ingredient in *Sitopaladi Churna*, and its oil is used as an application in toothache, headache and impotence (carefully!).

Coriander

Coriander leaves and fruit are not very pungent and are very cooling. The fruit is used like other carminatives to improve appetite and to relieve *vata* and *kapha*, especially in treatment of urinary complaints. Both the fruit and the leaves help to remove heat from the system, especially in the intestines and the eyes, and the leaves are applied to hot skin eruptions.

Cumin

Known as 'the Digester' in Sanskrit, cumin is pungent, slightly hot, and pungent after digestion. It controls both *vata* and *kapha* without aggravating *pitta*, except in excess. It is often used in combination with coriander or fennel and is an ingredient in numerous Ayurvedic recipes. A common folk remedy is a teaspoon of roasted cumin powder at bedtime to regulate the digestive function.

Dill

Dill leaves are cooked as a vegetable in West India and are used in poultices, as are the seeds, which are pungent and bitter, hot, and pungent after digestion. They relieve gas, colic and hiccups, especially in small children, and with fenugreek they control diarrhoea. Like anise, they increase breast-milk and medicate it to strengthen the baby's digestion.

Drumstick

All parts of the drumstick tree, *Moringa oleifera*, are used to increase the body's fire. They reduce *vata* and *kapha* and increase *pitta*. The leaves (a rich source of carotenes), flowers and the long, thin, green fruits from which the tree gets its name are all eaten as vegetables. The fruit purifies the liver and spleen and reduces joint pain; the flowers are said to be aphrodisiac; and *Bhavaprakasha* advises decoction of the root bark in ascites, enlargement of the liver or spleen, urinary stone, fever, and paralysis. Internally, it is a tonic to the heart and circulatory system, and calms the nerves and the gut; externally, it is applied to inflamed or rheumatic regions. The gum is used as temporary filling for dental caries, and with sesame oil in the ear for earache. Research has shown that the effect of drumstick extracts resembles that of adrenalin and ephedrine, and that it inhibits the growth of moulds and fungi.

Fennel

The fresh young succulent shoots of fennel are used as a vegetable in India, as they are in southern Italy. Fennel seed (sweet, pungent and bitter, slightly cooling, sweet post-digestively, decreases all the *doshas*) is chewed after meals to prevent gas and gallstones, and women take it, especially as a decoction, to increase breast-milk, alleviate pre-menstrual tension (PMT) and regularize menstruation, as it shows demonstrable oestrogenic activity. Its oil is decongestant and improves coughs.

Fenugreek

Like garlic, when eaten as a vegetable the odour of fenugreek appears in the sweat of its eaters and makes the body repel insects, which is why it is sometimes fed to cows and horses. Fenugreek is pungent, bitter and sweet, hot, and pungent after digestion, and reduces *vata* and *kapha*; in excess it increases *pitta*. It improves the digestive, respiratory and nervous systems, regulates the menses, purifies the skin and tones the whole organism. Fenugreek tea promotes sweating in fevers (especially those, like influenza, that are due to *vata* and *kapha*), purifies breast-milk, is decongestant and improves dysentery and arthritis. With valerian, it is given for relief of insomnia, depression and neuroses. The sprouts strengthen the liver and improve the semen, and the seeds are made into a confection given to women after childbirth to strengthen them and to promote milk production. Its seed paste purifies boils and abscesses, and it has been used as a shampoo to prevent premature hair loss.

Mustard

Seven species of *Brassica* are commonly used in India, most notably the black, red and white mustards. The seeds are made into poultices and are widely used in cooking legumes. The greens are eaten mainly in North India with corn *roti* (tortilla-like bread) to provide heat to the body during winter.

Nutmeg

Nutmeg is the nut and mace the aril (a fibre covering the nutshell) of *Myristica fragrans*, an evergreen tree that grows wild in parts of South India. A Portuguese physician found nutmegs growing luxuriantly in Indian soil some centuries back, but those that grow there now are *M. malabarica*, which lacks the delicate aroma of the other species. Nutmeg and mace are effectively interchangeable (pungent, bitter and astringent, hot, and pungent after digestion; reduce *vata* and *kapha*, and increase *pitta*) as spices, and are commonly used in medicine to calm the nerves of the lower abdomen. *Jatiphaladi*

Churna, literally 'Nutmeg Etc. Powder', which actually has less nutmeg than it has cannabis, is an exceptional remedy for diarrhoea, dysentery, sprue and other intestinal dysfunctions. On its own nutmeg can control, though not necessarily cure, almost any form of diarrhoea. It is given with buttermilk for diarrhoea, and with milk to induce sleep and control premature ejaculation. Its powder has also been used to treat urinary incontinence, and it is an ingredient in many aphrodisiac mixtures.

Saffron

The dried stigmas and the tops of the styles of the saffron crocus, *Crocus sativus*, picked early in the morning when half open, then gently dried on a slow fire, form saffron; 75,000 to 100,000 flowers are required to produce one pound of it. In the chill of an early November morning the sight of a saffron field in Kashmir covered with mauve saffron crocuses waiting to be plucked is truly unforgettable.

Saffron is pungent, bitter and sweet, hot, and sweet after digestion. It controls and balances all the *doshas*. Being a reproductive organ it is mainly used on the reproductive tract. It regulates the menstrual cycle, relieves dysmenorrhoea and PMT, and promotes fertility. It is widely regarded as an aphrodisiac for both sexes, especially when dissolved in milk, and is also digestive and relieves respiratory congestion. Saffron and opium dissolved in brandy and painted on the cheeks drives colds from the head; for children the opium is dropped and the brandy is replaced with milk. Saffron is used in pastes to adorn the skin and improve the complexion, both of humans and of deities in temples; ancient texts hail saffron paste as the supreme cosmetic for a woman's breasts. Saffron is also said to purify the mind.

Turmeric

Nine species of *Curcuma* appear in India. *C. amada* (white turmeric) is eaten fresh in season as a blood purifier, and is applied to the skin over contusions, sprains, skin blemishes and acne, while *C. angustifolia* and *C. zeodaria* are used as substitutes for arrowroot. The most used and most familiar of this family is *C. longa*, the turmeric that makes American-prepared mustard yellow. A native rhizome of India, turmeric is bitter, astringent and pungent, hot, and pungent after digestion. It balances the *doshas*, though in excess it can aggravate *vata* and *pitta*. Turmeric is used externally and internally to purify both blood and mind; in this regard it is the poor man's saffron. Every dish of dal (split legumes) cooked in India has turmeric added to it to protect the blood.

Turmeric's antiseptic actions have been scientifically confirmed. Applied to wounds, it slows bleeding. Its paste is used on bruises, bites, stings, open wounds, boils and breast disorders, and, with sandalwood, to purify and beautify the skin (brides and grooms are anointed with this mixture before they are wed). It is used in eye drops for conjunctivitis, and its smoke is employed to treat fainting, hiccups and asthma. As a natural antibiotic, it protects rather than destroys the intestinal flora, and it promotes the production of bile. It is effective, in combination, in the control of diabetes and several varieties of skin disease.

Turmeric is also said to have the power to dispel evil influences, and so it is an essential ingredient in many forms of ritual worship.

6

PATHOLOGY

_____

In short, everything in the world has only two conditions, abnormal and normal, and both of them are dependent upon a cause. Nothing can happen in the absence of a cause.

CHARAKA

Tibetan medicine, which has borrowed much from Ayurveda, including the Three *Doshas*, the Seven Tissues and the Three Wastes, recognizes four classes of disease: those due to the strong influence of karma from previous births; those that are caused earlier in life and manifest later in life; those that involve spirits; and those that are superficial. Superficial diseases are caused, and can be easily corrected, by diet and behaviour, while the first three classes need spiritual treatment as well. In only the last class of diseases is the causative action of the *doshas* primary; otherwise they act only reflexively, as it were, in response to other, more powerful and more subtle causes, most notably the Law of Karma.

The Law of Karma, otherwise known as the Law of Action and Reaction, is Newton's Third Law of Motion: 'Whenever one object exerts a force on a second object, the second exerts an equal and opposite force on the first.' The Law of Karma extends this physical law to the non-physical realms of existence: whatever action of any sort, even mental, a being performs in the world will be returned in kind. Jesus said it in this way: 'Do unto others as you would have them do unto you' for 'as you sow, so shall you reap.'

The doctrine of reincarnation was important to the lawgivers of India's Classical Age for political as well as doctrinal reasons. Aiming to protect their privileges by legitimizing the rule of the nobility over the trading class and the peasantry, the priests found it convenient to believe that one's condition in this life is a direct result of one's actions in a past life, and that abject acceptance of one's plight now is the only way to ensure a better rebirth next time round. Extension of this premise led to the conviction that the karma of past lifetimes is the only cause of health and disease, and that such past karma is immutable in this lifetime. Because all is predestined, medical treatment is useless; destiny alone determines if a patient survives or succumbs, just as destiny determines who governs and who is governed.

Ayurveda, while also espousing the doctrine of reincarnation, accepts the fact but not the immutability of the Law of Karma. Charaka devotes a whole chapter to the theory of karma and its application in medicine, concluding that while the influence of past karma is important, the efforts of the present life are also important, and that rational therapy is useless only if the patient is medically incurable. Jesus taught that one's sins, or past karmas, can be redeemed; Ayurveda applies this teaching to physical existence, maintaining, as does Tibetan medicine, that karmic diseases disappear as soon as the force of the karma is exhausted, and that some such diseases can be eliminated by careful medical treatment over a long period of time.

Charaka avers that all treatises on the subject of medicine unanimously conclude that 'there are causes, there are diseases, and there are means of remedying the remediable diseases', suggesting that the idea of disease as a consequence of wrongdoing in a previous existence is acceptable in medicine only when no other explanation is possible, just as *prabhava*, or special power, is invoked when a substance shows actions in the body that cannot be predicted by its taste, potency or post-digestive effect. *Prabhava* is inexplicable by reason, as is karma. Of all accepted logical methods of proof in Ayurveda, direct perception (*pratyaksha*, literally 'before the eyes') is regarded as the most reliable and therefore the most important, while the authority of the scriptures was relegated to a secondary position. Karma therefore had to take a back seat to what was visible and, as such, more controllable by a physician's efforts.

The importance of non-apparent causes still persists in Ayurveda, however, because of the many conditions that cannot be explained by recourse to *dosha* imbalance alone, their causes existing deeper in the organism than the level at which the *doshas* operate. There are seven main types of disease:

genetic or hereditary – including tendencies that may or may not fully manifest, such as leprosy, piles, diabetes and asthma;

congenital – such as deformities;

metabolic – due to disturbance of the *doshas* by excessive or insufficient intake of food and other nutrients;

traumatic – physically or mentally;

temporal – failure to follow seasonal or other regimens or to protect oneself against the weather or adverse astrological influences;

divine – disobedience to the guru, curses, magic or epidemics;

natural – hunger, thirst, sleep, fatigue, other urges, decay, senescence and death.

Of these, only one type is directly due to the machinations of the *doshas*. The fundamental cause of all these diseases, direct or indirect, and the cause of all human karma-producing activity, is the passionate attachment of living beings to the things of this world. We call it desire.

THE FEVER OF DESIRE

Vagbhata's treatise *Ashtanga Sangraha* commences with the words *ragadi rogah*: 'all diseases, beginning with *raga*'. The word *raga*, which is cognate with the English word 'rage', means desire, passion and heat. Desire is that force which creates both pain and, that receptacle of pain, the human body. Just as it disturbs the primeval equilibrium to permit the cosmos to evolve, so desire disturbs an individual's equilibrium and allows diseases to evolve. Desire is called the first of all diseases because it disrupts contentment and drags the mind away from balance. Charaka says, 'He who wishes to protect from harm that great organ, the heart, those great-rooted ones, the channels, and *ojas*, should scrupulously avoid anything that afflicts the mind.'

Satisfaction creates calmness, and so coolness, in the consciousness. The agitation generated by dissatisfaction, especially with regard to selfish desires, generates the heat of passion, an abnormal heat that disturbs all layers of the organism and manifests as physical or mental fever. Charaka notes,

All living beings come into the world with fever on them and likewise with fever on them they die. It is the great delusion; enveloped by it, creatures do not recall any action done in their previous lives. It is fever alone that in the end takes away the life breath of all living beings.

By heating up body, mind and senses, the fever of fervour 'diminishes wisdom, strength, lustre, liveliness, and enthusiasm, induces physical and mental exhaustion and delusion, and obstructs nutrition'. Longevity requires coolness of mind, senses and body; fever, and the passion that is its source, incinerate the organism. 'The body itself is fire' says a verse, and fever is the entry into the *Rasa* Channel of heat that belongs in the gut. *Kapha* is fundamentally cold and unctuous, *pitta* hot and unctuous, and *vata* cold and dry. The combination of hot and dry that occurs in fever represents the action of the fire and air elements on the body's juiciness (which is composed of water and earth), resulting in obstruction to the channels and aggravation of the *doshas*. Since cold is merely lack of heat and since we cannot conversely define heat as 'lack of cold' (while absolute zero is truly absolute there is no theoretical limit to heat), the cause of all disturbance of the *doshas* is heat imbalance, and fever is the only true disease.

DISEASE PERSONALITIES

Charaka's list of external causes for fever includes exhaustion (for example, after childbirth), assault or other injury, sorcery and witchcraft, curse, possession by evil spirits, infection by micro-organisms, poison, romantic passion (which causes mental imbalance, stupor, lethargy or languidness, refusal to eat, pain in the heart and emaciation), fear or grief (which creates delirium), or intense anger. Anger, grief and fear are said to aggravate the Sweat Channel. They may do so directly, by affecting the physical digestion, or indirectly, by impeding the mental digestion, but the result is still fever, which usually obstructs perspiration.

Physical digestion is ruled by taste, and mental digestion by emotion; what is taste on the physical level translates into emotion on the mental level. Each emotion produced by the achievement or non-achievement of desire generates its own taste pattern in the body. Sometimes it is these tastes that disturb the *doshas* and manifest ailments, while at other times the ailment develops directly; fear of diarrhoea, for example, can actually cause diarrhoea. One full section (*sthana*) of Charaka's treatise is filled with discourses on the pathology of the eight diseases that are caused mainly, directly or indirectly, by greed, malice and anger: fever, *rakta pitta* (haemor-rhagic diseases), *gulma* (phantom tumours), diabetes and other uri-nary disorders, skin diseases (especially leprosy), consumption, insan-ity and convulsions.

Charaka provides a mythological origin for each of these eight great diseases. Fever is said to be a malevolent, potentially murder-ous being born from the congealed anger of Rudra, the god of death known better as Shiva, when he was insulted by Daksha ('The Adept'). This myth suggests that anger can cause fever directly or it can cause *pitta* increase, which then causes fever; it is also a warning not to insult influential or powerful people lest they curse, bewitch or otherwise 'broil' you. Fever, then, is a being that possesses its hosts; in simple fevers the possession is quickly termi-nated, while in periodic fevers, such as malaria, it recurs, the patient becoming temporarily 'free' of the possession when the fever dies away and 'bound' by it again when the fever returns.

Since fever is of divine origin, worship is a valid treatment for it. While few know how to employ Atharva Vedic incantations that can invoke and expel fever from the body, even today in much of India a person with chickenpox, measles or other fever with a rash is considered to be possessed by a goddess, who is worshipped carefully until the sickness departs from the house.

A disease is a living being, a creation of your own mental and physical wastes, which has come alive by the fortuitous combination of desire, seasonal influence, mental perversity, and dietary and other indiscretions. Some diseases have physical presences, such as those caused by bacteria or viruses; they possess a single 'consciousness' even though they live in different bodies, as do bees, ants or termites. Mental diseases are possessions by alien personalities, either 'pre-existent' or generated out of one's own personality. It hardly matters whether such beings really exist or not, since they act as if they exist. And, asks the Indian philosopher, what really does exist?

Facile Western theories of personality are finally being shaken by the phenomenon of multiple personalities. 'Timmy' does not suffer from hives, but his dozen other personalities do. Hives appear if 'Timmy' drinks orange juice and a personality allergic to orange juice emerges while it is being digested. If 'Timmy' returns while the allergic reaction is present, the itching immediately disappears and the hives start to subside. The abrupt appearance and disappearance of rashes, welts, scars and other tissue wounds have been documented in patients of multiple personalities, along with switches in handwriting and handedness, selective colour blindness, epilepsy, eating disorders and differences in visual acuity, shape and curvature of the eye and its refraction, including even squint.

The differences observed in the responses of child and adult personalities to drugs reflect those seen in actual children and adults, independent of the patient's chronological age. When one personality shifts into another, the individual's heart rate, breathing rate, blood pressure and other physiological rhythms, including the patterns of blood flow in the brain, become disorganized, and new patterns develop as soon as the new personality is properly 'seated' in the organism. These facts and others like them support Ayurveda's contention that human personality is a group of qualities brought together and forced to operate as a unit by *ahamkara*. Change *ahamkara*'s self-identification to a new set of qualities, and *voilà*! you have a new personality.

Most of us 'normal, functional' people have several sub-personalities, which surface at different times. Because these sub-units are all relatively coherent with one another, and because they each have the same name, we 'average' humans do not display the extreme variations in behaviour that sufferers from multiple personalities do. However well we can function in society, though, most of us cannot claim to enjoy the thorough integration of consciousness and intention that characterize a saint or a madman, two beings who have proceeded to the logical end of personality development. The saint subsumes his or her entire consciousness to the divine will of Nature, while the psychopath ruthlessly replaces all traces of altruism with allegiance to a self-centred, diseased vision of reality.

Every disease has its own independent personality. Like a shadow brought to life, it lives a temporary, parasitic, shadowy existence, feeding off your physical and mental wastes, and then it dies, sometimes dragging you along with it. The strength of a disease is proportional to how well it possesses you; a good 'fit', which happens when your own personalities do not 'fit' well in your body, makes it easier for the disease to enter and remain inside you, its consciousness possessing your consciousness and skewing the way you think, feel and act.

While your disease possesses you it also takes over your internal clock. You then live on 'disease time', the time it takes for the illness to be born and live within you before it dies. Some diseases do not completely 'die' but only 'die away', like those plants that die back to their roots in winter and come back to life in spring. Such ailments have two states: *vega* ('urge' or 'momentum') during which it manifests, and *avega*, during which *vata* 'hides' it in the tissues, where it remains dormant until its season rolls around again.

Jaundice, a condition in which bile turns the skin, eyes and urine yellow, is also possession by a malignant personality; in this case it is the colour yellow that comes to life and takes over the patient's being. In jaundice the mind 'yellows' too, and the patient sees the world through 'bile-coloured glasses'. Modern medicine's strictly materialistic eyes see inflammation of the liver as the 'cause' of jaundice; Ayúrveda, concerned with deeper causes, sees the liver only as the place of the disease's manifestation and sees jaundice as being due to *pitta* in the body and to 'hot' emotions in the mind. Vedic medicine sees the organism's imbalance at a level on which symbol is more real to the organism than is the so-called reality we inhabit, and treats jaundice by directly invoking and extracting the yellowness.

Differences in principles of classification cloud one-to-one correspondences between Vedic diseases, Ayurvedic diseases and modern diseases. It is also possible that people have changed over the past five thousand years. Perhaps Vedic-era humans actually were more aware of different levels of reality than we are today, and perhaps this awareness made them more prone to certain diseases. Maybe Vedic jaundice, Ayurvedic jaundice and modern jaundice are actually three varieties of the same condition, which differ according to where the organism holds its consciousness and how it perceives itself. If the Vedics actually were exceptionally aware of the contents of their minds and the movements of *vata* and prana in their bodies, that very awareness when disturbed by an abnormal thought may have more quickly set the disease process in motion and brought it to resolution than could happen in the Classical period, when people had become more aware of the material world, or today, when we hyper-materialists have polluted our bodies and dulled our minds by every excess.

In the absence of substantive proof such ideas remain speculative; but the amazing control that some yogis display over their physiological processes makes one suspect that such control could once have been more common in the populace, and that those people would have lived truly different lives than we. Their nervous systems, endocrine glands and thought processes would have been connected together in ways that might seem incomprehensible to us now, and their diseases would also have developed, manifested and subsided in unfamiliar ways. Some of their diseases may have vanished over time, which is why we can no longer identify them clearly, and some diseases familiar to us that do not seem to appear in the texts may have arisen more recently, as has AIDS in our own time.

Though diseases come and go, the fact of disease remains. The mind, which tends to believe itself immortal, often ignores the ticking time bomb that is the body. One of the Sanskrit words for 'body' literally means 'that which decays', suggesting that the body, whose fuse starts to sputter the moment it draws its first breath, is itself a disease. Though the body is only a temporary haven for an individual's consciousness, and though everyone sees death around them regularly, most people are too immersed in the world of desire to be able to conceive of their own deaths, to notice the ingress of alien intelligences or even to pay attention to the deterioration of their own bodies.

CRIMES AGAINST WISDOM

The mental attitude that permits an organism to act contrary to its own self-interest is known in Sanskrit as *prajnaparadha* (literally, 'crime against wisdom'), a word that reflects the importance of *prajna* (transcendent wisdom) to Buddhist philosophy. On the most obvious level *prajnaparadha* is a 'violation of good sense', both mental and physical, as, for example, failing to protect oneself against the cold or the rain when one goes outside. Such failings are due to allurement, the selfish desire of a microcosm to try to ignore the inherent rhythm of the universe (*rtam*) and the transcendent wisdom that arises from it, and rearrange the macrocosm to suit itself. Charaka says, 'Whatever act is done by one who is deranged of understanding, will or memory is to be regarded as a volitional transgression (*prajnaparadha*). It is the inducer of all pathological conditions.'

A 'sin' is also a 'volitional transgression', the difference between sin and *prajnaparadha* being that sin implies guilt. *Prajnaparadha* is an impartial assessment of one's unwillingness or inability to remain in a state of harmony with the cosmos. Until you become enlightened, you are bound to be out of rhythm with the universe from time to time, and your responsibility is simply to take responsibility for your condition and to work to improve it one day at a time, examining your past indiscretions that you may avoid repeating them in the future. Guilt plays no part in Ayurveda because, by reinforcing your limitations, it discourages you from making progress and learning to take Nature's advice.

The mythological origins of certain diseases remind the reader of the grave consequences inherent in failing to heed the warnings of the 'gods' of the body and mind. Fever had not existed in the universe at large before Rudra's wrathful outburst, nor does it exist in the microcosm before anger's birth; but after its manifestation fever gives birth to other ailments. *Prajnaparadha*, which is universal (it afflicts even the gods), is an outpouring of energy in an inappropriate direction. When this energy gets trapped in an archetypical 'mould', which may be a bacterium, virus, metabolic pattern, mental aberration or other self-propagating 'parasite', a disease springs into manifestation as soon as the proper microcosmic conditions occur.

Raja yakshma is such a disease mould. *Raja yakshma*, which means variously 'the king's disease', 'the king of diseases' or 'the disease of King (Moon)', entered the universe when the Moon was cursed by his father-in-law, Daksha, that same Daksha who suffered from Shiva's ire, with loss of his 'unctuous element' (*shukra, ojas*). The Moon attracted this curse because he spent too much time dallying with Rohini and neglected her twenty-six other sisters (the *nakshat-ras*, or lunar constellations) who were also his wives. Daksha's curse generated the *raja yakshma* disease mould, and now anyone who gets carried away by lust risks attracting its attack. *Raja yakshma* is sometimes translated 'consumption', a wasting away of the tissues, which includes, but is not limited to, tuberculosis. The story of Daksha's curse is at once an object lesson (never mistreat your wives!) and a statement of two major causes of consumption: exhaustion of *ojas* and the tissues by excessive sexual activity, and rashness of behaviour.

This wasting away of the microcosm resembles the wasting away of the flora and fauna of a region beset with drought. Any earthly ruler who neglects his duties and abandons himself to lust (astrologically, the moon represents emotion, especially romance) is likely to be laid low with consumption, and because the health of the ruler and the health of the ruled are inextricably linked, such a king's kingdom will suffer drought, the 'wasting away' of the kingdom. Drought in the macrocosm is land deprived of rain; in the microcosm, it is the 'field' of the body deprived of 'juice'. Drought is a particularly appropriate metaphor, as the Moon is the Lord of Water (he causes the tides), and in his role as King of Plants he is in charge of keeping all plants well filled with sap, and the wasting away of the one leads to the wasting away of all the others.

Although kings and princes no longer rule in either India or Sri Lanka, many people in both countries still believe that a good government makes a nation healthy, and that a corrupt, cruel or otherwise evil government transmits its corruption to the nation's workplaces, schools and homes, and even to the land itself. A corrupt, heartless government corrupts those it governs; people pattern themselves after their rulers, even when such patterning may be fatal to them. Like those they lead, village, municipal, national and international leaders are led into wrongdoing by the force of *prajnaparadha*. The curses attracted by their unrighteousness include epidemics, insect plagues and other catastrophes. When the ruled imitate the ruler's failure to follow the path indicated by the cosmic *rtam*, disorder (cosmic lawlessness) supervenes, disturbing the winds, the water, the land and the seasons, resulting in drought, epidemics, wars and affliction by diabolic powers.

When *ahamkara*, which rules the microcosm, is laid low by lust, consumption blasts the fields (tissues) of the body-land with drought. Ayurveda's emphasis on altruism and the restraint of selfishness was not grafted on later by orthodox editors; it sprouted logically from the Classical physician's attempt to minimize *prajna-paradha*, the true cause of disease, and its varied devastations.

CAUSES OF DISEASE

'Perversity of mind' is the ultimate cause of every disease. It can affect any activity of speech, mind or body directly, or can work indirectly through improper conjunctions of the senses with their objects or inattention to the changes in diet and lifestyle necessitated by the evolution of time cycles (daily, seasonal, digestive, age, etc.). Time itself becomes improper when the macrocosm is imbalanced, such as when there is too much or not enough rain, or abnormally high or low temperatures during a given season. Examples of underuse, overuse, misuse and abuse of the sense organs include stopping up one's ears and refusing to use the organ of hearing, exposure to intensely loud noise, and listening to sounds that frighten or otherwise disturb body or mind. Neither the senses nor their objects cause either pleasure or pain; the real cause is the unwholesome contact of the senses with their objects. Neither microcosm nor macrocosm is at fault when the fault lies in an unhealthy relationship between the two.

Both improper use of the sense organs and inattention to time are subsidiary to *prajnaparadha*'s subversion of awareness by desire, resulting in vitiation of the *doshas*. Though the *doshas* do not even appear as such in the Vedas, they had by the Classical Age supplanted other causative factors in most Ayurvedic thinking about pathology because of their ability to vitiate all elements of the body, both stationary (the already-created tissues) and mobile (the digested nutrients ready to nourish the tissues), the vitiation spreading from one to the other. Disturbed channels spread their corruption only to other body channels, and polluted tissues only to other tissues, 'whereas *vata, pitta* and *kapha* when vitiated pollute the entire organism, being, as they are, of a vitiating nature'. This vitiating nature makes them dangerous, unstable, Trojan-horse-like forces, which the strong stresses that afflict city dwellers call into such prominence that they cannot be ignored.

The tissues and wastes are taken together as *dushyas*, things that are vitiated by the *doshas*. According to the law of cause and effect as espoused by the Nyaya system of philosophy, the Three *Doshas* are the instrumental cause of disease (the effect), but remain always separate from it. Indiscretions in diet and activity are the supporting causes, which enable the *doshas* to become aggravated. The *dushyas* form the inherent or material cause, which is inseparable from the effect (the disease exists in the tissues and wastes); loss of this disturbance means elimination of disease. The invasion of the tissues or wastes by the *doshas* is the non-inherent cause; removal of the *doshas* from the *dushyas* will alter the disease, but may not be enough to eliminate it.

Causes are also classified as:

Being weak or strong, and being 'near' (quickly resulting in disease) or 'distant' (taking time to demonstrate their effects). When improper diet aggravates the *doshas*, the effect is seen immediately from head to toe and then slowly ebbs, like a flood. When *dosha* imbalance is due to seasonal change, as in the accumulation of *kapha* in winter, which produces ailments only in spring, the effect is delayed.

Exciting the *doshas* in general (for example, the sweet taste causes *kapha* increase), creating specific diseases (like straining at stools, which causes piles) or both.

Being primary or secondary, internal or external, 'natural' (*kapha* disease in spring, its natural season for aggravation) or 'unnatural' (*vata* or *pitta* disease in spring), independent or dependent, and 'constitutional' (*vata* diseases in a person of *vata* constitution) or 'unconstitutional' (*pitta* or *kapha* diseases in a *vata* person).

Our high-tech world provides us with plenty of strong external causative factors – including imbalanced diets, pervasive pollutants (chemical, radiological, electrical, magnetic, noise, artificial light), overactivity, the side-effects of medical treatments, high-speed travel, overdependence on humanity-destroying machines, inharmonious architecture and interior decoration, and the weight of all the negative thoughts being broadcast by millions of humans in all directions – which continuously drain our energies as we attempt to come to grips with them and with the internal causes that steer our minds towards *prajnaparadha*. The usual result is aggravation of the *doshas*.

How much any particular substance or activity disturbs a *dosha* depends upon its relative affinity for that *dosha*. A substance that has three *vata*-causing qualities (say, dry, cold and light) will disturb *vata* more than one that is merely dry and cold, which, in turn, will vitiate more than one that is merely dry. Asafoetida, which is hot, pungent and intense, deranges *pitta* more than does sesame, which is only hot and oily, and so on. When two or three *doshas* come together, the symptoms produced can either be similar in nature to them both or entirely different from what one would expect, according to how their own individual qualities interact. All this also holds true for the two *doshas* that directly afflict the mind, namely *rajas* and *tamas*, and for the interactions between the mental and physical *doshas*.

The *doshas* can be normal, increased or decreased in strength. Most people today, especially in the West, suffer from increased *doshas*, since most people take in many more 'things', such as food and information, than they can hope to digest. The *doshas* do not automatically aggravate each other, nor, though they are mutually antagonistic, do they negate one another, because they have a mutual natural immunity – they are 'naturally *satmya*' to their fellow *doshas* – just as a snake is not killed by its own poison, which is part of itself and to which it is habituated.

Ama

How the *doshas* affect the body and mind is expressed in a verse from Charaka: 'The balance and aggravation of the Doshas is at all times due to the relative strength or weakness of the digestive fire. Therefore one must always protect the digestive fire, and prohibit all activities which might weaken it.'

All diseases are due to *agnimandya*, weakness of the digestive fire (with the exception of one condition, in which this fire becomes exceptionally intense). *Prajnaparadha* is a sort of weakness of the mental digestion, which is transmitted via various paths to the body. The body's digestive fire is normal when there is normal desire for food, no discomfort after eating, no belching and no heaviness or other symptoms during digestion; when a sense of well-being and satisfaction (indicating proper nourishment of *rasa*) occurs; and when all wastes have normal consistency, do not contain undigested food and are excreted at normal times. The mind's digestive fire should be examined in a similar way; *prajna-paradha* is clearly indicative of weak mental digestion.

Like all fires, the body's digestive fire changes from moment to moment. It becomes weak as a result of overuse of cold and liquid substances, especially ice water, especially in winter; overeating or undereating; overconsumption of heavy food, such as meat; eating before the previous meal has been digested; improper food combining; restraint of natural reflex urges, which causes *vata* to move in improper directions; disturbances of sleep; consumption of food to which one is not habituated; consumption of food at the wrong time, according to the seasons, the climate, one's age and health, and so on; overactivity (especially sexual) or underactivity; and mental causes, especially envy, fear, anger, greed, anguish, wretchedness, misery and sorrow.

All these causes are stresses. Stress can be good (eustress), such as the effect of gravity on our bones, or it can be distress; the difference between the two often depends upon how we interpret its effects on us. All the flows of body and mind feed, directly or indirectly, the desires of the embodied ego; welcome to inputs from outside depends on the strength of the immune system, which depends, in turn, on the integrity of the identity. Dys-stress leads to *agnimandya*, which leads to the production of *ama* ('raw, uncooked, unripened'). *Ama* is a generic term for food that is absorbed into the system without having first been properly digested. Such partly digested material cannot be used by the system, and acts mainly to clog it, eliciting an immune reaction. Stagnant pools of *ama* in an organism breed disease as surely as a stagnant pond breeds mosquitoes.

Ama is more sinister than simple stagnant water, however, because it is generated from food essence that should have gone to form healthy *rasa*. Ayurvedic purity is the purity of the body's 'juices'. Though the foul-smelling, sticky *ama* that pollutes *rasa*'s purity still maintains its power to nourish even when it can no longer be utilized by the tissues, this perverted nourishing power provides a culture medium for every parasite in the neighbourhood. *Ama* is the juice that nourishes disease, just as *rasa* nourishes its fellow tissues. Mental *ama* arises when the mind becomes unable to come to grips with disorienting sense perceptions, thoughts, emotions or opinions and leaves mental nutrients sitting undigested, polluting the mind with *prajnaparadha*. Both forms of *ama* reinforce one another: selfish thoughts pollute the body, which, in turn, disturbs the consciousness. The fundamental cause for all *ama* is indigestible desire.

The concept of *ama* is not limited to Ayurveda. In the Egypt of 1500 BC healers believed that most disease was due to an 'ill wind' (*vata*) or to toxic body wastes, which they called *whdw* (pronounced 'ukhedu'), produced by overeating, drunkenness, evil spirits or emotional disorders. Closer to home, intestinal toxaemia, a condition in which the internal milieu of the intestines, especially the colon, changes so that toxins are generated during digestion, was a diagnosis popular in the West before the Second World War. It was accepted by many main-line physicians and articles on it were published in leading medical journals. Evidence of intestinal toxaemia was found in asthma; allergies; arthritis; irregular heartbeats; ear, nose and throat diseases; the toxaemia of pregnancy; eye, skin and breast diseases; low-back pain and sciatica; cancer and mental illnesses, including schizophrenia and senility.

Intestinal toxaemia develops mainly from overconsumption of protein, especially meat. The human gut is too long for us to be healthy carnivores, and high-protein foods tend to become stagnant in the intestines; this stagnation encourages proteolytic and putrefactive bacteria to grow in the colon and convert the ingested food into *ama*. *Ama* includes all abnormal molecules produced by improper digestion of any foods, especially those high in protein and fat, which pass through the walls of the digestive tract into the general circulation and evoke a strong immunological response.

Complex carbohydrates can also produce *ama*, but are less likely to do so because they burn more cleanly and because their large amounts of natural fibre discourage intestinal stasis. This is one reason they are the main ingredient of a healthy diet.

Charaka stresses that 'the use of a wholesome diet is the main factor that promotes the healthy growth of man; and the main factor that makes for disease is the indulgence in unwholesome diet.' Elsewhere he adds: 'The wise man, by constantly avoiding all avoidable causes of diseases in the matter of diet, escapes blame at the hands of good people, and it behooves him not to lament on falling victim to those pathogenic factors which it is not possible for anyone to avoid', blame and lament being two emotional factors that predispose to *prajnaparadha*.

Pathology

Ama is the immediate cause of most human afflictions; exposure to disease-causing microbes results in disease only in those people whose internal conditions are ripe for colonization. Louis Pasteur and Claude Bernard argued for years over the primacy of infective agents versus internal conditions, and it was only on his deathbed that Pasteur finally admitted that Bernard was right, and that the *milieu intérieur* is more important than exposure to a pathogen. This is especially true of diseases in which no 'pathogen' can be detected. Nine times out of ten, specific causes for high blood pressure cannot be determined because it arises as the sum (*yukti*) of complex interactions between environmental, social and psychological stresses, the individual's constitutional tendencies, the central nervous system, the endocrine glands and the circulatory system.

Ayurveda was not unaware of infectious disease. Sushruta recognized leprosy, fevers, consumption and conjunctivitis as being contagious, 'caused by intimate contact', such as sex, physical contact, contact with expired air, eating from the same dishes, sleeping in the same bed, and the common use of clothing, garlands, unguents and so on. In the tenth century A D Dalhana added smallpox to this list. Charaka mentions that some blood-borne parasites are round, legless and too minute to be visible to the naked eye, and certain Vedic passages also allude to micro-organisms. While some people argue that without modern equipment such tiny beings could never have been seen, others maintain that the five senses are not the only means of perception open to those who, like the seers who cognized Ayurveda, have adequately trained their consciousnesses.

Microbes were, however, never particularly important to Ayurvedic pathology, because the principle of *yukti* discourages any attempt to find single causes for effects. Ayurveda teaches that the growth of any system, be it a single organism, a village or an epidemic, is caused by the same mechanism. Sushruta compares this process to the fermentation of yeast, and Charaka describes it with an agricultural metaphor: season, field, seed and water. Good crops are produced when healthy seed is sown in the proper season in a well-tilled, well-irrigated field. A good human is produced when healthy parents with healthy seed unite during the proper portion of the woman's monthly season, when the womb-field is well irrigated by *rasa* and blood.

Likewise, when a viable seed (bacterium, virus, pathological emotion or selfish thought) is sown in an appropriate season in the field of a body or mind that has been thoroughly watered by *ama*, the result is a 'disease-being'. 'Season' can refer to any of the time cycles that affect humans: daily, yearly, age-related, digestive, astrological or other. Diseases are especially produced at the junctions or 'joints' of the seasons, those periods when one season is not quite over and the next has not quite begun, and the environment is in a state of upheaval. This is especially striking in temperate climates during the period between winter and spring, when the weather vacillates for days or weeks, unsure of its proper direction. Puberty, that turbulent season during which the adolescent is neither a child nor an adult, promotes imbalances of all sorts, as do menopause and male mid-life crises.

The usual process by which disease develops is known as 'Obstruction to the Pathways'. It begins with *prajnaparadha*, which leads to inappropriate behaviour, which results in digestive weakness, which generates *ama*, which obstructs some or all of the channels of body and mind. This obstruction prevents *vata* from moving in its normal direction, making its movements erratic; thus thwarted, it becomes *prakupita*, 'exceedingly angry', and like a tornado strews *pitta* and *kapha*, tissues and wastes in all directions until it finds a weak point where it can settle and generate a disease-being, which is invigorated by *vata*'s pseudo-life-force and nourished with the poison of *ama*. Though *vata* is central to the generation of such diseases, their symptoms often differ significantly from the symptoms of aggravated *vata*, because *vata* accepts the qualities of whatever it transports. Though *vata* is itself cold by nature, it causes both 'hot' and 'cold' diseases according to the tissues, wastes or other *doshas* that are its passengers.

Vata can also become aggravated in 'dry' conditions by two processes known as 'Wasting of the Tissues' and 'Emptiness of the Reservoir Organs'. When the body becomes emaciated, *vata* gains in strength because it has nothing to restrain its strength, nothing heavy and oily that can weigh it down and keep it under control. When a hollow organ remains empty for too long, *vata*, which is always looking for things to stimulate and move, stimulates the organ's fibres into excessive motion, causing spasm, which in the case of the colon is colic. In such cases the resultant disease is less a creation of *ama* (though most people have enough residual *ama* in their tissues after years of dietary indiscretions to nourish many an ailment) than it is 'possession' by the 'evil spirit' of a malign *vata*.

THE SIX STAGES OF DISEASE

Weakness of the digestive fire is the root cause of all diseases, *vata* is the chief cause of the development of all diseases of any variety, and *ama* is the principal nourisher of disease. All illnesses caused by whatever relative influence of the *doshas* follow a six-step programme of development.

Accumulation

As a result of exposure to causative factors, one or more of the *doshas* accumulates in its 'seat': *kapha* in the stomach, *pitta* in the small intestine, and *vata* in the colon.

Each produces its own characteristic symptoms: *kapha* creates lethargy, heaviness of the limbs, pallor, bloating, and loss of appetite with weakened digestion; *pitta* produces burning sensations, increased body heat, a bitter taste in the mouth, yellowness of the skin, acidity in the stomach and increased anger; *vata* causes weakness and dryness of the body, desire for warmth and hot articles, stiffness or fullness of the abdomen, flatulence and/or constipation, disturbed sleep and increased fear. The *doshas* are easiest to remove from the system at this stage. Seasonal purifications protect health by removing the accumulations of the *doshas* that occur naturally due to the inherent qualities of the various seasons.

Aggravation

In this stage, which literally means 'rage', the *doshas* continue to increase and put pressure on their reservoirs, intensifying the symptoms they have produced. It is still fairly easy to remove the *doshas* even at this stage, but while treating them, their reservoir organs, which have been stressed by their ire, need also to be strengthened.

The *doshas* do not always accumulate before they become 'enraged'; if the causes are strong enough, aggravation may occur directly. A salient example is the common cold. While some colds arise from mucus build-up caused by accumulated *doshas*, others occur when sudden exposure to intense cold – such as when one steps out of a warm house into a cold winter night – slams shut all the channels of circulation in the head and allows the *doshas* there, usually *vata* and *kapha* in this case, to become immediately irritated even if they are in a balanced condition in their respective reservoirs.

Overflow

If aggravation is permitted to proceed unchecked, the *doshas* escape their homes, wandering about the body like vagabonds searching for a place to camp. All the previous symptoms worsen, and *kapha* may produce vomiting; *pitta*, diarrhoea; and *vata*, colicky pain in the colon and painful defecation, with the liberation of copious quantities of gas. Overflow can also occur without previous accumulation or aggravation of the *doshas* in their reservoir organs if they are displaced by the force of an aggravated *vata*, which may be directly disturbed by exposure to strong imbalancing causes such as excessive desire (especially sexual), sleeplessness, excessive talking and activity (especially on an empty stomach), sudden vomiting or diarrhoea (particularly if self-induced), intense joy or sadness, and the restraint of any of the natural reflex urges.

Disruption of *vata*'s natural direction or rhythm is sufficient to initiate many disease processes. Under the influence of a misdirected *vata* the *doshas* may move up, down or sideways, wreaking havoc with the system wherever they roam. Misdirected *vata* is called *pratiloma* in Sanskrit, literally 'against the hair', referring to the direction in which body hair grows. Body hair, a waste product of bone (the one tissue in which *vata* predominates), is the external display of the underlying movement of *vata* in the body. Ayurvedic surgeons are warned to avoid incising the skin against the direction of hair growth, as that will interfere with *vata*'s normal direction, causing increased pain and slower healing. So long as *vata* is *pratiloma*, its momentum creates functional obstructions to the movement of various substances in various channels. Treatment aims to make it again *anuloma*, flowing 'with the hair'.

Suppose that you, like many modern people, live too much in your head, denying your body the attention it deserves. This forcible concentration of energy at your upper pole weakens the downward motion of *apana* (the form of *vata* that controls excretion), making it *pratiloma*. Since *pratiloma apana* can no longer properly perform its functions, constipation, retention of urine, colic, accumulation of gas, impotence or even endometriosis (caused by menstrual blood flowing up and into the abdominal cavity instead of down and out of the body) develops. *Pratiloma apana* can also cause headache by disturbing the other *vatas*, illustrating just how circular the chain of causation is: energy in the head angers *apana*, and *apana* can vitiate the energy in the head, both tending to reinforce one another until the cycle of causation is broken.

Vata's direction becomes disturbed when its natural rhythm of movement is lost. Good *samskaras* train up body and mind to live in harmony with both internal rhythms and the external *rtam*, making imbalance and disease less likely. Poor *samskaras* leave one open to the depradations of every parasite on every plane of existence. Good health requires 'grace under pressure', a commitment to act according to the exigencies of both season (*rtu*) and cosmic rhythm (*rtam*) even under the most trying circumstances so that *vata* will continue to move in the right rhythm in the proper direction.

Vata's *gati* is both its way of moving through the body, and the direction taken by this movement. The upward movement of *prati-loma apana* is an example of abnormal *gati*; which tissues this misdirected *apana* disturbs depends upon its *marga*, the path it follows through the body. The word 'path' is derived from the Sanskrit *patha*, whose meaning is identical; from *patha* is derived *pathya*, 'that which is appropriate to one's path'. When treating a disease, *pathya* is the specific set of diet and activities that return the wandering *doshas* to their own proper bodily paths and the individual to his or her proper life path. Like Dr Bernie Siegel's 'path report' (a pun on 'pathology'), Ayurvedic pathology reports on how well an individual is following his or her own proper path through life; it does so by reporting on the paths taken by the system's *doshas*.

Every disease follows its own particular path. In Tibetan medicine disease is said to reside and spread in the skin, develop in the flesh, move through the channels, adhere to the bone and descend to the vital or reservoir organs. In Ayurveda the system is divided into three disease *margas*, or pathways: Internal or Visceral, External or Peripheral, and Medial or *Marma*.

The Internal Pathway, which is the digestive tract and the tissue *rasa*, is usually the first to be affected by the *doshas*, which naturally concentrate in the major digestive organs. If the *doshas* are not expelled by active purification or reduced in strength by more conservative treatment, they eventually change their direction (*gati*) and start to flow into, instead of out of, the body, entering the Peripheral Pathway, which consists of the other six tissues. If the imbalance is further suppressed with stimulants or strong allopathic drugs or by repressing emotion, both *ama* and the *doshas* dive deeper into the tissues and enter the *Marma* Pathway, which contains all the essential organs, particularly the heart and brain. Though the three pathways represent deepening penetration of the disease process into the system, disease manifestation tends to confine itself to a single pathway at a time; when more than one pathway becomes involved, treatment becomes more difficult.

Whatever their direction and momentum in whichever pathway, the *doshas* eventually discover a convenient locale for their depredations.

Location

The *doshas* usually find their location in a previously weakened body region. Charaka compares this process to the falling of rain from a cloud; the cloud floats through the sky until it encounters appropriate atmospheric conditions, which induce it to release its burden of water. Likewise when the circulating *doshas* find the right location in which to concentrate themselves, they do so, initiating the specific illness by physically or functionally obstructing the local channels. No matter how intensively the tissues or wastes may be involved, they are not the immediate cause of the ailment; every illness is caused by the presence in the tissues or wastes of aggravated *doshas*, just as a burn received by touching a hot iron ball is caused by the ball's heat, not the ball itself. All ailments, even those known to be due to pathogenic organisms, are classified according to the underlying causative *dosha*.

At this stage begin the premonitory symptoms, which herald the ailment's arrival. Pulmonary tuberculosis often first shows itself as an evening rise of temperature with burning of the hands and feet; diabetes first causes increased frequency of urination, especially at night; diarrhoea is often preceded by constipation; and incipient fever should be suspected when there is changing desire, first for heat (hot food, warm environment) and then for cold.

Once the *doshas*, *ama* or *rasa* is located, the ailment can develop fully and display its qualities.

Manifestation

At this stage the illness is recognizable as such; for example, when *vata*, by its dry quality, changes the taste of *ojas*, which is naturally sweet, into astringent and carries it to the urinary organs, the result is diabetes.

Specialization

The specific variety of the illness results from specialization, which is usually indicated by the predominance of the *dosha* involved. For example, oedema is a swelling of the skin, flesh or other tissues, usually as a result of accumulation of fluid. Oedema caused mainly by *kapha* pits on pressure; that caused by *vata* does not do so; and *pitta* oedema is very tender. Most diseases have several varieties.

CLASSIFICATION OF DISEASES

There are basically three types of disease: endogenous (breakdowns from within), exogenous (attacks from without), and mental, any one of which can lead to any other. In exogenous disease – which includes infections, epidemics, occupational disorders, iatrogenic disease, accidents, adverse planetary positions and possession by spirits – the symptoms arise first, followed by imbalance of the *doshas*. In endogenous disease it is the other way round.

Mental disease can arise from an imbalance in either the mental *doshas* (*rajas* and *tamas*) or in *vata, pitta*, or *kapha*, or because of intense emotions or misuse of intoxicants. It can manifest in the mind (as does anxiety), in the body (as may asthma) or both; constipation, for example, may be a purely mental condition, caused by intense mental attachment and 'tightness'.

From another perspective there is only one type of disease, which comes from within as a result of *prajnaparadha*. According to this theory, even such seemingly uncontrollable events as accidents are due to long-term accumulating stress, which periodically releases itself into the consciousness, like an earthquake, and causes one to put oneself, knowingly or unknowingly, into harm's way.

Diseases are also classified according to severity, curability, etiology (especially cold versus hot), symptoms, location, time (for example, worse during the day or night or during a certain season or stage of digestion), prognosis and management. Iatrogenic disease, which is caused when a patient is treated for another ailment, is a separate category; Tibetan medicine delineates twelve types of such side-effects, which can arise from both successful and unsuccessful treament.

Diseases may be primary (arising independently) or secondary (occurring as a complication of some previously existing disease). Madhava observes that sometimes one disease eliminates itself in giving rise to a new disease, while at other times it causes a new disease and continues to co-exist with it. *Rakta pitta* (haemorrhagic tendency) can come from fever or cause it, and both together may cause *shosha* (emaciation; literally, 'drying out'); diarrhoea, malabsorption syndromes and haemorrhoids can all cause one another; and the common cold when neglected can develop into cough, which, if neglected, may deepen into consumption, which can then 'dry out' the patient.

All diseases are due either to undernourishment (drying out of the body) or overnourishment (making it too wet). Substances or activities that dry out the body – such as dry, stale food; excessive exposure to wind or sun; worry; fear; sorrow; fasting from sleep; old age; and excessive loss of blood, semen, faeces or other tissues or wastes from the body – weaken the digestive fire in the same way that lack of fuel starves an external fire. When the body is too dry, sufficient *rasa* to nourish the tissues properly cannot be formed, reducing the production of *ojas*, which weakens both the mental and physical digestive fires. Because dryness is a quality of *vata*, the drying out of the body is also a direct cause of *vata* aggravation, and usually leads to *vata*-type diseases.

Substances and activities that cause the 'wetness' of the system to increase weaken the digestive fire in the same way that wet fuel weakens an external fire. Because most of the diseases of affluent people are a result of excess, this wetness-increasing quality (*abhishyandi*) is a major cause of ill health. When the Ayurvedic seers elected to colonize relatively arid areas, and warned of the plethora of diseases that strike inhabitants in humid areas, they were thinking of this quality of *abhishyandi*, which everything in a humid climate, being perpetually drenched in wetness, comes to possess, and which naturally *abhishyandi* substances such as yoghurt, pork and salt possess regardless of their source.

IMMUNITY

Now that modern medicine has the ability to suppress most common acute human diseases, people can avoid purifying themselves for years while continuing to shove huge amounts of *ama* and *doshas* into their tissues, making any resulting diseases chronic almost from their onset. The sort of chronic degenerative disease that affects so many of us who live in modern societies seems to have been less common in the past, at least in India, where for centuries people have believed in regular physical purification. Many such diseases, including especially gout, obesity and diabetes, are grouped together under the rubric 'diseases of affluence', diseases of overnutrition, which arise in people who have too much of everything.

While it is quite possible that people were actually wired together differently in the past, it is true that no century before ours has had access to our volume of consumables, nor has any other culture been exposed to our unique and powerful pollutants. These two factors ensure that our diseases, on average, penetrate deeper into our beings than did the diseases from which our ancestors suffered, and now they attack the roots of our immunity and identity. Amyloid, a waxy sort of substance derived from immune cells and deposited in various tissues during the course of many degenerative diseases, is a form of internally created *ama*, an indigestible mass of material whose essence should have been used to nourish the tissues but instead was expended on combating immuno-insult.

Ahamkara, the ego or 'I-former', controls the millions upon millions of cells of the immune system, which safeguard us from potential mental and physical parasites, cells empowered to discriminate between that which *is* the body and that which wishes to enter the body. Only if there is a clear memory of who one is on the personal identity level will the immune cells on the body level be able to distinguish between self and not-self, and know which cells to kill and which to heal. If the immune system's defensive operations are routinely interrupted, as when antibiotics are routinely given to deal with minor problems, the immune system begins to confuse its friends with its foes, and as it weakens, degeneration supervenes. Degenerative disease strikes at the source of an individual's identity.

7

DIAGNOSIS

Modern medicine's 'objective' approach to health and disease is especially evident in its diagnostic technique, where chemical testing and machine imaging have largely taken over from the traditional 'signs and symptoms' approach. Objective tests are, however, usually unable to allow for test values that stray from the range generally accepted as normal. Any healthy person has a significant chance of having one 'abnormal' value show up when multiple tests are performed, because most people even when healthy do not fall precisely within medicine's metabolic norms. When such tests are used for random 'screening', such 'abnormal' values may lead to useless and potentially dangerous treatment. Some doctors overtest their patients in order to appear vigilant and to guard against malpractice suits, and many patients insist on overtesting. As a result, vast resources are wasted to achieve very little.

Ayurveda's diagnostic tests, being more subjective, are limited to the context of the patient being tested, and concentrate on the individual as a unitary whole, investigating its 'state', the pattern of relationships existing among organs and channels, instead of over-emphasizing the importance of a single tissue, organ, channel, *marma* or *chakra*. Your 'state' is the sum of where you have been, where you are now and where you are going on all levels of existence. Widowhood is a state, as are poverty, marriage, impurity and other such conditions of being. Your present state of existence, which is the sum of all your past experiences, determines your possible future states. Ayurvedic diagnosis is not limited to what is 'wrong' with you, but is rather an expression of where you are now, how much and in what direction you are changing, what influences are affecting that change, and what can be done to make your state harmonious and your life momentum rhythmic.

Ayurvedic diagnosis begins with what is *right* with you, namely how well-nourished, perfectly toned or 'excellent' your tissues are. The skin discloses the state of the underlying *rasa*. Skin that is unctuous, smooth, soft, clear, thin, full of lustre and covered with short, deeprooted delicate hairs indicates happiness, good fortune, power, pleasures, intelligence, knowledge, health, cheer and long life. When *rasa* is well nourished, it adeptly performs both its physical and psychological functions, generating a harmony in the microcosm that manifests as prosperity in the macrocosm. It is no accident that people with *pitta–kapha* or *kapha–pitta* constitutions achieve success more easily than others; their consciousness resonates better with prosperity.

Each tissue has its own signs of excellence. Blood, which gives vigour and vitality, is also usually examined through skin. The conditions of flesh, fat and bone are obvious to the discerning eye, and excellent marrow is seen through the lustre of body parts such as the eyes. Men who have excellence of *shukra* (semen), says Chaaka,

are gentle and possess gentle light in their eyes, which appear as if full of milk, and are full of cheerfulness. They have unctuous, round, firm, close and even teeth, a clear unctuous complexion and voice, and are lustrous and large-hipped. They are coveted sources of enjoyment for women, and are strong and possessed of happiness, power, health, wealth, honour and offspring.

Women whose *artava* (female reproductive 'juice') is excellent possess similar qualities. Excellence of *shukra* tends to produce excellence of *ojas*, that essence of immune power, which creates a powerful aura, which attracts others like flowers attract bees.

Those few people in whom all the elements are excellent and in perfect tone are very strong, able to bear troubles, self-confident in all enterprises and given to good pursuits; have firm, well-knit bodies, are firm in tread and have resonant, mellow, deep, strong voices; and are happy, powerful, wealthy and honoured, enjoying all pleasures. Both they and their offspring are slow to age or to be attacked by disease, and live long. Such people are 'endowed with joyful circumstances'; they are the recipients of that marvellous boon known as 'good health', and the metabolic joy each of their cells feels overflows into their outer environment and makes it healthy as well. Just to live in the aura of such people improves one's own health, happiness and peace of mind, because such well-balanced, excellent individuals uplift any society of which they become part.

These excellences are a good measure of a person's strength and vitality, and so provide good indications of life momentum. It is easy to be deceived by a body's appearance unless you examine its excellences. Major diseases may seem minor in people who have 'richness of spirit, vitality and body', while minor disease will seem major in a patient with 'poverty' of those things. Robust people with big bodies are not necessarily strong, for some giant-sized people are blown up like balloons of *vata* and, like balloons, are ready to burst with the slightest pinprick. People who are emaciated or have small bodies are not necessarily weak; they may be like the ant, who can carry loads far larger than itself. In all things size is not as important as proportion. 'Long life, strength, vitality, happiness, power, wealth and other desirable qualities depend upon the proper proportion of the body', Charaka tells us.

Excellence of mind is shown by strong memory, devotion, gratitude, wisdom, purity, great energy, skill, courage, prowess in battle, freedom from sorrow, firmness of tread, deep intelligence and character. Such people are given to good pursuits, even if their bodies are not perfectly healthy. People with strong minds, even if weak in body, appear unaffected when afflicted by severe ailments, while those whose mental power is moderate, seek consolation for their inadequacies by comparing themselves with others, and seek consolation from others in order to compose themselves. Weak minds cannot be calmed and composed either by themselves or by others.

Weak-minded people, even if strong in body, are incapable of bearing even small ailments stoically; their minds quickly go unhinged when exposed to fear, sorrow, temptation, delusion, disgrace, horror stories or shocking sights, such as that of flesh and blood. The stronger a person's mind, the more likely it is that he or she will be able to 'digest' such experiences and emerge from them even stronger.

JYOTISHA

Like a good astrologer, a good physician tries to discover first his patients' strengths and then their weaknesses, hoping to use those strengths, wherever possible, to counteract the weaknesses. An expert Indian astrologer can generate a horoscope by any of three separate methods: by calculation, palmistry or mere facial examination. Vimalananda was able to accurately read people's horoscopes simply by reading their features. Even fingerprints tell stories: for example, people who have one or more arches in their fingerprints display from childhood a tendency to constipation and other gastro-intestinal symptoms. Astrology is important to diagnosis because of what it can reveal of the inner and outer forces affecting a person and the effect of such forces on his or her existence. Knowledge of the movement of the sun, moon and planets is as important to medicine as it is to the martial arts and to sexuality.

One of the most famous Ayurvedic physicians of recent times was Tryambakam Shastri, who lived about a hundred years ago in Benaras. Any patient who would come to see him would first ring the bell hung outside his door. As soon as the sound of the bell reached him, Tryambakam Shastri would note the time, make a few calculations and select three possible medicines. Then the patient would enter and be diagnosed by other methods, but almost invariably the proper remedy would be one of the three medicines selected by the astrological route.

Judy Pugh of the University of British Columbia detects three separate arts in Indian astrology: the art of dialogue, the art of prediction and the art of remedy. Ayurvedic physicians work with patients in much the same way: establishing a base of communication, suggesting the likely course of the disease and providing remedies that can ameliorate the problem and ease the suffering involved. Astrology, medicine and spirituality are three different disciplines whose shared purpose is to help people understand their own states and learn how to relate to them. For this purpose the practitioners of these disciplines construct images of reality, a guru using gods or cosmic principles, an astrologer using the planets, and a doctor using the Three *Doshas*.

These processes require the subjective time of the individual to be put into relationship with the objective time of the temporal system involved (cosmic time in spirituality, calendrical time in astrology, and seasonal and 'disease time' in medicine). A clearly defined relationship shows the client how he or she fits into the system and breeds a confidence that itself, like the cellular confidence engendered by excellence of the tissues, makes good things happen. The amulets a guru gives to his disciples, the gemstones an astrologer prescribes for his clients and the medicines a doctor administers to his patients all exert their own independent effects according to their innate qualities, and all also function as mnemonic devices, perpetual reminders of the advice and reassurances given and the predictions made.

Like a guru or astrologer, a physician must at all times, especially during the diagnostic process, broadcast curative energy toward the patient; there is no place for objectivity in diagnosis. Diagnosis can no more be divorced from treatment than effect can be divorced from cause. The very naming of the disease can either start the patient on the road to recovery or propel him or her past the point of no return, depending on how the physician names it. 'Where there's life, there's hope' is no less true for being a cliché; faith and hope, the physician's allies, must be reinforced whenever possible.

METHODS OF KNOWING

A physician can use any of four methods to thoroughly know a patient's condition. Direct perception is the best method, though it is sometimes unreliable due to defects of perception. Whatever cannot be known directly must be elicited through the other means, namely logical inference, analogy and the testimony of experts. Prior to the nineteenth century even allopathic diagnosis was based on clinical dialogue, the same inspection, palpation and interrogation through which Ayurvedic doctors obtain data about their patients.

An Ayurvedic doctor is expected to use all his or her sense organs except the tongue to evaluate the patient; some Tibetan physicians even use the tongue to taste secretions or discharges. The sense of smell usually suffices, however, to know whatever one can know by taste, since *ama* is malodorous, certain *dosha* imbalances (especially those of *pitta*) have odours, and some diseases have characteristic smells (like typhus, in which the patient's odour is 'mousey'). The senses provide direct perceptions for logic and intuition to process, particularly as applied to the eight important diagnostic factors: faeces, urine, tongue, sound, touch, sight, face and pulse. Few physicians are expert in all the diagnostic arts, each usually becoming expert in one or two methods.

Inspection

Traditionally, patients come to Ayurvedic physicians early in the morning before consuming anything, having avoided all stimulants the night before. The doctor then begins with inspection, the examination of all parts of the patient that can be seen with the eyes. Astrological diagnosis is a kind of inspection, as is diagnosis from the face, iridology and, today, all the various imaging systems. An Ayurvedic doctor inspects tissues first, noting their fullness or emaciation, and then studies the skin more closely, examining the wastes that fill the body spaces and inspecting the 'Nine Doors' (two eyes, two ears, two nostrils, mouth and throat, anus and penis or vulva) and their secretions, paying particular attention to the tongue. Like the irises, the palms of the hands, the soles of the feet and the external ears, the tongue is a map of the internal organs. Careful examination of the tongue provides information on the condition of the digestive fire, the load of toxins in the body, the efficiency of *vata*'s movements or lack thereof, the conditions of the channels, and more.

Faeces examination discloses the condition of the digestive tract, especially the presence or absence of *ama*. Urine examination, which some experts suggest was introduced into India around 1100 AD, is often more extensive, and has been elevated into an art by the Tibetans. A midstream sample of the first urine of the morning is taken for testing, and the Tibetans examine it thrice: first when it is hot, then when it has become lukewarm and finally once it has cooled. In a healthy person everything should be moderate: colour, vapour, odour and froth.

Urine is usually very clear or light blue or pinkish in *vata* conditions, very yellow or orange in *pitta* (unless the patient has swallowed B vitamins, eaten beetroots or taken something else that might colour it!), and milky white in *kapha*. The presence of cloudiness usually indicates a heat disorder, and the urine may smell of ingested food in conditions in which *ama* is present in the digestive tract. The Tibetans also use urine analysis to diagnose tumours, determine whether or not a patient will survive and diagnose possession by spirits. They determine whether a particular drug is good for a patient by sprinkling it on the patient's urine: if it sinks, it will be ineffective; if it spreads quickly, it will be quickly effective; and if it spreads only over a limited area, it will be effective but slowly.

Palpation

Any method by which the patient is touched comes under this heading. Palpation includes examination of the pulse, estimation of the body's relative heat or coldness, and testing of the hardness, softness or roughness of the skin. Of these, pulse diagnosis is most important. Some traditional Ayurvedic physicians refuse to ask questions of their patients, preferring to take the pulse silently and then inform the patient of his or her symptoms. Pulse diagnosis was apparently first introduced into Ayurveda by Sharngadhara, though there is some evidence to suggest that it was already present in Siddha medicine and possibly even earlier among the wandering yogis and sadhus who dedicated their lives to the study and worship of prana.

Examination of the pulse is examination of the movement of prana in the body. All mobile beings have their own style of motion. The inherent qualities of each species produce a characteristic rhythm of *vata*, which manifests as a characteristic gait (*gati*): ducks waddle, frogs hop, flies flit and elephants mosey along regally. Each combination of the *doshas* imprints its own characteristic gait on the pulse, but fundamentally all gaits are due to *vata*, the only mobile *dosha*. Pulse diagnosis is the examination of these gaits, coupled in some cases with examination of the conditions of specific organs.

Any of the body's arteries can be used for pulse diagnosis, including the *dorsalis pedis* on the foot, which is sometimes used to test for imminence of death, and the ulnar on the wrist, which is said to indicate one's potential life-span. The most commonly used pulse is the radial pulse, sometimes called the 'soul's witness'. One hundred and eight separate pulse gaits have been described, of which the most important for *vata* are those of the leech and snake; for *pitta*, the sparrow, crow and frog; and for *kapha*, the swan and pigeon. The quail and partridge describe conditions in which all three *doshas* are aggravated.

The pulse is tested early in the morning before food or drink is consumed. Usually the physician tests a male's right arm first and a female's left arm first, since the right side of the body is the male side in most humans and so is ordinarily predominant in men, while the left side, the female side, ordinarily predominates in women. Both sides of the body should be examined to detect potential imbalances in prana. The examiner's index finger is placed about half an inch away from the crease of the wrist, towards the elbow, with the middle and ring fingers close to it; the ring finger is thus closest to the elbow. The index finger tests the strength and condition of the body's *vata*, the middle finger tests *pitta*, and the ring finger tests *kapha*. The little finger is used to test spirit possession alone.

A *vata* pulse is usually relatively irregular, weak, fast, empty, cold and changeable; it slithers under the fingers like a leech or a snake. A *pitta* pulse is hot, strong, full, regular and of medium speed; it bounces underneath the fingers like a hopping sparrow, crow or frog. A *kapha* pulse is cool, strong, full, regular and relatively slow; it swims under the fingers like a swan. The overall tenor of the pulse must be carefully evaluated before drawing conclusions. For example, though some modern evidence suggests that subtly irregular heartbeats may be a sign of health, and monotonous regularity of the heartbeat may indicate danger of sudden death from cardiac arrest, conclusions can be drawn from a particular pulse only after examining its other characteristics.

Pulse diagnosis, though usually used to detect disease, can also disclose other consequences of the movement of *vata* and prana. The Tibetans describe the Seven Wondrous Pulses:

the Family Pulse, by which one tests the senior member of a family to know the whole family's condition;

the Guest Pulse, which indicates the location of a guest who is about to visit the family by testing the pulse of that family member whose relationship with the guest is closest;

the Enemy Pulse, to determine the consequences of attacking an enemy;

the Friend Pulse, examination of the head of the family to know how many friends the family will have;

the Evil Spirit Pulse, taken on a healthy person whose life-situation has changed strangely, to determine what kind of spirit has caused the problems;

the Substitutional Pulse, examination of a loved one when the patient is unable to see the doctor (used for prognosis rather than diagnosis);

the Pregnancy Pulse, to determine if a woman is pregnant and, if so, what sex the child will be.

Every influence on the system shows its traces in the pulse, on the skin and in other body parts of the patient. Pulse diagnosis requires at least the touch of the physician's hand on the patient's arm, while the esoteric form of diagnosis called *svarodaya* does not even require touch; instead the physician examines the subtle differences in the direction and rate of flow of the breath in his own nostrils, which indicate the condition of the flow of prana in the patient's *nadis*. Vimalananda was an expert at this method of diagnosis, which requires extreme sensitivity.

Even the doctor influences the pulse; the accuracy of pulse diagnosis, like that of radionics devices, depends on the sensitivity and objectivity of the practitioner. Unconscious pressure variations, inaccuracies of perception and mental preconceptions make it easy to find what you are looking for even if it is not there, and so the Tibetans insist that on the day before pulse diagnosis both the patient and the physician should avoid very hot, or very cold and very heavy food, should neither fast nor overeat, nor eat anything they are not habituated to, nor indulge in strenuous activity or sex, nor go without sleep, nor talk too much, worry or argue.

The prowess of expert pulse diagnosticians in India is legendary. One tale from the days when women of the court were kept in strict seclusion concerns a royal physician who was occasionally called upon to diagnose a queen or princess. The woman would sit behind a curtain and tie a thread to her wrist, and the physician would then take her pulse via the thread. One day the king decided to test the doctor by installing a pregnant buffalo behind the screen. The doctor came, sat concentrating intently on the thread for some moments, and then declared, 'The patient is hungry. Please feed her some grass, as she will be delivering a calf in a few days.'

Interrogation

Interrogation may involve auscultation, listening to body sounds, including the heartbeat, the breathing sounds and any sounds of injury or disease, such as the crepitus created when two ends of a broken bone creep across one another. Most interrogation, however, is done verbally to elicit the patient's medical history, to determine possible causative factors, to elicit past and present symptoms, and to learn how the patient views his or her condition. Some doctors even diagnose solely by the tone of the patient's voice. When a patient talks, a good doctor listens to the sincerity or lack of it behind the words. A patient who sincerely wants to get well and one who is not really sure whether he or she wants to get well will have two very different responses to treatment; unless the physician is sure of the patient's intentions, problems are certain to arise during therapy. A doctor who can read body language and hear the messages between a patient's words will not be misled about the true state of the organism.

Sometimes differences in time of arising can help distinguish the pathology involved. The pain of rheumatoid arthritis is usually worse in the morning after the joints have been immobile all night; movement lessens the stiffness and pain. Osteoarthritis, by contrast, usually worsens later in the day after movement. Sometimes a symptom in one area can provide information on conditions in another area; for example, tightness in the hamstrings or upper calf muscles generally indicates tightness in the colon as well. Also, wherever there is a tumour in the body, the skin above that area tends to get bluish-blackish and gets dirty quickly.

Symptoms merit careful evaluation so that the pattern of *dosha* involvement can be determined. While, as Vagbhata says, 'there is no pain without *vata*, no inflammation without *pitta*, and no pus formation without *kapha*', the other *doshas* can modify the effects of the principal *dosha* involved in producing the symptom. Pure *vata* pain is intense, breaking, tearing, pricking or stabbing, like intestinal, renal or biliary colic (colic being a spasm in a tubular organ, and *vata* ruling tubular, hollow organs). The sudden intense pain you get when you eat cold things too fast is also due purely to *vata*, created by sudden increase in its cold quality. *Pitta* pain is a burning, pulling or sucking pain, like the pain of a sunburn or ulcer, while *kapha* pain, which is caused by pressure, is dull, heavy and annoying, such as the pain of a stuffed-up nose.

Inflammation due to *vata* or *kapha* is relatively mild, whereas *pitta* inflammation is fiery red and burning. *Vata* pus is small in amount, thin and flows with difficulty; *pitta* pus is hot, yellow or green and bloodstained; and *kapha* pus is large in amount and white or whitish green with an offensive, rotten odour. A cough that produces abundant clear or white phlegm is probably due to the cold and damp of *kapha*; one with yellow or green phlegm and inflammation is likely due to the damp heat of *pitta*; and a dry cough, especially with chills, particularly if chronic, is usually due to *vata*'s cold dryness.

The common cold can be caused by excess *kapha*, which creates more mucus than the channels can handle, or by *pitta* or *vata*, which, by obstructing the free flow of mucus through its channels, causes mucus to accumulate without actually increasing. *Pitta* obstructs by its heat and intensity, which inflame the mucous membranes and squeeze the channels shut, while *vata*'s dry, cold and astringent qualities throttle the channels. These three different colds produce three different sets of symptoms: in the *kapha* variety discharge predominates; in the *pitta* type, tenderness and perhaps fever; and in the *vata* version, constricted breathing passages and pain, possibly including headache.

Typical *vata* symptoms in the body include increased movement (diarrhoea, tachycardia, tics, giddiness, insomnia), decreased movement (bradycardia, slowed circulation, paraplegia, cramps, infertility due to poor sperm motility, deafness, fainting, numbness), perverted movement (yawning, hiccups, convulsions, aphasic speech, tremors, choreas, delirium, hallucinations, mania and the like), and the separation of one tissue from another (cracking of the skin, split hair ends, dislocation of the joints, fractures, deformities, prolapses, atrophy, amnesia, rheumatism, etc.).

Pitta symptoms include indigestion, diarrhoea, hyperacidity, fever, inflammations, increased sweating, burning sensations, fainting, gangrene, ulcerations, bleeding, redness, rashes, jaundice, anaemia, moles, freckles and so on. *Kapha* symptoms are basically the symptoms of *ama*: atherosclerosis, goitre, pallor, cough, pressure, drowsiness, coldness, dullness, heaviness, whiteness and oiliness of the body, excess mucus, obesity, itching and the like.

AMA

A distinction must be drawn between those symptoms caused by the aggravated *doshas* alone and those caused by the *doshas* in partnership with *ama*. When the *dosha* are vitiated without *ama*, they can be quickly eliminated from the body by purification; when *ama* is present, it must first be digested before purification is attempted, lest the stimulation of *vata* before the channels have been cleared enrages *vata* further and makes the obstruction worse. Acute accumulation of *ama* in the system may produce some or all of the following symptoms:

obstruction to the channels;

destruction of strength;

heaviness in the body, head and mind;

abnormal movements of *vata*;

lethargy due to the blockage of the *Rasa* Channel;

indigestion;

expectoration (the mouth waters and patient constantly wants to spit);

retention of wastes (relative or absolute constipation or retention of urine; inhibition of sweating is a sure sign);

experiencing food as tasteless, or experiencing unusual tastes for common foods;

fatigue without exertion.

When *vata* is associated with *ama*, it causes obstructions and swellings all over the body, for example in the joints or the abdomen. When *pitta* joins forces with *ama*, its vehicles in the body, such as blood and sweat, become foul-smelling, heavy, thick, dark and acrid. *Kapha* and *ama* working together make its vehicles like mucus, saliva and synovial fluid sticky, opaque and ropy or stringy. *Ama* can also cause body aches, insomnia and other obstructive symptoms. *Ama* in the urine makes it turbid, foul-smelling and dark. Healthy faeces have the consistency of a ripe banana and little odour; stools with *ama* are sticky and heavy, filled with pieces of undigested food, and foul-smelling. A coated tongue usually indicates *ama* in the digestive tract, especially if the breath smells 'unripe'.

PROGNOSIS

There are four common prognoses:

Curable with ease   An acute disease without complications, whose causes and symptoms are mild; caused by a single *dosha* that is not reinforced by the season, local climate, patient's constitution or tissue involved; disturbing only one channel and one disease pathway but no vital part; in which the body can withstand any medication and all four factors of treatment (physician, attendant, remedy and patient) are optimal.

Curable with difficulty   Chronic afflictions, or those that affect vital body parts, or diseases in pregnant women, the aged and small children, or those involving two *doshas* or *pathways*, or those in which some qualities of season or constitution reinforce the *dosha* involved, or in which complications are present.

Ameliorable   Such diseases, which are very chronic, need surgery, affect vital bodily parts or whose symptoms conflict with one another, improve only as long as treatment is given and relapse when treatment is stopped. Treatment supports the patient in the same way that pillars support a collapsing structure.

Incurable   Those diseases that involve all three *doshas*, all three pathways, all sense and motor organs, and in which there is excessive weakness and restlessness, causing excitability and eventual coma. Congenitally incurable diseases are to be treated so that patients may attract healthier bodies in their future incarnation.

Because prognosis is not always clear, Charaka dedicated a twelve-chapter section of his treatise to the problem of how to determine when a patient is going to die, a section called, appropriately, the Section on the Senses, as the clever physician must press all his senses into service to determine treatment's likely outcome. Unfavourable signs relating to sensory observations by both the physician and the patient, dreams, forebodings and changes in the patient's shadow and aura are included, as are ways of predicting the time of death.

Chapter Twelve deals with omens concerning the messenger sent to call the physician to the patient's bedside. Omens have no particular power in and of themselves; instead, they are, like the excellence of tissues, the gait of the pulse and the flowing of the breath in the nostrils, suggestions of synchronicity, indications of prosperity's gait, which can indicate 'how the winds are blowing'. For example, if the messenger arrives in a dishevelled state or when the physician is in a state of ritual impurity, one concludes that the forces of life and prosperity are flowing away from the patient, making a terminal outcome likely. When, however, the messenger is well-dressed and has an air of auspiciousness about him, and arrives at an auspicious moment, then the omens are propitious and treatment is likely to have a favourable outcome.

The doctor should also see good omens on his way to the patient. Good omens include yoghurt, rice, bulls, a king, jewels, pots full of water, a white horse, fruits, little children seated in the laps of elders, a single tethered animal, upturned earth, a blazing fire, sweetmeats, white flowers, sandal paste, attractive articles of food and drink, a carriage full of people, a cow with her calf or a mare with her colt or a woman with her child, the common mynah, swan, blue jay, peacock and a few other birds, elephants' tusks, the swastika, conch shells, a mirror, Vedic recitations and umbrellas.

Like omens, dreams symbolize the gait and momentum of the various forces that swirl about both physician and patient. Dreams, which have been used in Western diagnosis since well before Aristotle, are important to Indian diagnosis because it is believed that one can actually do something about bad dreams. Inauspicious dreams are definite indications that something has gone terribly wrong with one's direction in life, but with enough will-power and through penances such as fasting, praying and giving alms, the trend of the impending tendencies can be shifted and their qualities changed from bad to good.

According to Charaka, dreams of the moon, the sun, gods, kings, living friends, Brahmans (possibly a later insertion!), cows, a burning fire or a place of pilgrimage bring health and happiness in their wake, and dreams of gaining victory over foes, travel toward the north-east, ascending a palace or a mountain or riding a bull or elephant bestow health. Dreams of flowers, clean clothes, meat, fish or fruit, or of being bitten by leeches, bees (honey or bumble) or serpents yield relief from disease, if one is sick, or gain of wealth if one is healthy. Even the performing of a forbidden act, covering yourself with a paste of filth, weeping, dying or eating raw flesh in a dream supposedly presages the gain of both wealth and health. An example of an inauspicious dream is to ride a large black buffalo in a southerly direction at dusk.

When the prognosis is grave, the physician must be careful not to communicate it until it is clear that such knowledge will not shock the patient and distress the family; besides, the patient might by some miracle pull through. Physicians are also expected not to waste medicines and the family's money treating dying patients, whose deaths will soil the doctor's good name, simply because the patient is desperate to prolong life. Doctors ought not to eat food or even drink water in the household of a dying patient, since the surroundings are tainted by the inauspiciousness (or rather, the negation of worldly prosperity) that is death. An incurable patient's mind and body no longer can or will respond to health-giving energy. When the time for death arrives, such a patient should be permitted to prepare for it with a calm, clear mind undisturbed by any sort of external activity, therapeutic or otherwise.

8

TREATMENT

The art of medicine consists of amusing the patient while Nature cures the disease.

VOLTAIRE

Voltaire expressed a Hippocratic principle, that imbalances return to normal naturally when permitted to do so, which was also shared by the seers of Ayurveda; in Charaka's words, there is a cause for the manifestation of beings but no cause for their annihilation. A disease-being, which manifests because of *yukti*, the coming together of many causes at an appropriate time and place, is annihilated by change of time or place or by withdrawal of the causes. Charaka probably had a more philosophical meaning in mind here as well: causes are needed to manifest human beings, but metabolic chaos is sufficient to annihilate them.

Therefore 'the essence of treatment is removal of the cause', and avoidance of causative factors is the best way to stay healthy. *Prajnaparadha* being the ultimate cause of all disease, its elimination is the ultimate treatment: 'the remedy for all miseries', avers Charaka, 'is the elimination of the allurement of desire.' Francis Zimmermann notes that this is Ayurveda's expression of the conviction, held by most major Indian philosophies, that all desires are fundamentally illusory, producing frustration when they are not fulfilled, and addiction and intoxication when they are. The salient difference between Ayurveda and other philosophical systems is that Ayurveda concentrates upon the effects of desire on health, the ability to function harmoniously in the relative reality of the world, rather than upon one's relationship to the Absolute Reality.

The destruction of desire and removal of delusion eliminate the root cause of disease and should theoretically destroy all ailments produced therefrom, though, practically, most people require more than spiritual therapy for their illnesses because their minds are too muddled even to locate the roots of their foolhardiness, much less uproot them. So long as delusion remains, so will disease, as it does in those people who neglect their bodies as a result of excessive study or ritual practice, or in order to curry favour with influential people, or out of preoccupation with business, or because they sell their bodies or minds to gratify customers – in short, anyone who puts career before health. As soon as one disease in such a patient is cured, another takes its place. Charaka calls such people the Ever Sick.

The Ever Sick are afflicted to an extreme degree with the same delusion that we all share. Gautama Buddha, the Compassionate One, allowed his monks the use of medicines and purificatory and surgical techniques because he realized that medicine, by helping to preserve the physical body, also helps to clear the mind of delusion, encouraging it to weed out *prajnaparadha*. How powerful a medicine needs to be depends upon the extent to which the patient's mind is deluded. No therapy can make you well if you are determined to remain sick, and if you develop the conviction that you will get well, that conviction alone is enough to make you well. Though there are some things that are very improbable, nothing in life is impossible.

When a woman I know, whom we can call Mary, finds herself out of sorts, she sits down, gives herself a serious talking to, and 'sends her shadow self packing'. Her shadow self, which is generated from the petulance and selfishness that motivate her to perform 'crimes against wisdom', is her own personal disease-being. Sending it packing removes from her consciousness the cause of her problems. This is a superior method of disease control, which requires, however, sufficient objectivity to be able to identify old sick beliefs and habits and to distinguish between them and the valuable parts of your personality. You also need sufficient energy and courage to resolutely 'send them packing', and sufficient sobriety and patience to gird up your loins and replace those old sick habits and beliefs with new, healthy ones, which avoid the paralysis of guilt for past indiscretions.

Those rare people like Mary who can fearlessly gaze at their demons and order them out generally need medical assistance only in emergency or when they need a new perspective on a particularly difficult problem. Most people need more assistance more often. Vimalananda used to enjoy saying that if you are sick and you want to get well, you have only two alternatives: you can develop faith in yourself, in your own healing capabilities, or you can find a physician, healer, guru or other authority figure in whom you can place your faith, following their instructions without question. If your faith is dwarfed by doubt, your healing will take time. Everything works well when you have true faith that everything will work. Despite the incipient chaos that often seems ready to take it over, India remains intact, held together by the faith of millions of people that it will hold together. Because faith is often difficult to come by, particularly when one is in pain, therapists exist.

THE IMPORTANCE OF PHYSICIANS

Charaka identifies four factors that are essential for successful medical treatment: the physician, the remedy, the nurse and the patient. The physician should be expert in theory and in practice, skilful, and pure in body and mind. Easy availability, appropriateness, utility in a variety of forms and high quality characterize the optimal remedy. The best nurse is knowledgeable, skilful, sympathetic and pure. The ideal patient is courageous, able to describe what he or she is feeling, and remembers all the physician's instructions and follows them carefully; all these qualities help the patient get well more easily.

Gautama Buddha proposed five qualities that make a patient easy to treat, and five attributes of a good nurse; his lists closely resemble those of Charaka. Pride of place in this scheme is assigned to the doctor, who must know both the disease and the remedy, must instruct both the nurse and the patient, and must prescribe both the medicine and the dietary regimen. Deficiency in any of these factors impedes the progress of treatment. A skilful, ingenious physician who can make do with what is available can compensate for any deficiencies in patient, remedy or nurse, while an incompetent physician will prevent treatment from being successful even when the other factors are optimal. Charaka, who observes that 'one may survive the fall of a thunderbolt on one's head, but one cannot expect to escape the fatal effects of medicine prescribed by an ignorant physician', calls incompetence 'the best cause of fear'. Only a competent doctor can inspire in patients that faith which is a prerequisite for the courage needed to endure the rehabilitation process.

In the Rig-Veda a doctor is compared to a warrior; Charaka compares a physician to a conqueror, a cook and a potter. The latter two lowly vocations, disapproved of by the lawgivers, produce practical results, namely food and the pots for food, which are essential for embodied life, Ayurveda's declared field of interest. Sushruta compares a therapist to the chief priest at a sacrifice, a very Brahmanical allusion, though one that is appropriate to the general theme of 'life as sacrifice'. Zimmermann calls medicine a 'cooking' of the world, to make it palatable and digestible to the patient, and a form of politics or statecraft, a balancing act between the needs of the microcosm and the rights of the macrocosm. Any *yukti*-related allusion, such as the production of music from an orchestra, is a fit metaphor for medicine.

Cook, potter, general, priest; a physician must be different things to different people. Doctors must learn how and when to be passive and let Nature take its course, and how and when to act, though all medical activity should be limited to assisting the action of the organism's natural forces which are working to return it to order. Sometimes a physician must take control of a being whose innate wisdom has become disturbed, but even then the physician's role should be limited to eliminating the disturbance and restoring that innate wisdom. The physician must also consider whether a patient deserves to be treated or not. Charaka advises that treating those who fancy themselves doctors, those who hate doctors, kings and good people, those who are fatalists, are devoid of faith and who refuse to carry out the doctor's orders, and those who are fickle, rash, cowardly, ungrateful, envious, fierce-tempered, cruel or vicious earns for the physician 'opprobrious odium' and potential punishment.

Modern medicine also throws the burden of treatment on to the physician's shoulders, but, disbelieving in Nature as an intelligent being, also adds the burden of cure. Vimalananda once made a pun on the word *upadhi*, which means both 'a college degree' and 'a complication'. Medical degrees complicate doctors' lives when doctors are made to feel a greater necessity to act, to be busy 'doing', invading the system even when unnecessary, simply because they must be seen to be doing something. While Vagbhata emphasizes that the truly 'pure' treatment is that which cures without creating a new disorder, iatrogenic illness has become prominent in modern medicine, in part because both doctors and patients, like our society as a whole, value action, often violent, over observation and 'masterly inactivity', which is sometimes the best therapy available.

Violent action is characteristic of modern medicine, whose armamentarium includes antibiotics, drugs that are literally 'against life'; radiation and chemotherapy, which slay normal and abnormal cells alike; and forcible extraction of body parts that refuse to comply with our plans for them. Surgery is an important limb of the Ayurvedic tree, but, like acupuncture in traditional Chinese medicine, it is the last resort for a good doctor and the first resort for a poor one. Some people say that meat eaters will always prefer surgery because the idea (chopping flesh) is already so familiar to them. Most surgeons certainly tend to look at every problem surgically, as did Sir William Arbuthnot Lane, an eminent British surgeon of the early twentieth century, who advocated removal of the colon in chronic constipation and the intestinal toxaemia it produces. One really must be very balanced to be a surgeon, to maintain love and compassion for your patients while slicing them apart.

A good doctor avoids actively delivering a pregnant woman, instead encouraging and relaxing her to help her through a natural childbirth; a poor doctor gives in to impatience and induces labour or performs an unnecessary Caesarean section, which is often violence for the sake of convenience. Unnecessary violence in medicine is a poor way to teach health. Physicians who use such heroic treatments without knowing whether or not they are necessary are scathingly denounced by Charaka; of such ilk were surely the physicians who bled George Washington seven times in a single day. They were probably surprised when he died soon after.

Violence of any sort always breeds more violence; if you minimize violence in your life, less violence will come to you. Even visualizing immune cells tracking down and killing the cancer cells is a violent image that does nothing to rebuild the body. Treatment requires re-education, replacement of negative disease-causing messages with positive health-producing messages. A good doctor is careful to send only messages of health to patients. The idea that one can will one's patients to health appears even in modern medicine in the 'halo effect', an enhancement of the placebo effect caused, especially with regard to experimental therapies, by the intense interest, desire and hope of the researchers and clinicians working with the new therapy.

Re-education begins with right use of language. A doctor curses you who tells you you have 'X' months to live. He does so on the basis of statistics, not because he knows what is actually going on in your body, because he has been taught to think in terms of statistics, not individuals. Diseases, however, are not statistics; they progress through individuals in individual ways, to which statistics can only be pointers. Nor are people statistics; their hope or hopelessness sometimes depends on as little as a single word. Sometimes a single word at the right moment works wonders on a problem that has resisted many other attempts to rectify it, if the doctor knows that moment at which it will work. Naming the disease can damage if, like 'cancer', it is believed to be a death sentence; and it can help to heal, as in the Atharva-Vedic hymn to fever, which states accusingly 'your name is Hruudu!' ('Hruudu' has no known grammatical meaning; its power was incantational), if there is a chance that the disease can be cured or at least managed.

Uncertainty is often more unsettling than an inaccurate certainty, and patients and their physicians today also use incantations to weaken a condition by confining it within the walls of a word. 'Chronic fatigue syndrome' is such an incantation; it reassures partly because of its mysteriousness.

The meaning of a doctor's message to a patient is the response it elicits, not the intention with which it was given. The patient's interpretation of disease and therapy is always more important than any objective criteria, and there is every chance that a patient's definition of cure differs from the doctor's. Communication with patients is crucial to good doctoring, especially nowadays, when many people exist in a semi-permanent somnambulistic trance brought on by overexposure to all sorts of stimuli. It is always the responsibility of the physician to ensure that communication with the patient is clear and precise, and that no misunderstanding mars the therapeutic process, particularly because sometimes the different levels of the patient's being cannot communicate with one another. The physician must teach such patients how to communicate with themselves.

A patient suffering from a serious illness who has a cooperative, communicative personal physician and who, with that doctor's help, develops a workable plan of recovery, and who follows that plan with faith, increases the likelihood of his or her recovery. A plan helps to re-create that 'gait' that a patient needs to stroll comfortably through life. A good physician is a good teacher; the word 'doctor' is itself derived from a Latin word meaning 'to teach'. A physician is a patient's temporary guru, whose life must set a good example of health for the patient to emulate. Every Ayurvedic physician worthy of the name lives Ayurveda in his or her life; as Zarrilli observes, speaking of *kalarippayattu*: 'The authoritative text in the living tradition is the master's embodied practice.' A sincere physician must have a healthy relationship with Nature, and must therefore be something of a shaman.

A shaman is a magician, and it has always been difficult to draw a firm dividing line between medicine and magic, especially today when animals are being trained to respond to innocuous substances such as camphor and saccharine with changes in their immune activity. Orthodox medicine regards such research as 'voodoo' because, as with homeopathy or the placebo effect, there is seemingly no 'physical' explanation for the results produced. Such methods have, however, been used in India for many centuries, and some physicians still train people to use specific smells, tastes, sights, sounds and touches therapeutically, choosing the therapeutic substances and activities according to their ability to resonate with and balance the patient's *doshas*. This system has worked well in India because patients traditionally trust their doctors implicitly, and doctors traditionally do not hesitate to use this trust to the patient's advantage, though this is now changing.

Ayurveda also sometimes employs the opposite approach, the use of active remedies disguised as inactive substances. In his discussion on consumption Charaka states that if there is a medical need to give the patient a variety of food that he might object to or be disgusted by, such as fried earthworms, the physician should, if necessary, lie about its true origin and give it anyway to ensure cure. This sort of paternalism would attract a malpractice suit in the United States today, and even in Charaka's day physicians who treated their patients wrongly were fined by the state, but the system worked well (and sometimes still works well) in India because of the seriousness with which both doctor and patient accept their roles and the fidelity with which they carry them out.

TYPES OF THERAPY

No treatment is a true panacea, although, thanks to the vast time and effort invested by Tantric alchemical researchers, some mineral preparations come close to being cure-alls. Otherwise everything has its place in treatment, even maggots, which can destroy healthy tissue but can also save life by eating away necrotic tissue. Nothing is absolutely bad or good: though white sugar can be devastating when eaten in excess, it soothes inflamed surfaces and helps heal wounds when used externally; cabbage juice can cure ulcers, but excessive indulgence in raw cabbage can cause goitre. Nothing is a cure-all, not even 'nothing'. 'Doing nothing is also a medicine' a text advises, and restraint is advised in many diseases. Knowing how to treat is fundamentally a question of knowing what to do or not to do, and when to do or not do it, always seeking to use the simplest method first.

Dozens of alternative therapies compete for attention today; many of them are effective, but none is effective in all conditions at all times. Except for moderation (which is always good) and for crimes like rape (which is always bad), there is no 'always' or 'never' in Ayurveda; every individual has a different path. The many possible permutations of mental and physical imbalance in individuals of varied constitution living in varied climates during varied seasons require varied therapeutic response. To help balance the *doshas* Ayurveda employs all five senses, including, in context, purification techniques, surgery, drugs, cautery, diet, herbs, minerals, massage and other body work, acupressure, manipulation of the *marmas*, exercises including yoga, Indian classical music, aromatherapy, flower and gem essences, potentiated remedies such as those of homeopathy, colour therapy, meditation, visualization, chanting and ritual worship. While acupuncture as such does not seem to appear in classical Ayurveda, it does fit neatly into the Ayurvedic scheme of things.

Some treatments have become less common in India than they probably once were, such as what is now called polarity therapy, a system developed from knowledge of the *nadis*, which has been popularized by Dr Randolph Stone. Other treatments are becoming more common, such as yoga, which has been used therapeutically by yogis for centuries but is now being codified into 'yoga therapy' by some Ayurvedic physicians, who have begun to use it in non-traditional ways. Other manipulations of the life-force include procedures such as the 'laying on of hands', or therapeutic touch. Mantras (words of power), which were popular in the medicine of the Atharva-Veda, are still employed by some therapists; their use is limited to those who know how to use them properly. A mantra must be pronounced with a particular resonance in a certain area of the body with an appropriate intention and intonation if it is to do any good. All substances, 'real' and 'unreal', can be used therapeutically, if only you know how to use them.

AYURVEDIC TREATMENT

Disease therapy is a sort of spiritual advancement. Your visit to your healer is a pilgrimage, at the culmination of which comes the healing ritual performed by the doctor-guru, which helps remove your 'sins', dietary and otherwise, from where you have stored them, deep within you in the form of *ama*, so that the body's fire element can cleanse you of them. Every moment your body creates your past as it absorbs the products of digestion. By dealing with your past in your present, you can proceed confidently towards your future, a future of righteousness, in which your tissues will be pure and healthy, your wastes quickly and efficiently excreted, and your *doshas* balanced.

Most of us have many levels of toxins accumulated over a lifetime of indiscretions, all of which cannot be released at once lest they overwhelm the excretory organs and ravage the mind. Your mind and body have become habituated to these poisons, which have become part of your equilibrium equation. Removing them all at once would seriously imbalance your physical body and confuse your mind so that you no longer felt like 'yourself'. Should you try to force the process, your system would, of its own accord, resist you. You must respect your body's wisdom and permit it to release its toxins at the rate that pleases it. Purifying the system is a long, slow process, requiring many cycles to expunge the many layers of dirt. You must be patient with the process and with the newly developing you, just as you would be patient with a slowly growing tree. When you backslide and return temporarily to your old unhealthy ways, you must learn to always pick yourself up, like a child learning to walk, and begin again.

Ayurveda favours gradual over sudden cure to protect your identity, which controls your immune system. If it is possible for you, gradual elimination of your addictions, by substituting less dangerous ones for more dangerous ones and then weaning yourself from those lesser evils, is better for your immunity than is the immediate, 'cold turkey' procedure. Even medical treatment should never be stopped abruptly, but only gradually, to give the system time to acclimatize itself to living without a medical crutch. If the change and self-redefinition are sufficiently gradual, at the end of the programme you will find yourself transformed without being able to point to any 'crisis' that did the transforming. The 'healing crises' that some medical systems encourage are really only occasionally necessary; Ayurveda tries to avoid crisis with well-managed physical and mental catharsis.

Rather than get bogged down in concern over a particular organ, gland, energy centre or *chakra*, unless that area is seriously devitalized, it is better to see the big picture with an overall master plan for your development that you are not afraid to change whenever the need for change arises. A plan gives you direction and produces strategies to deal with health fluctuations. Sometimes it is not possible to make a firm diagnosis, since some illnesses do not fit neatly into commonly accepted disease categories; and sometimes, because of the large number and variety of stresses to which we are exposed, no one factor can be pointed to as *the* cause. When either disease or cause is unsure, treatment can still proceed according to the general treatment for the *dosha* involved, since the *doshas* are the prime causes of physical health and disease. Even in diseases of non-physical origin, such as those fevers that are caused by the planets, curses or black magic, the *doshas* must still be identified and rebalanced.

There are three therapies with regard to their location of action: 'scientific' therapy, which uses the *yukti* of proper diet, activities and remedies according to season and climate, at the level of the physical body; 'conquest of the mind', involving restraint of the mind from the desire for unwholesome objects; and 'divine' therapy, including all sorts of spiritual ritual and penance. Medical intervention at the physical level is of four types: diet, activity, purification and palliation. Accumulation of the *doshas* should be treated with changes in diet and activity; when they become aggravated, palliating or pacifying them with substances of opposite qualities is best. Once the *doshas* escape their reservoirs, however, it is best to remove them from the system; if this is impossible, they must be neutralized with medicine. Should the *doshas* localize in a weak part of the body, that part will need local treatment as well.

Charaka uses agricultural metaphors to describe this incrementally more invasive approach to treatment. For mild diseases, control of the diet, including fasting, is enough, just as a puddle of water is quickly evaporated by sun and wind. For an ailment of medium strength, dietary control and pacifying medications are required, just as the adding of sand and ashes to a well or pond helps wind and sun to dry it out. For a strong disease, active purification is necessary, just as a flooded rice paddy is easily drained by breaching its *bund* (retaining wall). Note that these allusions are to the presence of excessive fluid in the system, a condition generated by diet and activities that are 'moisture producing' (*abhishyandi*). This sort of medicine is drainage of the body, comparable to the draining of a swamp to make it fit for cultivation. When the body has been well drained and good seeds are planted in its fields in the right season, and watered with good *rasa*, the result is a bumper crop of health.

Diseases due to 'drought' are usually treated by precisely opposite principles, namely nourishing, oiling and stabilizing therapies. Treatment usually requires the use of substances and activities whose qualities are opposite to the disease and/or its cause, but there are cases in which similar qualities must be administered, such as a hot poultice applied to an abcess due to *pitta*, an emetic given to cure vomiting, small amounts of medicinal wine given to treat alcoholism, and shock treatment or threats used on a patient of mania due to *vata*.

The basic principles of Ayurvedic treatment are immutable; how they are applied differs from case to case. 'Treatment is rooted in measure': the effect any particular therapy has on any particular patient depends on its dosage, which depends upon the patient's species (since Ayurveda is not limited to humans), the climate, the *doshas* involved, the strength of the patient versus the strength of the disease, the patient's age and constitution, the specific syndrome, the patient's social environment, the goal of treatment, the physician's preferred methods of treatment and so on. Time cycles, including 'disease time' and the 'joints' of the seasons, are especially important, because the *doshas* are controlled differently at different times, depending upon both external time and the disease's 'momentum' within the microcosm. Treatment is supposed to be totally individualized, and so different diseases may sometimes share a single therapy, while a single disease may be treated differently in different patients according to the 'measure' of the factors involved.

When more than one *dosha* is involved in a disease's pathology, some authorities teach that they should be conquered from the head down (first *kapha*, then *pitta*, then *vata*), because when the organs are coated with *kapha*, there is loss of appetite, which inhibits intake of food, which interferes with our ability to control the *doshas*. Sushruta and others say that because of the importance of the digestive fire, *pitta* should be controlled first, then *vata*, and finally *kapha*, especially in fever and diarrhoea. There is also the view that since *vata* is by nature the strongest *dosha*, and *pitta* the next strongest, that *vata* should be controlled first, then *pitta* and only then *kapha*, the least powerful among the three.

Vagbhata maintains that the most disturbed of the *doshas* should be attended to first, and this approach is generally accepted, even by Sushruta, who qualifies his previous position by explaining that all severe complications must be treated first. Sometimes it also happens that a *dosha* weakened by treatment produces powerful symptoms as it leaves the body, like a flame, which burns brightest just before it goes out, or like the top position of a slender tree, which sways violently if even a tiny monkey jumps out of it. The skilful physician must not be deceived by such deceptive signs.

General treatment for the doshas

Vata

The main remedies for *vata* are heat and oil, externally and internally, to counteract its dry and cold qualities. Any purification should be mild; the best is enema. Salty is the most important taste, both in medicine and food, since it improves appetite and digestion and is anti-spasmodic and slightly laxative; next comes sour and then sweet. Medicinal wines are beneficial, as are medicines that have been potentiated 100 or 1,000 times. Massage of all sorts is desirable. In certain cases shock treatments, 'de-memorizing therapy' (something like de-programming), and binding are used. The patient's anxieties should be eliminated and he or she should enjoy plenty of entertainment and total relaxation. When *vata* is aggravated, the patient requires 'good space' in the form of freely flowing channels, which produce happiness of body and mind.

Binding promotes free flow in the channels by supporting and calming the nerves, which is why strait-jackets are used on maniacs and why babies are swaddled to make them go to sleep quickly. Women in India have their abdomens bound with a cloth after delivery to prevent accumulation of *vata* in the newly emptied womb, and it is often possible to quell a headache due to tension or exhaustion by tying a bandana tightly around the head.

Pitta

Pitta must be cooled. Purgation and blood-letting are the preferred purifications for *pitta* because they quickly draw excess heat from the two places it is most concentrated: the digestive tract and the blood. Bitter is the most important taste, followed by sweet and astringent. Sweet-smelling scents (perfumes, incense, flowers) help to overcome *pitta*'s own intense odour, especially if, like sandalwood, lotus or rose, they are also cooling. Cool showers, moon bathing, pearl necklaces (especially chilled), white clothes and residence in green gardens amid fountains are other means to refrigerate the system. Anything that reduces *pitta*'s native intensity will also help, including soothing music and meditations to keep the mind calm and cool. Because fire is so strong, the patient should keep his or her internal fires busy; a raw food diet may help, or a job or hobby that requires plenty of problem-solving to keep the mental fire engaged.

Kapha

Kapha requires intensity and action to break up its natural inertia and lethargy. Pungent, composed of the fire and air elements, is the most important *kapha*-controlling taste, followed by bitter and astringent. When *ama* is present, however, bitter should be used first to clear the channels and only then should pungent, to reawaken the digestive fire, and astringent, to expel excess 'moisture', be employed. Emesis (therapeutic vomiting) is the main purification, though purgation may also be used, and all medicines and foods should be hot, intense and dry. Aged wines and liqueurs in small doses; nights without sleep; sexual intercourse; vigorous exercise, such as wrestling, running and jumping, to cause copious sweating; fasting; smoking; rough, dry, warm clothes and extremely hot baths all decrease *kapha*. Patients should, when possible, be saddled with responsibilities and prevented from indulging in their normal recreation, 'the giving up of the comforts of life with a view to eventual happiness'.

Palliation

Before treatment begins, the physician must ascertain whether or not the body is filled with *ama*. If it is, the patient must fast for a day or two until the major portion of recently produced *ama* is digested and expelled from the body. Afterwards, or immediately if *ama* is not a major factor, the strength of the patient must be measured against the strength of the disease. If the patient is relatively strong and the disease relatively weak, active purification by the method known as *panchakarma* (see p. 204) is indicated. When, however, the patient is relatively weak and the disease relatively strong, active purification is unwise, because the purification methods all extract material, albeit morbid, from the body, thereby weakening it to some degree. This weakening, and the emptiness of the 'reservoir organs' that causes it, may increase *vata*, potentially enhancing the disease process instead of resolving it.

After purification, or instead of purification when the disease is strong and the patient weak, or in those people – such as pregnant women – whose bodies are not fit to undergo purification, palliation, or pacification, of the aggrieved *doshas* is the route to be followed. Seven methods make up the traditional pacification regimen: 'cooking' the body's accumulated *ama*, enkindling its digestive fire, fasting from food, fasting from liquids, exercise, sunbathing and wind bathing. Of these, fasting is called 'the first and most important of all medicines'. Fasting can be without either food or water, on water alone, on liquids such as soup or juice alone, on a single food, such as the rice and mung bean preparation known as *khichadi*, or on a number of different foods selected for their utility in treating the condition in question.

Fasting permits the body to digest *ama*, reawakens the digestive fire, clears the channels and eliminates excess 'moisture' from the tissues. Though a wonderful medicine, fasting in excess, particularly for weeks at a time as some 'natural therapists' recommend, can cause degeneration of the tissues and disturb mind–body cohesion, encouraging the production of new and more powerful diseases. Like all other medicines, fasting must be used in the 'dose' appropriate to the individual patient. Absolute fasting from food or even water is usual in Ayurveda for a maximum of two days when a person is thoroughly clogged with *ama* and has lost all appetite. As soon as some desire for food returns, rice or barley gruel is commonly given, followed progressively by mung-bean soup, mung beans cooked with rice, and a return to other foods as the system's fire flames up and demands more nourishment.

Once the acute stage of the disease has passed, the patient is given a pacifying regimen to follow in which diet plays a central role. Medicine is administered at various times during the day according to the condition to be treated:

first thing in the morning for *kapha* disease or for rejuvenation;

half an hour before food for disturbances of *apana*;

the middle of the meal for disturbances of *samana* or *pitta*;

half an hour after lunch for *vyana* and half an hour after supper for *udana*;

at the beginning of the meal for delicate patients or strong medicines;

between meals for *vyana* and diseases of the head;

at the beginning and the end of the meal in severe *vata* disturbances;

whenever necessary for asthma, cough and the like;

with each morsel of food to increase the digestive fire and for aphrodisiac effect;

after each morsel of food for heart disease and other grave conditions.

Every medicine is always given with an *anupana*, a vehicle that prevents possible side-effects, encourages quick, efficient absorption, and causes a synergistic effect so that the dose of the drug can be reduced. Ayurvedic medicines do not produce their desired effects unless they are given with proper *anupana* and diet. The best of all *anupanas* is honey, which penetrates the tissues without needing digestion, since it has already been digested by the industrious bees who created it. Poison shares this quickly pervading quality with honey, but honey is sweet in taste, while the system can neither comprehend nor withstand the taste of poison. Water is the simplest *anupana*, hot water always being used in conditions where *ama* is present. Other common *anupanas* include medicinal wine, herbal decoctions, fruit juices, medicinal jams, hot and unctuous food, butter, ghee, raw sugar, and meat soup.

Change of *anupana* can make the same drug useful in a variety of diseases; psyllium husk, for example, is given with milk for constipation, and with buttermilk for diarrhoea or dysentery. Sometimes the *anupana* changes along with the season; *haritaki* is given with jaggery in summer, rock salt during the monsoon, sugar in autumn, ginger powder in early winter, long pepper in late winter and honey in spring. Alternatively, it may be given with salt in diseases of *kapha*, with sugar for *pitta* problems, with ghee for *vata*, and with jaggery if all three are aggravated.

After the disease is eliminated from the body, a period of convalescence is enforced, during which dietary and other restrictions continue for at least the length of treatment; that is, if it took you a month to recover from your disease, your period of convalescence should last not less than a month. Relapse is possible if any of the rules of convalescence are violated by excess, such as excessive or forceful talking, travel (especially long-distance), excess walking, continual sitting or lying in one position, overeating (especially when it leads to indigestion), inappropriate diet with wrong food combinations, daytime sleep except summer, and any kind of sexual activity.

Unctuous therapy

The external application and internal consumption of oil, fat, bone marrow or ghee is used to prepare patients for purification and as a curative treatment for some *vata* conditions, especially those caused by emaciation. Unctuous therapy is also good for people who have enjoyed too much alcohol or sex, who have too many worries, who are very old, very young, very thin or have lost much blood or semen, and who have certain eye diseases. *Sneha*, the umbrella term for unctuous or oily matter, also means 'love'; fatty substances actually transmit a sort of chemical love to the body, which can be therapeutic particularly for those people who cannot find or accept love elsewhere.

Internal unctuous therapy, which is especially necessary before therapeutic vomiting or purging, is often performed by administering sesame oil or cow's ghee, the dose and variety depending upon the patient's requirements, twice or thrice a day for three to five days. One can be sure that the digestive tract has become thoroughly oiled when the oil starts to pass out undigested in the faeces. Unctuous treatment must be avoided or modified in conditions of *kapha* increase and when *ama* is present in large amounts in the body. Internal and external unctuous treatments are rarely given simultaneously.

Sweat therapy

After unctuous therapy the patient must be made to sweat. Sweating leads the *doshas* into fluidity, making it easier for them to leave their locations and flow out of the system. There are two principal ways of inducing sweat: external application of heat or retention of body heat, the latter including exercise, heavy clothes or blankets, fasting, the judicious use of alcohol and even anger. Active heating can be done by a well-heated residence, medicated steam, sauna, hot-water bottle, sunbathing, exposure to fire (or an infra-red lamp), plasters of hot substances such as mustard, hot baths or showers (especially with medicated oil or water), and hot packs – for example, bolus bags of rice cooked with medicinal herbs or of *kulattha* and rock salt to relieve joint pain and swelling.

Plants like castor root, *punarnava*, barley, sesame, *kulattha*, black gram, jujube and the drumstick plant all encourage the body to sweat more easily. Therapeutic sweating is contraindicated in pregnancy, bleeding disorders, recent use of intoxicants (especially alcohol), intense anger, hate or jealousy, for people who are very fat or very thin, and in diarrhoea, jaundice, anaemia, consumption and recent food-poisoning. Excess sweating must be avoided in patients suffering from fainting, dizziness, nausea, fever and other such ailments.

Panchakarma

The ancient Egyptians tried to purge the body of toxins with vomiting or laxatives. We use these methods in Ayurveda also, along with enema and nasal medication, grouped together as the *panchakarma*, or 'five actions'. There are two different lists of the five actions: Charaka includes two varieties of enema, evacuative and oily, in his list, while other writers take these two varieties together and append blood-letting as the fifth. The latter list is accepted by the majority of Ayurvedists today. *Panchakarma*, which is indicated only when the patient is strong relative to the disease, is divided into two sorts, according to whether it depletes the system (emesis, purgation, evacuative enema, evacuative nasal medication, blood-letting) or nourishes it (oily enema, nourishing nasal drops and the like).

Like the seasons, sacrificial rituals and life itself, *panchakarma* has a clearly defined beginning, middle and end. Children are educated to perform the tasks assigned to them during their adulthood, after which they retire to rest and advise others. The prime action of life occurs during adulthood, but adult life cannot be lived to its fullest without the preparatory run up and the wind down thereafter. *Panchakarma* is punctuated into the preparatory stage, the principal purification and the post-treatment care.

Preliminary rituals before a sacrifice include purification of the ground on which it will be performed, pacification of all ethereal beings in the neighbourhood, including the planets, and the setting up, at an appropriate astrological time, of the structure in which the sacrifice will take place. Preparation for *panchakarma* involves oiling and heating the patient to return the *doshas* from the limbs to their proper reservoirs in the digestive tract, from which they can be expelled. After their return, the *doshas* are brought to a state of 'excitement' by a procedure called *utkleshana*, to make them ready and anxious to emerge from the body. For example, heavy, oily food such as meat juice is used for *utkleshana* of *kapha*. When the signs of good *utkleshana* occur, for example watering of the eyes with belching when *kapha* is increased, the body is ready to be purified.

Suppose, says a text, you take an old, dried stick and try to bend it; it will probably break in your hands. But if you first soak it in oil and then warm it gently, it will regain the suppleness of its youth, and you can then bend it with ease. Likewise, if one tries to administer purification to someone whose limbs are filled with *doshas* without first opening the channels and liquefying the wastes by oiling and heating, purification may merely weaken the organism and convince it to clutch its accumulated *doshas* to its tissues even more tenaciously. Those modern 'natural therapists' who administer colonic irrigations weekly for months to their patients to purify them, often succeed mainly in creating severe aggravation of *vata*.

Before trying to purify, you must take your past, in the form of the *doshas* you have trapped in your body, back into your present; it is no coincidence that *vartma*, one of the words for 'channel of circulation', also means 'present time'. Your present is what flows in your channels; as soon as it is deposited somewhere it becomes your past. Once the *doshas* are flowing again in your 'present', they are expelled by *panchakarma*. The texts testify that originally such purifications were highly ritualized, with invocations to various deities and initiation of treatment at an auspicious moment. This ritualizing helped to realign macrocosm and microcosm to regenerate a harmonious life-rhythm. Such attention to cosmic time is rarely lavished on Ayurvedic treatment any longer, which is more a comment on the current state of Ayurveda in India than it is on the efficacy of such measures.

After a sacrifice's main offerings are concluded, the priests complete the process with various closing rituals to speed the gods back to their homes. After Ayurvedic purification, procedures are performed to remove any remaining excess *doshas* (after vomiting, for example, smoking is prescribed), followed by pacification treatment to rebalance the *doshas* and protect the system until it returns to normal. Thereafter, therapy is given to strengthen the body part affected by the illness to encourage it to resist further illness; this is a sort of rejuvenation.

Emesis and purgation

Vomiting, which is usually induced in the morning, is used especially to treat fevers and respiratory complaints due to *kapha*, loss of appetite, certain tumours and upward-moving 'sour' *pitta* (which causes heartburn). The most important emetic in Ayurveda is *madana*, which is identified in Kerala as *Catunaregam spinosa* and in most of the rest of India as *Randia dumetorum*. *Madana* is prepared in different ways according to the specific condition of the patient to be treated. In upward-moving 'sour' *pitta*, for example, it is simmered in milk, and in *kapha* excess that milk is made into yoghurt. For other conditions it is made into ghees, jams, oils, suppositories, powders, potions, decoctions and sweetmeats. For delicate patients, its powder is applied to a lotus, which the patient is then made to smell. It is also sometimes used in potentiated form, prepared by rubbing it in its own decoction three to twenty-one times. Other substances used for emesis include calamus root, liquorice root, mustard seeds, common salt and loofa.

The purgatives used in Ayurveda include *triphala* (see page 220), urine (especially cow's) and, in sensitive patients, raisins or milk. Castor oil is used especially in conditions of excessive ama. *Trivrt* (*Ipomoea turpethum*) is Ayurveda's most regarded purgative; it calms *kapha* and *pitta*, but aggravates *vata* because of its dryness. Like *madana*, *trivrt* is made into various preparations, including powders, jams and demulcent drinks, and, like *haritaki*, it is prescribed with different vehicles according to season. *Aragvadha* (*Cassia fistula*) is especially good for children, the aged, the weak and the delicate, as it is mild. The most powerful Ayurvedic purgatives are made with *Croton tiglium*, which is so strong that a purgative effect may follow application of its oil to the skin. Its oil is occasionally used in modern medicine to suddenly lower the pressure of blood or cerebrospinal fluid in certain disease conditions.

Many possible complications of therapeutic emesis or purgation are listed in the texts with advice on how to correct them. For example, if an emetic is taken by someone who purges easily or does not react well to vomiting, or is hungry, or whose *kapha* is not much increased, or if the dose is too intense or too cold or too small, or if it is taken before the previous meal has been fully digested, then it will go downward and act as a purgative. In this case one must give unctuous treatment and then again give the emetic. In other conditions sometimes the dose only agitates the *doshas* without being able to eliminate them, producing oedema, hiccups, faintness, thirst, pain in the calves, weakness in the thighs, etc. In this case you should anoint the patient with oil mixed with salt, induce sweating, administer a strong evacuative enema followed by a meal consisting of the soup of the meat of animals from arid regions, then give an oil enema, then unctuous treatment and, finally, repeat the purifying dose. Overintensive purification leads to continuous vomiting or diarrhoea; these conditions are treated basically as they would be had they arisen on their own.

Enema

Some authorities suggest that enema is the only treatment a physician needs to know, and others assert that it is 50 per cent of treatment, even for animals, for whom specific enema recipes are provided in Charaka's text. Besides herbs, which make up the bulk of enema recipes, meat soup is used in enemas to create strength as is, occasionally, medicinal wine and even raw blood. Recipes that are now little used include the boiling in milk of such meats as peacock, partridge, monitor lizard, mongoose, jungle cat, porcupine and bandicoot rat, and the use of fish soup without milk. Enema is different from emesis and purgation in that it does not deplete the system of digestive juices and can be used to nourish the system as well as to purify it. To preserve the body's strength and prevent *vata* aggravation due to emptiness in the organs, one should eat a small meal of solid food before an enema, and consume a light meal of a hot, light substance, such as soup, after the procedure is done.

The maximum dose of enema material, including all liquids and pastes, is about 1 pint. Usually a maximum of about 4 ounces of paste is used, and some authorities reject the use of paste altogether. Honey is often added, and one-fifth to one-sixth of the total amount should be fatty substance; vegetable oils, ghee, animal fat and bone marrow can all be used. Fat is included because herbal decoctions used alone dry out the colon and aggravate *vata* all over again. Therapeutic enemas are sometimes given in courses of eight, fifteen or thirty in total, according to the intensity of *vata*. Such courses, which begin with an enema of oil alone (usually between 4 and 8 fluid ounces) separate each purifying enema (containing herbal decoction) with an oil enema. The specific type of enema to be given is determined after considering the strengths of the patient and the disease, the time cycles and the *doshas* involved in both the patient's constitution and condition.

Nourishing enemas should not be given to those who need to have their excess 'moisture' depleted (as in obesity, diabetes and many skin diseases), nor should depletive enemas be given to those in need of nourishment. Aphrodisiac herbs, such as long pepper, make enemas aphrodisiac, and rejuvenating herbs make them rejuvenative. Adding such things as cow's urine, *chitraka*, salt, barley alkali or mustard intensifies an enema and makes it better able to remove an obstruction, while milk, ghee and mild, sweet drugs make it milder and so more nourishing. Mild enemas are usually 26 fluid ounces in volume and have fewer dietary or other restrictions than do other enemas, whereas that enema consisting of only 4 fluid ounces or less of oil has no restrictions whatsoever, and can be used regularly for individuals emaciated by overwork, overexertion, excess sex, excess travel and excess *vata*. One popular enema recipe is the so-called Oil and Honey Enema, made with those substances plus decoction of castor root, rock salt and dill; it requires few restrictions and gives great benefits.

An enema given to someone without proper preparatory heating and oiling, or given cold, or with insufficient unctuous material or drugs, or too thick will aggravate the *doshas* but fail to eliminate them. Neither will the enema fully emerge from the patient, causing pain, distention and digestive weakness. Heating and oiling, suppositories and enema with cow's urine or medicinal wine rectify this condition. Overintensive enema usually causes diarrhoea instead of obstruction, and its treatment is like that for purgative overdose. Strong enema is used to cure the stagnation caused by an enema that is too mild, and an unctuous, sweet, mild enema is given to reverse the excessive depletion caused by too strong an enema. Massage, breath control and even shock treatment are also used to control the ill effects of improper enema.

Several other treatments are included in the category of enema. Vaginal douche is used to reduce menstrual cramps, vaginal dryness and other such conditions, and is often made of oil alone. The ears are filled with oil for earache, tinnitus (ringing in the ears), deafness and in certain infections, and the eyes are soothed, strengthened and relaxed by constructing dams around them with flour paste and filling the 'ponds' thus produced with oil or ghee.

Despite its name, head enema is quite different from ordinary enema. First the patient's hair is cut short and a tall leather or plastic 'hat' without a top is firmly fixed above the ears and eyebrows and sealed with cloth and flour paste. Oil is then poured into the apparatus until it is standing an inch or two above the crown of the head, and is kept there about half an hour in *vata* disease, less for *pitta* and even less for *kapha*, or until mucus oozes from the patient's eyes, nose and mouth. This procedure is usually done in the evening for three, five or seven days. After removing the oil from the head, the soles of the feet, palms of the hands, the shoulders and the area behind the ears should be gently rubbed until they are warm. Then the patient is oiled and bathed.

Head enema is given mainly for *vata* diseases of the head, including loss of sensation especially with 'pins and needles', facial paralysis, insomnia, headache, hair loss and even insanity. I have seen head enema produce amazing calm in people who otherwise found it difficult to settle down. It is uncertain whether the oil penetrates into the brain or not, but considering that the rabies virus, which is vastly larger than the average molecule of vegetable oil, can move along the nerves from the brain to the very roots of the hair, there is no reason why oil could not traverse the same path in reverse.

Nasal medication

Nasal medication is the preferred purification for all diseases of the head. It is of various types, according to *dosha*: purgative (using dry powders such as black pepper) for *kapha*, nutritive (using mainly medicated oils) for *vata*, and pacifying (usually oil or ghee) for both *vata* and *pitta*. A good daily routine includes the introduction of a couple of drops of medicated oil or ghee into the nose and the massage of its mucous membrane with the little finger.

Blood-letting

Sushruta, who opined that half of all surgical problems could be successfully treated by blood-letting, was well aware of its dangers. He mentions twenty types of faulty punctures, and emphasizes that excessive blood flow, causing weakness to the patient, must never be allowed. Blood-letting is used mainly for abscesses and other infections, for congestion of blood in the liver or spleen, for some types of chronic headache, for varicose veins and in some cases of head and neck tumours, sciatica, hydrocele, ascites and lymph stagnation. Leeches are used mainly for local ailments and venepuncture for systemic problems. Blood-letting can be done on all parts of the body according to need, even under the tongue and on the penis (the penis should be erect before its veins are punctured).

Treatment with fire

The use of heat or alkali to brand or cauterize parts of the body is often attempted in order to avoid surgical intervention in ailments such as ulcers, caseated lymph nodes, piles, new growths (such as cancers), hernia, inflammation of the joints and even sinusitis. Fistula-in-ano, an abnormal tube-like tract that connects the anal canal with the outer skin, and of which there are five types, has a unique treatment: a thread is soaked in a mixture of alkalis, dried, passed into the tract and tied at both ends. The alkalis chemically cauterize the scar tissue that prevents the fistula from closing. Unlike surgery, which is tedious and usually ineffective, this procedure, which almost always succeeds, is standard in many Indian hospitals.

The more superficial forms of treatment with fire used in diseases such as paralysis involve burning medicinal substances over a *marma* point, something like the Chinese moxa treatment. Branding, by heating such substances as goat dung, cow or ox tooth, arrowpoint, metal probe or even honey, jaggery, ghee or oil, is resorted to for ascites (dropsy) and for spurs on bones; the shape of the burn is important. Frequently there is a graduated escalation in the intensity of treatment. For example, in chronic enlargement of the liver and spleen sweating is tried first, then application of alkali-containing paste and ingestion of alkali, and finally application of oil of *bhallataka (Semecarpus anacardium)* to blister the overlying skin. If these are futile, the second-last resort is branding the abdomen, followed by surgery.

MEDICINAL SUBSTANCES

PLANTS

Charaka taught, and Buddha's physician Jivaka demonstrated, that there is no substance in the world that has no medicinal value, provided you know how to use it. About six hundred different medicinal plants are mentioned in the principal Ayurvedic texts, selected for inclusion from the thousands of species of plants growing in India by the seers on the basis of unknown criteria, some probably because they are easily available, others because they are useful in a wide variety of conditions, and still others because they have unique properties.

Plants have played an important part in Indian society, and even in these days of polyethylene and styrofoam millions of people still use natural plant products in their daily lives; for example, eating off disposable plates made from banana or other leaves, smoking cigarettes rolled in *tendu* leaves, cooling their houses with vetiver (cuscus) roots tied to fans, and offering flowers, fruits, roots and seeds to gods and goddesses. The study of Indian plants cannot be limited to an examination of their therapeutic properties, but must extend to their place in Indian culture.

Western interests

Indian plants have been attracting foreign interest for thousands of years. Dioscorides mentions many Indian plants, including datura-smoking for treating asthma, nux vomica for paralysis and indigestion, and croton as a purgative. Pliny complained of the heavy drain of Roman gold to India to buy costly Indian drugs and spices. Today Western pharmaceutical companies are scouring the Third World, including India, for rare herbs that are fit for commercial exploitation. Some Indian plants or their extracts have already been adopted into modern medicine, including psyllium seed for bowel problems, and reserpine, the alkaloid extracted from *Rauwolfia serpentina*, which is used to reduce blood pressure. *Cissampelos pareira*, which is used in Ayurveda to stop diarrhoea quickly, has been found to contain a powerful, smooth muscle relaxant. It has been used in China as an anaesthetic and muscle relaxant, and is used in folk medicine in Rajasthan for snake-bite.

Many other plants that have been used almost exclusively in folk medicine are now attracting the attention of various researchers. The allopaths are looking at herbs like *Cassia fistula*, *Elephantopus scaber* and *Pristimera indica* (= *Hippocratea indica*), which show antibiotic activity; *Pergularia extensa* (= *Daemia extensa*), which has an effect on the uterus like that of pitocin; *Jatropha glandulifera*, which shows immunomodulatory activity; and *Butea superba*, which has a marked oestrogenic effect. Ayurvedic doctors have recently discovered *Tylophora asthmatica*, which is not mentioned in the standard Sanskrit or *unani* texts but is now often used to treat bronchitis and asthma. Possible contraceptives for males, including bamboo shoots, *neem* fruit, betel leaf, *bibhitaki*, and three varieties of tomato, are also being investigated, the most promising being papaya seed, which immobilizes sperms; its effect is reversible (two to three months after stopping consumption of the seeds the man again becomes fertile). It seems to have a similar effect in females also, and may induce abortion.

The most intensively investigated plant of recent years has been *Coleus forskohlii*, from which a substance called forskolin has been isolated. Forskolin has been shown to activate cyclic adenosine monophosphate (AMP); used in Ayurveda for treating heart disease, it has duly been found to be cardiotonic by modern methods of investigation. It also reduces blood pressure and is anti-spasmodic, which has led to its use in relieving abdominal colic, painful urination, respiratory disease, insomnia and convulsions.

Some plants are noteworthy for their unusual properties, such as *Cocculus hirsutus*, whose leaf juice when mixed with water forms a jelly that is used externally and internally for cooling. *Laportea crenulata* causes high fever and enlargement of the glands should you happen to touch it – even elephants in the forest give it a wide berth – but its seeds are said to be as cooling as those of coriander and are used for the same purposes, and its root juice is used in long-standing fevers. *Canavalia virosa* seed, which is said to be narcotic and poisonous, is rubbed raw on one side and applied over a scorpion or centipede sting; it remains attached there for five to seven hours, and when it falls off, on its own, all the poison has been extracted from the tissues.

Many herbs that have medicinal properties are better known for their other uses, such as the birch tree, whose bark was, and occasionally still is, used for drawing *yantras* (mystical diagrams). Powdered teak wood (*Tectona grandis*) can be used as a cooling plaster in 'hot' headaches and swellings, and its infusion 'cools' the stomach when taken internally. Its leaf juice is red, and has a mild antiseptic effect. *Shorea robusta*, another timber tree, yields a resin used in treating dysentery, for fumigations and plasters, to strengthen the digestion and as an aphrodisiac. The resin of *Pinus longifolia*, the chir pine, which yields turpentine, is used internally to tone the stomach and externally as a plaster to help abscesses to suppurate. Cedar (*Cedrus deodara*) oil, gum, bark and needles induce sweating in fever and relieve flatulence, rheumatism and respiratory disease. Today *Sapindus trifoliatus*, the 'soap nut', is used more to wash the hair or body and to clean silver than as an emetic, its classical Ayurvedic use.

Many plants that are commonly used in Western herbology grow wild in India but never became popular in classical Ayurveda, though most of them are used in folk medicine. These include agrimony, belladonna, buckbean, burdock, cleavers, red clover, coltsfoot, ephedra, eyebright, hawthorn, horehound, hyssop, kudzu, lemon balm, marigold, mistletoe, motherwort, mugwort, mullein, nettles, oregano, plantain, reed-mace, rhubarb root, St John's Wort, tarragon, verbena, violets, wormwood and yarrow. Juniper does appear in the texts, but is not much used. Such herbs commonly find the same sort of application in Indian folk medicine as they do in the West, such as mullein, which is used in respiratory disease and as a poultice in inflammations.

Senna (*Cassia angustifolia*), a popular laxative in the West, was never popular in classical Ayurveda, though its cousin *aragvadha* (*Cassia fistula*) is much used as a mild, sweet laxative and in relieving fevers and treating skin diseases. Other cassia species are used in treating coughs and asthma. Mint does not even have a Sanskrit name, although at least half a dozen species grow in India, but it has become a popular domestic remedy to relieve gas and colic, stimulate the circulation, control headache and relieve nausea, cough and congestion. Mushrooms and lichens are not much used; ferns are used sparingly. Galls, which are tumours created on trees by insects, are used as astringents for diarrhoea and dysentery, and as expectorants in respiratory problems.

Some herbs that were originally alien are now cultivated and used in popular medicine, many of them introduced by Arabian or European physicians. These include wintergreen, whose oil is almost pure methyl salicylate and is applied externally to ease aches and pains, and eucalyptus, a tree that has been widely planted by state forestry departments and has become controversial, as it apparently lowers the groundwater level where it grows. Eucalyptus oil, however, has caught the imagination of the public and it is widely sold, even by itinerant pedlars on trains, as a remedy for rheumatism and upper respiratory tract ailments, and as a mosquito repellent.

Some imports from abroad have had more sinister histories. *Argemone mexicana* seeds yield an oil that is used to adulterate mustard oil; it produces 'epidemic dropsy' in those who consume it. The cocaine habit began in India as early as the 1890s, apparently in the city of Bhagalpur in Bihar, and spread extensively within a decade, mostly to the large towns along the main railway lines emanating from Calcutta and Bombay. It was used mainly as a sexual stimulant, added to the betel-nut–betel-leaf chewing mixture known as *paan*, and at the zenith of its use probably more than a million people had become addicted to it. Its use dwindled in the 1930s and is now limited to the major cities.

Opium has been cultivated in India for at least five centuries; it seems to have been first mentioned in Ayurveda by Sharngadhara. In the sixteenth century, when the Emperor Akbar made opium a state monopoly, it became an important article of trade with China. This monopoly eventually passed into the hands of the East India

Company and was the cause of the notorious Opium Wars fought by the British to force the Chinese to import Indian opium for their addicts. For many years the British government's attempts to keep China addicted were mirrored by Indian nursemaids, who gave small amounts of opium to their charges, especially during teething, to keep them quiet. Dried ripe poppy capsules, whose narcotic properties are mild, were used in medicine well before the milky sap was recognized as being narcotic, and the drinking of an infusion of such capsules was very common between the sixteenth and eighteenth centuries; Akbar himself frequently indulged in it. Today its use is restricted mainly to rural areas of Rajasthan, Madhya Pradesh and Punjab.

Tobacco is also a relatively recent import to India, apparently having been brought by the Portuguese a few hundred years back, but it has been enthusiastically accepted into folk medicine for its purifying, dehydrating and anodyne qualities. Tobacco smoke is blown into the ear for earache and on to the gums for toothache, and is used to fumigate strains and sprains to relieve pain. Its charcoal is widely employed as a tooth powder and, with salt, as a remedy for whooping cough. The whole leaves are used as poultices in swellings and scorpion stings. The leaf paste is used with turmeric for treating skin diseases, and with slaked lime to draw out splinters and felons.

Although it is a deadly poison that can create many serious diseases when used habitually, when smoked or chewed occasionally in medicinal amounts tobacco tones the colon and sharpens the mind. Nicotine's unique effect is to alter the pattern of availability of brain chemicals. Tobacco can make task performance easier by enhancing alertness and concentration, improving memory (especially long-term memory), reducing anxiety, increasing pain tolerance and reducing hunger, all depending on how it is consumed: short puffs on a cigarette arouse the nervous system while deep drags calm it, allowing a smoker to 'fine-tune' his or her response to everyday life. These qualities and its anti-aphrodisiac effect have made tobacco use almost universal among wandering ascetics.

Some plants are used mainly as substitutes for rare or otherwise difficult-to-obtain herbs. Vidari, a strengthening and rejuvenating tuber, is usually identified as *Ipomoea paniculata*, but one survey of

South Indian medicine bazaars found *Pueraria tuberosa*, *Adenia hondala* and *Cycas circinalis* sometimes being sold in its stead. *Nagakeshara* (*Mesua ferrea*) stops haemorrhage; the common herbs sold in its place, *Calophyllum inophyllum*, *Cinnamomum wrightii* and *Myristica fragrans*, are all more likely to increase bleeding rather than stanch it.

Other plants are simply controversial; there is no agreement on their proper identification because they have been lost over time, like the soma of the Vedas. *Jivanti* is a semi-legendary herb whose sweet, cooling roots alleviate all *doshas*, revitalize, tone, nourish, rejuvenate and virilize the system, and strengthen the eyes. It has been variously identified as *Leptadenia reticulata*, *Holostemma annulare* or *H. rheedianum* and *Dendrobium macraei* (= *Desmotrichum fimbriatum*). *Varahi*, which Sushruta included in a list of eighteen 'highly powerful' medicinal plants, may be *Dosicorea sativa* or *D. bulbifera*, though *Curculigo orchioides* and *Tacca aspera* have also been proposed. *Ipomoea sepiaria*, *Mandragora officinarum* and *Smithia* spp. have all been used for *lakshmana*, which is a rejuvenator and aphrodisiac, and promotes fertility.

Some of these controversial plants are in common use, such as *pashanabheda*, which, as its name implies, breaks up urinary stones. *Aerva lanata*, *Rotula aquatica*, *Homonoia riparia*, *Bergania ligulata* (= *Saxifraga ligulata*) and *Coleus aromaticus* or *C. amboinicus* all have some lithotryptic activity, and all have their supporters for the title of *pashanabheda*. *Parpataka*, which is used in fever and cough, has variously been identified with *Rungia repens*, *Oldenlandia corymbosa*, *Fumaria officinalis* or *F. parviflora* and *Peristrophe bicalyculata*.

Frequently the differences of opinion take on a regional cast. *Caniscora decussata* is used for *shankhapushpi* in Bengal and parts of North India, as is *Clitoria ternatea* in Kerala, and *Convolvulus pluricaulis* elsewhere. In western India *Clitoria ternatea* is identified as *aparajita*, a laxative and diuretic, and *Evolvulus alsinoides* is used as *shankhapushpi*. Both western India and Kerala identify *Evolvulus alsinoides* with *vishnukranta*, which cures *vata* and *kapha* and is used to treat fevers. *Shankhapushpi*, whatever it may be, is renowned for its ability to improve intellect, epilepsy, insanity, insomnia, stuttering, stammering, weak memory, strength, digestive power, complexion and voice, and as a rejuvenative.

Chirabilva, which shows lipolytic activity and is a good scraper of *ama* from the tissues, may be either *Holoptelea integrifolia* or *Pongamia pinnata* (= *P. glabra*). In North India *Caesalpinia bonducella* or other *Caesalpinia* species are called *latakaranja*, while in Kerala the same plant is called *kuberakshi*. Physicians in Kerala adamantly maintain that *rasna*, which Charaka calls the most important *vata*-controlling herb of all, is *Alpinia galanga*, a herb known as *galangal* in America, where it has been used to treat Hodgkin's disease. However, *Pluchea lanceolata* and *Alpinia calcarat* are also candidates for the title of *rasna*, some doctors now use *Polygonum glabrum* for it, and in much of northern and western India it is identified with *Vanda roxburghii*, while *Alpinia galanga* is referred to as *kulanjana*, which is mainly used for respiratory disease, nervous debility and impotence, as an antispasmodic, a treatment for rheumatic diseases and a purifier for the lymph system.

Qualities

Ayurveda is concerned with the qualities of herbs and the actions they produce after ingestion, so taxonomical classification is not as important as classification by quality. So long as a plant performs the same action as the plant mentioned in the texts, it will be useful for the purpose at hand regardless of its species. Vaidya Nanal, one of my teachers from Poona, visits Germany from time to time, and on one occasion wanted to prepare the compound known as *Tribhuvana Kirta Rasa*. He was able to locate most of the required ingredients, but drew a blank when it came to *tulasi*, or holy basil, *Ocimum sanctum*.

While it would have been simple enough to have some sent from India, Vaidya Nanal, who is a strong supporter of the Ayurvedic principle that one should whenever possible use the herbs growing in one's locality for one's medicine, perused books until he found a German herb that seemed to have *tulasi*'s qualities. He tasted the herb and found that it had *tulasi*'s pattern of tastes. After observing its effect on himself and on others for a few days, he decided that, indeed, this would be a satisfactory substitute for *tulasi*. He then used that herb to prepare *Tribhuvana Kirta Rasa*. Even within India there are occasions on which the proper herb cannot be located; in many cases the texts have anticipated this problem and suggest suitable substitutes.

How a herb is grown and collected affects its qualities as inevitably as how a child is grown affects its qualities. Soil and climatic conditions, season and pollution are all affecting factors. The texts suggest that plants meant for medicinal use should be collected from places where rainfall is moderate or scanty, on level ground where there is good soil that is soft to the touch. There should be no impurities nearby, and the location should be far away from any graveyard or cremation ground, place of worship or assembly, execution ground or place where sacrifices are performed. The ground should be covered with auspicious grasses, should not have been tilled, should be free of holes, cracks and ant or termite mounds, and water should flow nearby. The innate constitution of the region must also be considered; plants from the Himalaya are said to be mild and wholesome, and those from the Vindhyas (another mountain range), hot and intense.

Trustworthy, pure people (the texts say 'men') of virtuous conduct should collect the plants in the appropriate season after fasting and worshipping God or their gods the previous day. The plant must be told for what specific purpose it is being taken, and the collector must apologize for killing it. In Vedic times, before a branch was cut for a sacrifice, the priests would chant, 'O knife, do not cause any harm, O Lord of the plant, protect him.' Ideally, the collector should be intuitive enough to know whether or not the plant wishes to be collected, and will respect its wishes if it declines to be used. The plants selected should be deeply rooted, of normal taste, colour, smell and feel, not attacked by insects or affected by fire, drought or any other abnormal conditions, and well-tended by shade, sun and water. If a plant has been attacked by insects, its own immunity is undoubtedly weak; how then could it help you strengthen your own?

While a few individual doctors and yogis still wander about collecting their own plants, most Ayurvedic pharmaceutical companies hire members of a special herb-collecting caste to do the job for them, people who have grown up learning where and when each plant is ready for picking. Autumn is generally the best time for plant collection. Branches are best taken when they have sap (in India, usually during the rains or spring), while roots are best taken in the hot season or winter, before sap develops, when ripened leaves have been shed or when fresh shoots have appeared. The best time for bark, bulbs, tubers and latex is autumn, and for sap or heartwood, winter; flowers and fruits are collected when they appear. The root bark of big trees is taken, and the whole root in plants with tender roots; likewise the outer bark of big trees and the wood of smaller ones. Collected drugs, Charaka tells us, should be 'stored in houses whose door faces east or north, having a single window, where flower offerings and sacrifices are done daily, in clean containers sealed against the effects of fire, water, moisture, smoke, dust, mice and other quadrupeds'.

Below is a list of just a few of the more unusual, useful and unique herbs used as medicines in India that are either already available or rapidly becoming available in the West. The three most important medicinal plants in India – *amalaki, haritaki* and *bibhitaki* – which make up the combination known as *Triphala* (the 'Three Fruits'), are listed first. The remainder of the list is in alphabetical order by botanical name, followed by one or more Sanskrit names.

Amalaki (Emblica officinalis)

This plant has five of the six possible tastes (it lacks salty); its main taste is sour, but its potency is cold, and it, like its two friends, is sweet in post-digestive effect. It calms the *doshas, pitta* particularly. It makes a good conditioner or hair oil to retard greying and baldness, and a medicinal jam for treating respiratory complaints and rejuvenating. Charaka calls it the best medicine for preventing ageing. One fruit contains as much vitamin C as one to two dozen oranges in what is reported to be a heat-stable form which is not disturbed by processing. Its flowers, bark, root and seeds also have therapeutic value.

Haritaki (Terminalia chebula)

Like *amalaki, haritaki* has five tastes, lacking salty; its main taste is astringent, but it is hot in potency. It, too, calms the Three *Doshas*, but its main effect is on *vata*, though prolonged use may aggravate *vata*. It scrapes *ama* away from the tissues, especially from the digestive tract, and rejuvenates the body, especially the colon and lungs. *Amalaki* is its substitute when *haritaki* is unavailable.

Medicinal Substances

Bibhitaki (Terminalia belerica)

Mainly astringent in taste (with three undertastes), *bibhitaki* is hot in potency. It also calms all the *doshas*, its main effect being on *kapha*. The unripe fruit is laxative, while the dried ripe fruit stops diarrhoea, in which it is particularly effective. It is also of benefit in piles and skin diseases.

'When in doubt, give *Triphala*' could easily be the Ayurvedic motto. *Triphala* can be used to shampoo the hair and wash the body, as an emetic or a laxative, as nose, ear or eye drops, as a gargle or a snuff, and as a decoction for enema. Eaten, it gently scrapes *ama* away from, and rejuvenates, the membrane lining the digestive tract, helps reduce inflammation, scrapes excess fat from the body and balances the *doshas*. It is an ingredient in a large number of medicines and its three constituents are made into rejuvenators.

Acacia arabica: babbula

This tree provides gum arabic, which is used, especially as a medicinal wine, in treating diarrhoea, dysentery, diabetes and excessive menstrual bleeding. A sweet made from this gum is fed daily to women for four to six weeks after childbirth to help them regain their strength.

Acacia catechu: khadira

Another one of the dozen species of *acacia* in India, an extract of its bark is added to the postprandial digestive called *paan* (see *Piper betle*). Its other main uses are in skin diseases and as the principal ingredient of *Khadiradi Vati*, a pill for hoarseness and other throat afflictions. It has also shown some anti-fertility effects.

Acorus calamus: vacha ('speech')

Its characteristics are evident from its other names: 'auspicious', 'destroyer of spirits', 'intellect-awakener', 'harsh', 'intense odour', 'born from water' (it grows in damp marshy places) and 'success'.

In English it is called calamus or sweet rush. Being a 'hot' rejuvenator for the brain and nervous system, it reduces *vata* and *kapha* and increases *pitta*, and can act as an aphrodisiac. It enhances awareness, improves both the voice and the facility of speech, and is very effective in controlling epilepsy. Its powder is blown into the nose to return a patient in shock or a coma to consciousness. It has been used to control *vata* disturbances of the mind, such as bedwetting, sleepwalking and sleeptalking, and can help cure tobacco addiction. Its paste is given with gold and a little honey or ghee to babies to enhance the intellect and stimulate the immune system.

A paste of its rhizome is applied to the head in headache, to the chest in bronchitis and pneumonia, and to painful rheumatic joints. It can be used as an emetic and as an antispasmodic; it relieves hoarseness and cough, promotes expectoration of phlegm, improves digestion and relieves gas. It has been used to treat chronic diarrhoea and worm infestation, and, being insecticidal, it controls skin parasites such as scabies and lice. Although it grows in the United States, FDA restrictions (based on the supposed carcinogenic properties of its 'active ingredient', asarone) make it difficult to obtain there.

Aegle marmelos: bilva

This small thorny citrus tree is sacred to the deities Lakshmi and Shiva. Its root controls *vata*, its leaves are used as poultices in inflammations and gangrene; its leaf juice controls diabetes and can ameliorate both colds and fevers. The fruit is one of the few used in Ayurveda in an immature state; it is hot, unctuous, intense, stimulates digestion and cures *vata* and *kapha*. It is made into a medicinal jam, that works wonders in acute or chronic diarrhoea, especially where there is alternating diarrhoea and constipation; in malabsorption syndromes like sprue; and in ulceration of the intestines. The ripe fruit, which is heavy for digestion and tends to disturb the *doshas*, is laxative when fresh; it is usually made into a cooling astringent sherbet for the hot season. *Bilva* oil is used as ear-drops to treat deafness.

Aloe spp. especially *A. barbadensis* (= *A. indica*):
ghrta-kumari

The Sanskrit name suggest both that this plant contains the health energy of a young woman and that it tones the female organs. Fresh *kumari* gel (found inside the leaves) controls all three *doshas*. It is applied externally to burns, rashes, inflammations and other painful conditions; taken internally it cools *pitta*, particularly in the liver, purifies blood, balances the menstrual cycle and reduces excessive bleeding, cools the eyes, regulates the digestion (especially in an 'acid' stomach), and generally soothes and heals the whole body. It contains allantoin, a substance known for its healing properties. In Ayurveda it is most commonly used as a medicated wine, *Kumari Asava*. The leaf powder, which is used as a purgative or, in combination with myrrh, as a uterine purifier, may aggravate *vata* and shows anti-fertility effects.

Areca catechu: tambula

A handsome palm tree, its seeds are known as betel-nut. They contain arecoline, which strongly stimulates peristalsis, constricts the bronchial muscles and reduces the blood pressure; it depresses the heart like nicotine. Raw nuts produce dizziness and a sense of intoxication in most unhabituated people and so the nuts are usually roasted before use. While betel-nut has a mild anti-worm effect, its main action, as part of the mixture known as *paan* (see *Piper betle*), is to stimulate digestion and tone the intestines. It is also made into a jam that is tonic for the female organs.

Betel-nut enhances digestive strength and capacity when consumed after a meal; when it is taken without food, it calms the digestive fire, especially if tobacco is added. India's poor, whose diets are insufficient, often rely on betel-nut and tea to give them the energy to work. A like effect is seen with marijuana: used with food, it increases desire for food and sex; used alone or with tobacco, it decreases these two desires. These unusual effects are a property of the astringent taste.

Asparagus racemosus: shatavari

The root of this plant, a relative of the vegetable asparagus, controls all three *doshas*, especially *vata* and *pitta*; in excess it may increase *ama*. It rejuvenates the female organs and blood, helps to build up the body, strengthens the immune system, increases *rasa*, milk and sexual secretions and so is aphrodisiac, improves intellect, digestion and physical strength and cures urinary tract disorders. It can be used in any *pitta* condition in which *ama* is absent. It is usually given as a medicated ghee or is simmered in milk; when available, the juice of the fresh roots is used. Another species, *A. adscendens*, has many of its tonic actions but is not as beneficial for the female reproductive organs.

Azadirachta indica (= *Melia azadirachta*): *nimba*

All parts of this tree, called neem or margosa in English, are bitter and are used in medicine, especially the bark and leaves and the oil extracted from the seeds. *Nimba* reduces *pitta* and *kapha* and strengthens the immune system, but in excess may aggravate *vata*. A blood purifier, it can be used for any *pitta* problem. It is very 'cold', so cold that its overuse may actually cause a cold to develop in its user. This cold quality and its bitter taste make it strongly anti-aphrodisiac. Its main uses are in the treatment of fevers, liver problems such as hepatitis, ulcers (even gangrenous) and all varieties of skin diseases. Its special power is to cure itching of all kinds; it even seems to help cure syphilis. Since extract of *nimba* is a unique insecticide, which enters the tissues of the plants to which it is applied and makes the plants themselves poisonous to insects, animals who eat it probably become 'poisonous' to parasites such as worms, ringworm and scabies.

After one hundred years of life a *nimba* tree will, on a day that cannot be predicted, begin to secrete a sort of nectar or sap, which is its essence and can cure many diseases.

Bacopa monnieri (= *Herpestis monniera*): *brahmi* in Kerala; *Mandukaparni* in North and West India; see also *Centella asiatica*

Bitter, intense and hot, this herb none the less alleviates *pitta* and *kapha*, stimulates the heart and tones the nerves. Used in insanity, epilepsy and mental weakness, it contains an alkaloid related to strychnine but less toxic, which can be safely used over a long period of time to stimulate the intellect and the language faculty.

Bambusa bambos (= *B. arundinacea*): *vamsha, venu*

Young bamboo shoots contain cyanogenic glycosides; if they are eaten raw or improperly cooked, they can kill. Bamboo is used as a stimulant in fevers, asthma, cough and paralysis; the young leaves are used as an emmenagogue and are given to horses for coughs and colds. The silaceous deposit on the inside of its stem, known as 'eye of bamboo', or *tabashir*, is a key ingredient in the decongestant compound known as *Sitopaladi Churna*.

Berberis aristata (and nine other *Berberis* spp. *Coscinium fenestratum* is used in some areas): *darvi, daruharidra* ('tree turmeric')

The roots of this small bush, known in English as the barberry, contain berberine, an antibiotic alkaloid; being extremely bitter, they decrease *pitta* and *kapha*. *Darvi* is laxative and is used mainly to control *pitta* diseases such as jaundice, skin eruptions, inflammations such as gastroenteritis, gingivitis, laryngitis and conjunctivitis, and boils, abscesses and ulcers. Its solidified water extract, known as *rasanjana*, is used as a lotion for the eyes, usually applied with milk or honey. *Darvi* is especially good for piles, and has a 'scraping' action that helps to reduce enlargement of the liver and spleen and decrease body fat. If *darvi* is unavailable, turmeric is its substitute.

Boerhaavia diffusa (= *B. repens*): *punarnava*

Sometimes called pigweed, this weed flourishes during the rainy season, especially in peanut fields. It is astringent, bitter, sweet and pungent, and cures *pitta* and *kapha* diseases without aggravating *vata* unless used in excess. *Punarnava* is cooling, diuretic (perhaps because it contains plenty of potassium nitrate), laxative, digestive and appetizing. It is most renowned for its ability to relieve oedema and dropsy, but is also effective in many varieties of heart disease, cough, asthma, intestinal colic, haemorrhage, anaemia, some nerve diseases, haemorrhoids, urinary stone, alcoholism, rheumatism, consumption, hepatitis, biliousness, fever and poisoning. Its paste is applied to skin diseases and to treat oedema. In Rajasthan folk practitioners treat jaundice by tying one-inch pieces of *punarnava* root into a garland to which incense is offered. Then a coconut is offered and the practitioner, after making seven marks on his own hand, ties the garland on the patient, who should be cured within seven days.

Cannabis sativa or *C. indica: vijaya* ('conquest'), *siddhi* ('success')

Marijuana grows wild in the Himalaya. Of the three parts used (*bhang*, the leaves of both female and male plants and possibly the male flowers also; *ganja*, the flowering tops of the female plants; and *charas*, the resin), only *bhang* and *ganja* are commonly used in medicine. Marijuana is mentioned in the Atharva-Veda but became widely used in medicine only in medieval times. It aggravates all three *doshas* when used habitually over a long period. As a medicine it is extremely effective at lowering blood pressure and intra-ocular pressure (hence its use in glaucoma) and, especially with nutmeg, to control diarrhoea, dysentery, sprue and other intestinal conditions due to irritated *vata*. Usually *bhang* is used for these purposes, though *ganja* is sometimes used with nutmeg and honey in chronic dysentery and is applied externally in hydrocele and prolapsed uterus. The smoke of the leaves and flowers is used to shrink piles and hernias.

Marijuana's effect on the body varies according to the other herbs administered with it. With digestive herbs, it becomes an appetizer *par excellence*, good for increasing appetite and reducing nausea (it is better for cancer patients to take the leaves internally rather than to smoke the flowers), and becomes aphrodisiac when mixed with aphrodisiac substances. When taken with tobacco, it suppresses the appetite and becomes anti-aphrodisiac. Many wrestlers in North India take *bhang* by mixing it with a paste of almonds, pistachios, fennel, rose petals, black pepper and other such substances and then stirring the result into cold milk to give them the concentration to exercise for hours at a time, the appetite to eat large quantities of food and the ability to digest what they consume.

Centella asiatica (= *Hydrocotyle asiatica*): *brahmi* in North India; *mandukaparni* in Kerala

It is bitter but cool, and balances all three *doshas*. It stimulates the circulatory system, especially the blood vessels of the skin and the mucous membranes, and in very large doses has a mildly narcotic effect. Being rejuvenative, it revitalizes the nerves and brain, strengthens memory and intelligence, promotes longevity, and improves concentration, voice, physical strength, digestive power and complexion. It controls *pitta* and has been used in treating fevers, skin diseases and afflictions of the reproductive organs. It is usually given as a medicated ghee, especially with the addition of *shankhapushpi*; its rejuvenating effects are more pronounced if one to four teaspoonsful of its fresh juice are taken every morning just after arising, for three to four months. Oil medicated with it is used to promote hair growth and to 'refrigerate' the brain.

Cinnamomum camphora: karpura

Camphor can also be obtained from some species of *Ocimum* ('camphor basil') and *Artemisia*, but its traditional source is this large, handsome evergreen tree. Camphor is an important ingredient in ritual worship because the deities like its fire and smoke, and evil spirits do not. It is often added to liniments, medicinal oils and aphrodisiacs because it liquefies substances and causes them to flow. Because it is excreted in the breath, it cleans out the prana channel and so is used for respiratory complaints, particularly where *ama* is present. At least nine other *Cinnamomum* species also appear in India, including cinnamon and tamalapatra.

Commiphora mukul = *Balsamodendron mukul: guggulu*

This small tree, which grows in arid regions, produces a brown or dull green oleo-resin that is bitter, pungent, sweet and astringent, hot, and pungent after digestion. It controls and balances the *doshas*; excessive use might increase *pitta* but this is rarely seen. In the course of its excretion by skin, mucous membranes and kidneys, *guggulu* stimulates these organs and disinfects their secretions.

Guggulu scrapes *ama* and fat from the body, purifies blood, strengthens the nerves and rejuvenates the tissues. It is an excellent *yogavahi* (a compound that carries the other substances mixed with it deep into the tissues); when added to a compound, it potentiates its fellow ingredients. Its strong anti-inflammatory action makes *guggulu* the best medicine for many kinds of arthritis. It is also useful in treating hay fever and chronic bronchitis (in which its smoke is inhaled), consumption, emaciation, diarrhoea, colitis, chronic indigestion, hepatitis and leucorrhoea. Like its cousin, myrrh, it strengthens and purifies the gums and teeth and is added to poultices for swellings and boils.

Modern researchers, following a clue in a verse of Sushruta, found that *guggulu* reduces blood cholesterol, and an extract called guggulipid is now prescribed for this purpose by Indian allopaths. *Guggulu* has also been found to increase the number of white blood cells and to stimulate phagocytosis, the process by which the white cells engulf and devour alien invaders in the body, and to reduce myocardial necrosis (destruction of heart tissue, for instance, after a heart attack), to relieve pain, strengthen the thyroid and raise blood levels of thyroid hormone. It also seems to depress fertility and to counteract melatonin, the pineal hormone that is often implicated in depression.

More *guggulu* is used in preparing Ayurvedic medicines than is produced, suggesting that resins from the other four *Commiphora* species, and possibly even unrelated gums such as those of the drumstick tree (*Moringa oleifera*) and *karaya* (*Sterculia urens*), are being used in its place. *Guggulu* is purified by boiling it in decoction of *triphala*, *punarnava* or *kanchanara* (*Bauhinia variegata*) to extract the toxic fractions from the resin.

Commiphora myrrha: rasagandha

Myrrh is *guggulu*'s cousin. Like *guggulu*, it balances all three *doshas* but may aggravate *pitta* when given in excess. It can be used like *guggulu* in treating obesity, rheumatoid arthritis and other conditions of *ama* in joints and muscles, but its main action is to purify and rejuvenate the female reproductive tract. It makes a good astringent mouthwash or dentifrice, and is expectorant.

Cynodon dactylon: durva

Bermuda grass controls all three *doshas* and cures diseases caused by *pitta* and *kapha*. As it dries excessive fluids, especially lymph, blood, fat and urine, its main use is to stop bleeding. Its juice is used as nose-drops to stop nosebleeds, and as enemas for bleeding piles or colitis. It is taken internally, as much as an ounce of juice every fifteen minutes, in the above conditions, in the group of haemor-rhagic disorders known as *rakta pitta* and to reduce excessive menstrual flow. It is also helpful in diabetes, chronic diarrhoea, hysteria, epilepsy and insanity.

Cyperus rotundus (some use *C. scariosus*): *musta*

Nutgrass reduces *pitta* and *kapha* and regulates the menses; even the Romans used it as an emmenagogue. It digests *ama* without aggravat-ing *pitta*, especially as a weak decoction in water given during fevers, and is used as a medicinal wine to treat diarrhoea, dysentery, indigestion and piles, and its powder shows fat-reducing activity.

Datura metel: dhattura

Also known as *unmatta* ('intoxicated') and *kanaka* ('gold'), *datura* is a strong poison. Its seeds were smoked even during the Vedic period to relieve the respiratory spasm and expel the tenacious mucus of asthma, though now only the leaves or, occasionally, the flowers are used for this purpose, the seeds being too poisonous. Its medicinal wine is also used for asthma and cough. In appropriate amounts *datura* controls both *vata* and *kapha*, being anti-inflammatory and anti-spasmodic. A poultice of the leaves is applied to lumbago, swollen glands and swollen joints, and the oil made from the fresh leaf juice is applied in *vata* diseases. The fresh leaves are sometimes rubbed on the scalp to promote hair growth and remove dandruff.

Eclipta alba: bhrngaraja or *kesharaja* ('hair king')

Bhrngaraja balances all three *doshas* and is curative mainly for *pitta*. Taken internally, it purges the liver of bile and so is a trusted remedy for hepatitis, prevents ageing and helps rejuvenate bone and its subsidiary tissues, teeth and hair, improves sight and memory, and helps sharpen the intellect. Oil medicated with it is used to keep head hair healthy and prevent its greying.

Embelia ribes: vidanga

Vidanga eliminates intestinal worms, especially tapeworm and round-worm, and kills certain pathogenic bacteria, by destroying the *ama* on which the parasites feed. It is mild enough to be a safe home-remedy for children. It has been speculated that *vidanga* could also control the proliferation of those other microscopic wriggling creatures known as sperm, which, though created by the body, are alien to it (the body produces antibodies to sperm if they escape into the tissues). Efforts to convert *vidanga* into a safe male contraceptive are under way.

Ferula foetida or *F. narthex: hingu*

Asafoetida is the resin collected from the living rhizome and root of this small tree. It is exceptionally pungent, hot and foul-smelling, and cures *vata* and *kapha* while it increases *pitta*. Asafoetida is sometimes applied as a paste to swollen joints, but its strongest action is to free the downward movement of *apana*; Charaka says that no other herb is better for this purpose. Asafoetida is applied as a thin paste to a distended abdomen and is used with castor oil in an enema for distension and colic; both methods can help relieve painful or obstructed menstrual flow. Internally, asafoetida is given with jaggery to control *vata* during the rainy season and to relieve pressure on the heart from accumulated intestinal gases. *Hingvashtaka Churna*, which is used for indigestion, colic and any other ailment caused by an inhibited *apana*, is asafoetida's most popular compound.

Glycyrrhiza glabra: yashtimadhu ('the sweet stick')

The underground stem of the liquorice plant, which was much used in ancient China, Egypt, Greece and Rome, is sweet, bitter and astringent, cool, and sweet after digestion. It reduces *vata* and *pitta*, but increases *kapha* after long-term use by causing salt and water retention and potassium loss, comparable to the effects of cortisone. Liquorice soothes sore throats and eases hoarseness, dilates the respiratory tree to ease breathing and promote expectoration of mucus, regulates the menstrual cycle, quells haemorrhages, reverses the effects of poisoning and is an aphrodisiac. It can act both as an emetic and a laxative, improves the eyesight, strength, sexual power and complexion, and strengthens the hair. It increases the production of *shukra* and rejuvenates the system. Given with other herbs, it hides their tastes even while it catalyzes their actions. Its liniment is applied to injuries and its decoction or medicated ghee is applied to both accidental and surgical wounds to assist their healing. Chewing on a stem allays thirst, burning sensations, loss of appetite, cough, fatigue and emaciation.

Gymnema sylvestre: madhuvinashini ('killer of sweetness')

Sushruta called it 'killer of diabetes' because of its use in treating that disease. When chewed, it prevents the tongue from tasting anything sweet or, to a lesser extent, bitter for half an hour or more at a time. As the tongue fails to taste the sweetness of the ingested food, the body fails to overreact to it. Some sufferers from diabetes use it to permit themselves to indulge in sweets without danger, though their indulgence is also without much satisfaction since they cannot really taste what they eat.

Hibiscus rosa-sinensis: japa

The Sanskrit name suggests the plant's use in ritual worship. Hibiscus flowers are astringent and sweet, cool, and sweet after digestion, and reduce *pitta* and *kapha* without aggravating *vata*. The flowers, which are sacred to Ganesha, the god who removes obstacles, as well as to the Mother Goddess, remove heat from the body, as in fever, and control bleeding, especially excessive menstrual bleeding. Their infusion mitigates the heat of summer, cools the genito-urinary tract, purifies the blood and cools the mind, as does their oil, which also strengthens the hair when applied to the head. A hot infusion of the flowers or root is given to relieve coughs, and the fresh flowers are said to be aphrodisiac. Boiled and powdered hibiscus flowers administered to a woman thrice daily for a fortnight after her menses ends are reported to provide contraception for the whole month. A dozen other species of *Hibiscus* also occur in India.

Holarrhena antidysenterica: kutaja

The seeds, called *indrayava*, are pungent and bitter, hot, light and tonic. They alleviate all three *doshas*, purify the urinary and biliary tracts, strengthen the lungs, cure diarrhoea and dysentery (especially in infants), fever, bleeding piles, gas and colic, and are aphrodisiac. Its bark is pungent and astringent, cool and dry, and relieves diarrhoea, dysentery, bleeding piles, haemorrhages and skin diseases. *Kutaja* kills *E. histolytica*, the amoeba that causes most cases of amoebic dysentery, and is reported to be effective in slaughtering other intestinal parasites.

Inula racemosa: pushkaramula

Known in English as elecampane, this herb is common to Indian and Western herbology. It decreases *kapha* and *vata*, increases *pitta*, and targets the chest for its main actions. It removes *kapha* from the lungs and rejuvenates them, being the 'herb of choice' for pleurisy with effusion. It also tones the female organs and controls diabetes. Externally, its paste relieves muscle pain.

Myrica nagi: katphala

Bayberry bark reduces *vata* and *kapha* and can increase *pitta* even though it has a strong astringent effect. It purifies the respiratory and digestive tracts and the nervous system. Its most popular use is as a nasal purge for swoons, head colds and headaches, for which purpose its powder is snorted into the nose. It can also be smoked, or used as a mouthwash for mouth ulcers or toothache. A bayberry poultice purifies and heals wounds, especially of the mucous membranes; applied over the pubic region it relieves menstrual pain. Taken internally with honey or fresh ginger juice, it tones the voice and, as a decoction with ginger and cinnamon, it benefits asthma, cough and chronic bronchitis, diarrhoea and dysentery.

Nardostachys jatamansi (*Valeriana jatamansi*): *jatamansi*

Once called Indian spikenard, *jatamansi* balances all three *doshas*. It promotes awareness and strengthens the mind, and ameliorates epilepsy, hysteria, convulsions, heart palpitations (especially atrial fibrillation) and intestinal colic. It is a substitute for valerian.

Ocimum sanctum: *tulasi* ('matchless')

Holy basil is pungent and bitter, hot, and pungent after digestion. It controls *vata* and *kapha* but increases *pitta* unless *ama* is present in the body. *Tulasi* is worshipped as the embodiment of Lakshmi, the wife of Vishnu, the god who preserves life, and so it is planted around temples and in the courtyards of private dwellings to purify the air around them and invite the gods into the area. It also repels mosquitoes.

Internally, its main effects are on *rasa*, the skin and the digestive and respiratory tracts. Its special power is to cure fever produced by *ama*, for which it is often given with black pepper, ginger juice and honey. This mixture also protects the throat. *Tulasi* purifies, oxygenates and invigorates the body, is a heart tonic, removes the effects of poison from the body, and has been found effective in the first stages of many cancers. Its leaf juice is used as ear-drops and is consumed in colds, coughs, asthma, hiccups, pleurisy and bronchitis to cause the body to purify and expel mucus and to reduce spasm. Soaked in water, its seeds are demulcent for the digestive and genito-urinary tracts, like the seeds of its cousin, sweet basil (*O. basilicum*).

Piper betle: nagavalli

Betel leaf was mentioned in the Mahavamsa of Sri Lanka (504 BC). It is pungent and hot, and causes juices to flow freely, so its juice is given in cough and other respiratory ailments, it is chewed to promote salivation, and the paste makes a poultice for cough and asthma, headache, orchitis, mastitis and arthritis. It is also applied over the breasts to promote milk secretion.

Betel's main use, however, is in the preparation of *paan*, a mixture of betel leaf, betel-nut (*Areca catechu*), slaked lime, *khadira* (*Acacia catechu*) and other herbs and spices. *Paan* is prescribed in Ayurveda as a digestive and to sweeten the breath, for which purpose it is chewed slowly after meals. Because it makes juices flow, *paan* also acts as an aphrodisiac when aphrodisiac substances such as nutmeg, saffron and musk are added. *Paan* is an integral part of the welcome that guests, who are to be treated as gods, are given, and betel-nuts and betel leaves are important offerings in ritual worship.

Paan chewing creates a feeling of well-being and mild stimulation, mainly as a result of arecoline, the alkaloid that is betel-nut's most active constituent. The lime helps release the arecoline from the nut (and other alkaloids from tobacco, which has become a popular addition); and the betel leaf synergistically increases excitation. Occasional use of *paan* improves working capacity and mental efficiency, while addiction ruins teeth and gums, produces indigestion, palpitations and sometimes neuroses, slows the thinking process and encourages cancer of the mouth. Although *paan*'s intoxication is far milder than that of alcohol, its addiction, like that of tobacco, is almost impossible to break. Some Indians, especially the working poor, chew *paan* all the time that they are awake; the addicted rich may chew as many as 200 *paans* every day, a total of some twenty nuts or more.

Piper longum: pippali

Dried long pepper is pungent and hot, but its post-digestive effect is sweet and it reduces *vata* and *kapha*; when green, it increases *kapha*. Being unctuous, instead of drying like its cousin, black pepper (*P. nigrum*), it is virilizing and rejuvenative. Its main uses are in cough and asthma, as an aphrodisiac and as part of weight-gaining programmes. It is usually given with milk, ghee, sugar or honey for nourishing purposes, and soaked in salt water to enkindle the digestive fire. Charaka calls its root the best digestive stimulant, which also relieves abdominal distension.

Pippali fruit is frequently taken in gradually increasing doses to habituate the system to it. One method involves consuming the paste of three *pippalis* the first day and six the next day, increasing three daily until the daily dosage is 30, then decreasing three daily for the next ten days, for a total of 300. This method has been used to treat anaemia, rheumatic diseases, cough, asthma, loss of appetite, ascites, piles, consumption, certain fevers and other diseases of *vata* and *kapha*. *Pippali* fruit that has been ground to a paste in its own juice for eight days and then dried is given in cases of indigestion, respiratory complaints, diarrhoea, and enlargement of the liver or spleen.

Plantago ovata: ishadgola

This is the Indian species of psyllium. Only the husk of the seed is used, soaked for fifteen to twenty minutes in water or buttermilk as a remedy for diarrhoea or dysentery, and in milk as a treatment for constipation. Psyllium does not allow pathogenic organisms to grow in the gut, and its mucilage absorbs bacterial and other toxins there. Being demulcent, it tones and soothes the organs of elimination and so relieves colitis, but, being heavy, its overuse leads to weakness of the digestive fire, which may increase *kapha* or *ama*. To prevent this possibility it should be taken with medicinal wine.

Plumbago zeylanica (white flowers) and *P. indica* (red flowers): *chitraka*

The leadwort, most of whose Sanskrit names mean 'fire', is pungent and hot, decreases *vata* and *kapha* and increases *pitta*. The white-flowered variety is used mainly in northern and western India, and the red-flowered variety in Kerala. The fresh root has a vesicant (blister-producing) action and so its paste is sometimes applied to swellings as a counter-irritant. To prevent possible reactions during internal use, the roots are purified; in Kerala this involves washing and crushing them and then soaking them in lime water. As soon as the lime water turns red, it is discarded and fresh lime water is added until the water remains almost unaffected by the herb. Then the roots are thoroughly washed again in cold water and dried in the shade.

Chitraka is used alone or in combination in conditions in which the digestive fire needs to be enkindled. Charaka considered it to be unsurpassed as a remedy for piles and colic. It has its own pill, *Chitrakadi Vati*, a sovereign remedy for *vata* aggravation, particularly for intestinal gas, and to control *vata* during the rainy season. *Chitraka* is also an ingredient in a number of other preparations.

Ricinis communis: eranda

The castor plant is practically a pharmacopoeia in itself; Swami Shivananda of Rishikesh once wrote an ode to its greatness. Castor oil is sweet, pungent and astringent, hot, sweet after digestion and heavy, and reduces all the *doshas*, especially *vata* and *kapha*. Besides its well-known laxative use, it scrapes *ama* from the tissues, especially the joints, and in small doses over a long term scrapes away excess fat. Externally, castor-oil packs are reliable remedies for strains, sprains, menstrual pain and all sorts of inflammation, including those of the intestines and of other abdominal and pelvic organs.

Castor root reduces *vata* and *kapha* and increases *pitta*; it is used alone and in combination in *vata* conditions, including body aches, oedema, rheumatoid arthritis, certain types of chronic dysentery and diseases of the nervous system; it is also an aphrodisiac. A poultice of the seeds or leaves alleviates pain and swelling in rheumatic joints, and poultices of the leaves are applied to relieve headache or boils.

Rosa spp.: *taruni*

While wild hill roses (*R. moschata*) grow throughout the Himalaya, medicine uses mainly the cultivated variety. Roses are bitter, pungent, astringent and sweet, cool, and sweet post-digestively. They cool and soothe, balance all three *doshas*, and eliminate *pitta* from the mind and eyes. *Gulkand* is a preparation made by layering the fresh petals with honey and sugar and allowing the mixture to mature for a fortnight; it is taken before bed in water or milk as a mild anti-*pitta* laxative, especially for the heat of summer, and also helps relieve excessive menstrual bleeding. Rose water is used as drops in the eyes to cool them and to control inflammations such as conjunctivitis. Rose oil, especially in the form known as attar, is cooling and tonic to the sex organs and the mind.

Santalum album

A small tree, which is a root parasite, borrowing other trees' roots to nourish itself, sandalwood was known to the Egyptians as early as the seventeenth century BC, and it is mentioned in the earliest literature of both India and China. It is bitter, sweet and astringent, cool, and sweet after digestion. It controls the *doshas*, but its main physical effects are on *pitta*. It is used externally as a paste or powder to calm skin eruptions and internally to purify blood, cool burning sensations, cure hot fevers and quench thirst (as a weak tea). Its special power is to lighten and concentrate the mind; it is much used in ritual worship and by meditators, as incense or as oil or paste applied on the forehead. Only the heartwood is fragrant, and it can last almost indefinitely, as it is not eaten by termites or other vermin.

Pterocarpus santalinus: *raktachandana* Called 'red sandalwood', since it has many of the same qualities as *S. album* (though it belongs to a different botanical family), *raktachandana* reduces *pitta* and *kapha*. A paste of the wood in water is applied to skin eruptions.

Sida spp.: *bala* ('strength')

There are four plants in this group: *bala*, *atibala*, *mahabala* and *nagabala*. Identification of the latter two is quite uncertain. In northern and western India *bala* is *S. cordifolia* and *atibala* is *S. rhombifolia*, while in the south *bala* is *S. rhombifolia* subsp. *retusa*, *atibala* is *Abutilon indicum*, and *S. cordifolia* is not used at all.

All types of *bala* root are sweet, aphrodisiac, rejuvenative, unctuous and cooling, and strengthen the tissues and the nervous system. A special oil, called *Kshira Bala*, is prepared from *bala* root, milk and sesame oil and used for relieving facial paralysis and sciatica. It is also given with a decoction of *bala* root in milk for certain types of arthritis. Given with ginger, the root reduces fevers, and its powder, given with milk and sugar, strengthens the urinary tract and controls leucorrhoea and spermatorrhoea. Its seeds are aphrodisiac and are useful in treating colic and tenesmus (straining at stools). Ephedrine has been detected in *bala* (unusual, since ephedrine is otherwise found only in ephedra, which is a gymnosperm, while *Sida* is an angiosperm), making it very useful as a heart tonic, especially when given with a compound such as *makaradhwaja*.

Swertia chirata: kirata-tikta, bhunimba

A bitter substance that causes bile to flow, *kirata-tikta* was once used by European doctors in India as a replacement for gentian. Its main use in Ayurveda is to control *pitta*, especially as the main ingredient in *Mahasudarshana Churna*, a bitter powder given in chronic fevers like malaria and as a tonic, which is now also used to help control allergies.

Tinospora cordifolia: guduchi

This climbing shrub is especially fond of climbing *neem* trees, perhaps because of the qualities they share. *Guduchi* is bitter (it contains berberine among other alkaloids) and hot. It cures all three *doshas*, though it is used mainly for *pitta* problems – and there are few it cannot tackle. Its powder controls fever and is aphrodisiac; the juice of the fresh plant is diuretic and is given with honey for diabetes; and its *sattva* (starchy water extract) is used to relieve chronic diarrhoea and dysentery, fever, headache, urinary disease and debility due to *pitta*. *Guduchi* has been shown to stimulate the immune system.

Tribulus terrestris (T. alatus is also used): gokshura

Gokshura ('cow's hoof', relating to its shape) is sweet, bitter and cooling, and balances the three *doshas*. It rejuvenates the genito-urinary tract, particularly the prostate, and, being rejuvenative and aphrodisiac, particularly when given with milk, it helps to correct impotence. It relieves congestion in the body and revitalizes the tissues, and, being diuretic (it contains nitrates), it is given for pain on urination, for urinary stone, and for gout and kidney disease.

Valeriana wallichii: tagara

Valerian has been a common incense and perfumery material in India for centuries. Being bitter, pungent, sweet, astringent and hot, it balances the three *doshas* but may aggravate *pitta* if given in excess. It is used mainly as a sedative, nervine and anti-spasmodic for muscle spasms, menstrual cramps, colic, digestive upsets and nervous conditions. Being a natural tranquillizer, it has been used in treating hysteria, epilepsy and various neuroses; its incense balances the mind. It digests *ama* efficiently as a powder or decoction.

Vetiveria zizanoides: ushira

Vetiver, or cuscus, a grass that grows near water, is bitter, sweet and extremely cooling. It strongly reduces *pitta* and also reduces *kapha*. Its root relieves thirst and burning sensations, and purifies and invigorates blood, skin and the genito-urinary tract. It strengthens the digestive fire, digests *ama* and calms both vomiting and diarrhoea. It purifies sweat and urine; a strong decoction, cooled, is good for inflammation of the urinary tract or the reproductive organs, and a weak decoction, cooled, is sipped in high fevers. It is also used internally as a powder, a cold infusion and a medicinal wine. It benefits almost all *pitta*-caused inflammations, and its paste makes a good cooling application to *pitta*-induced skin diseases or in 'hot' fevers.

In the hot season many people soak bundles of vetiver roots in their drinking water to keep cool and to prevent *pitta* flare-up. Another popular practice is to tie the roots into large mats and wet them; a passing breeze (or a strategically placed fan) then wafts the cool fragrance of vetiver throughout the house. Incense or essential oil of vetiver cools the mind and can improve concentration.

Withania somnifera: ashvagandha

The Sanskrit name means 'horse smell', since the fresh root is supposed to smell like horse's urine. The root of this shrub, which is a member of the Solanaceae family, which includes henbane, belladonna and the tomato is unlike many of its relatives in being bitter, astringent and sweet, hot, and sweet after digestion. It reduces *vata* and *kapha*, but an excess may increase *pitta* or *ama*. It is aphrodisiac and tonic and is used mainly to combat debility due to old age, nervous exhaustion and simple overwork. It nurtures and clarifies the mind, calms and strengthens the nerves, and promotes sound, restful sleep. It rejuvenates flesh, marrow and *shukra*, rebuilds body and mind, and relieves such conditions as rheumatism, consumption, spermatorrhoea, impotence, paralysis, infertility, emaciation and diseases of the nerves, such as multiple sclerosis. In small amounts it is a good tonic for weak pregnant women, but it must be used with care, because large amounts have caused abortion. Its leaf infusion is given in fevers and the bruised leaves applied to boils and swellings, while the fruit and seed are diuretic. The seed is also said to be hypnotic.

KSHARA

Alkalis are prepared by burning plants, stirring their ashes in water, straining and drying them. They exert a burning and scraping action, are laxative, diuretic and digestive, are sometimes used as salt substitutes, and cause impotence. The most common *kshara* is that of barley, which, especially in combination, is used to treat urinary ailments – retention, pain, stone and gravel – digestive problems such as piles, malabsorption syndromes and acidity, and bronchitis or influenza.

SALT

Salt is hot, unctuous and intense, and is best used externally, as an application to reduce swelling and pain in *vata* diseases. Gargling with hot salt water and turmeric helps soothe sore throats. Salt is an ingredient in many compounds used internally, its job being to liquefy phlegm and relieve congestion. It is sometimes used on its own as a laxative and to treat loss of appetite, digestive weakness and indigestion, and it has been used in enemas for controlling *vata* and expelling threadworms.

Excess indulgence in salt causes oedema and other *kapha* diseases characterized by water retention, loss of firmness and strength of both body and mind, early wrinkling of the skin and greying of the hair, a tendency to excessive bleeding and other *pitta*-caused conditions, destruction of *shukra*, impotence and rise in blood pressure. Five types of salt are used in Ayurveda, including sea salt, but the one most used is the rock salt called *saindhava*, which supposedly does not to cause water retention like the other varieties, when used in medicinal quantities. It is also reputed to be cooling instead of hot, to calm all the *doshas* and to be good for the eyes.

SHILAJIT

Shilajit is a tarry blackish or brownish substance that is exuded from rocks, especially in the Himalaya but also in other mountain ranges, during the hot summer months. It appears in Arabic and Persian medicine under the name *Momiya*, and is a popular remedy in parts of the former Soviet Union. There is some speculation that it may represent the action of time and the elements on the latex of various species of *Euphorbia*, but its ultimate origin is still uncertain.

It is purified by dissolving it in water, filtering, and drying in the sun, or by heating with cow's milk, *triphala* decoction or juice of *bhrngaraja*. *Shilajit* acts mainly to purify and strengthen the genitals and the urinary tract; it is used in diabetes, ascites, urinary stone and reproductive disorders. It is a powerful aphrodisiac and stimulant, and is given as a rejuvenator to people suffering from consumption, chronic bronchitis, asthma, chronic digestive disease, diseases of the nerves and fractures.

ANIMAL PRODUCTS

Animals are more conscious than plants. Plants do feel terror and pain when they are attacked and killed, but the killing of an animal causes more misery. Because of the Law of Karma, a fraction of the pain suffered by the being sacrificed to make the medicine remains in the medicine and is partially responsible for its side-effects. Whatever may have been the Vedic opinion on this matter, the influence of the Buddhists and Vedantists certainly inhibited the use of animal products in Ayurveda, other than those that can be collected without slaughtering or maiming the beast, such as honey, ghee and deer antler, which promotes expectoration in cough, asthma and other respiratory complaints, reduces fever and is a heart tonic. Some folk remedies continue to use animals; from time to time I still see an entrepreneur on the streets of Bombay preparing oils to be used in treating weakness of the nerves and as a stimulant and aphrodisiac by slowly cooking live lizards, and, like the Native Americans, some people in India use fresh spider's web to treat chills and as a dressing for wounds.

The same standards of purity used for collecting plants also apply to animal products; for example, milk to be used in medicine should be collected from a cow well after the delivery of her calf so that it is less likely to aggravate *kapha*. Dung and urine should be collected only from healthy animals so that they are free of *ama*, and flesh, organs, horns, feathers and hooves should come from full grown, strong animals and birds so that they are well formed and well 'ripened'.

The most famous animal-derived Ayurvedic medicine is undoubtedly musk, which is the secretion of the preputial glands of the musk deer (*Moschus moschiferus*). The best quality of musk is reported to become available after the rutting season, when the animal breaks the gland's capsule open with its hooves and empties its contents on to the ground. The pod contains up to two ounces of musk; when fresh it is milky, then gradually turns viscid and brownish-red. One test for musk, which has a strong vasodilating (blood-vessel dilating) effect, is to hold it near your nose and inhale; if your nose starts to bleed, the substance is probably musk. Musk's fragrance is destroyed by exposure to other fragrant substances such as camphor, valerian, bitter almonds and garlic, but apparently not by asafoetida. An old test for musk purity involved passing a thread through asafoetida and then through the substance to be tested; if the smell of asafoetida remained, the musk was not genuine.

Being a strong vasodilator, musk is a stimulant and aphrodisiac. It is much used as a heart tonic and is also given in fever, chronic cough, debility and impotence. *Bhava prakasha* reported that the musk from Assam was best, that from Nepal was acceptable, and that from Kashmir was worst, but this is all academic now that the poor timid musk deer has been hunted nearly to extinction, and the availability of musk has sunk almost to zero. Fortunately for medicine, many other plants and animals have musk-like odours, including *Hibiscus abelmoschus*, the musk-mallow, whose seeds are sometimes used as a musk-substitute. Other substitutes include star anise, mace and clove, depending upon the specific effect desired. Similar to musk is castoreum, the dried preputial follicles of the beaver, which is used as a stimulant, emmenagogue and aphrodisiac; a like substance is also obtained from the civet cat.

Other fragrant substances used in medicine and perfumery include *gorochana*, purified ox-bile, which reduces body heat by purging bile from the system and is used to calm the nerves and mind in whooping cough, convulsions, hysteria, jaundice, asthma and intestinal disease; and ambergris, a substance secreted by whales. The sea is the source for many commonly used medicines, including pearls and coral, both of which control *pitta*; conch and cowrie shells, used mainly to regulate the digestive process; mother-of-pearl, a substitute for pearl; and *samudraphena*, or cuttlefish bone. *Samudraphena* is mainly used externally, as a paste with *datura* in earache and oedema around the outer ear, in skin diseases and to cool heat rash.

Back on land, animal products include elephant tusk (or tooth) charcoal, used in treating leucorrhoea, jaundice and conjunctivitis, and to promote fertility in women; peacock tail-feather charcoal, which quells vomiting; tiger or peacock fat, elephant dung oil and oil of bat for *vata* diseases like paralysis; and snake venom pills, used to stimulate the system in collapse and to treat nervous abnormalities like chorea. Elephant dung has also been ingested for contraception. Egg shells are an ingredient in at least two medicines, and lac, an exudation of the lac insect, appears in many more; it helps control haemorrhages and fills in holes in the body (cavities in the lungs, caries of the teeth, fractures of the bones). Urines are also popular medicines, especially cow's urine; human urine is mentioned only in *Sharngadhara*.

10

PHARMACOLOGY

Preparing an Ayurvedic medicine is a job for an expert cook, one who has mastered the arts of mixing various substances together and, by judicious use of processing methods (*samskara*), creating a coherently acting, 'tasty' product. Even a small dose of medicine can be made to give a powerful action, and a large dose can be made to give a mild action, by adding drugs to or removing them from a recipe (*yukti*), by processing and by judicious administration to the patient. The texts provide sample recipes for the physician of average intelligence to copy, and for the expert physician to use as a guide; the fourth chapter of Charaka's section on aphorisms, for example, lists 600 emetic and purgative prescriptions.

The principles of Ayurvedic pharmacology differ from those of modern allopathic medicine as much as they resemble those of Chinese medicine. Both Ayurveda and Chinese medicine lay emphasis on the innate characteristics of a substance's effect on a living system, with a view to enhancing positive qualities and eliminating negative ones, rather than on the 'active principles' that modern researchers seek to isolate from medicinal plants. Ayurvedic and Chinese prescriptions use assistant herbs and processing techniques to perfect the action of the main substance in a compound, rather than taking individual chemical fractions out of context and refining them to chemical purity at the cost of their life-force.

Reserpine causes side-effects and *sarpagandha* (*Rauwolfia serpentina*) does not, because *sarpagandha* is a living being and reserpine is not. Plants are made from the same five elements as we animals; like us, they also have channels of circulation as well as digestive fire (which performs photosynthesis). Substances that once lived have different effects on the system from those that either never have lived or have had their 'live' qualities effaced by drastic *samskaras*, such as those used to extract active principles. Reserpine is not as benign a medicine as its parent plant because it no longer *supports* life. It has become, at best, indifferent to life as it goes about its molecular way in the body; under certain circumstances it even becomes anti-life.

Modern medicine likes to 'do' things to the patient, to force the system to respond. Ayurveda tries instead to induce the system to balance itself. The duty of an allopathic drug is to alter the patient's metabolism; the duty of an Ayurvedic drug, first and foremost, is to protect the tissues from the attack of the *doshas*. Because of the deeply held belief that living tissue can be objectified, most modern researchers ignore the likelihood that a plant's active principles may exist in the plant in a more complex form than the one in which they are studied. They also often ignore the other molecules in the plant, which may enhance its efficacy and reduce its toxicity, and ignore the influence of diet, activities and mental state on the patient who consumes the extracts. New research of all kinds is going on in Ayurveda, based often on textual references, but much of it is this sort of active-principle extraction, compounded by the further violence to living beings involved in animal experimentation, dragging the medicines further and further away from that life which their use is intended to protect.

Just as the ancient seers listened to plants, we must listen to and speak to the substances that we take into our bodies and from which we continuously re-create our bodies. Every medicine is also a food, and only the very strong can profitably consume poison for very long without knowing how to neutralize it. There is no denying the strides modern medicine has made in certain directions, nor can we deny the need to return to more life-friendly therapies and to 'live' medicines, medicines still filled with living prana.

The physicians of Kerala take most of their recipes from Vagbhata's *Ashtanga Hrdaya* and from a local text called the *Sahasrayogam*, 'the One Thousand Yogas'. Here 'yoga' is used in the sense of a group of live substances combined together synergistically to produce an efficient effect. For example, *arjuna* and *punarnava* are not particularly impressive heart tonics when given individually, but together they can be very effective. Instead of isolating active principles, Ayurveda enhances them by combination and processing, *yukti* and *samskara*.

For success in this endeavour the actions of each plant on each part of the body must be well known. Various Ayurvedic texts have classified drugs according to source and uses, though these lists often disagree with one another, since differences of opinion are frequent among Ayurvedic physicians. Enough is common, though, to permit logical conclusions, though translation into English does crimp the multiple levels of meaning that pervade Sanskrit. The word '*hrdya*', for example, means, depending upon how one chooses to interpret it, 'good for the central part of the torso', 'good for the heart' or 'hearty, cordial'. A substance that is *hrdya* could be any or all of these things; it might relieve intestinal gas and thus relieve pressure from below on the heart, it might directly improve the condition of the heart muscle and it might literally be 'hearty' or 'cordial' to the whole system. Likewise, an herb that is *jivaniya*, like liquorice, promotes life in many or all spheres of the organism, including the mental sphere.

Such multi-meaningful words enable us to perceive otherwise hidden connections between body parts. For example, most of the *hrdya* substances listed by Charaka are non-*pitta*-aggravating sours, such as mango and pomegranate and *kokum* (*Garcinia indica*). The sour taste is 'hearty' because it enhances both the digestive fire and the appetite, which may improve heart function either by some obscure metabolic pathway, or by improving the emotional state, or both. Some of the main plant actions are listed below.

Balya   Provides strength to body and mind; examples are *ashva-gandha*, *bala* and *vidari*.

Bhedaniya   Breaks up the stools into pieces, and thus is laxative; examples include *trivrt* and castor oil.

Brmhaniya   Increases the strength of the solid tissues, usually by causing the system to add more juice or 'sap'; the word suggests expansion. Examples are *ashvagandha* and *bala*.

Dipaniya   Enkindles the digestive fire; examples are long pepper fruit and root, *chitraka*, fresh ginger, black pepper and asafoetida.

Kanthya   Good for the throat and, by extension, for the things that live in the throat, such as the voice, and, by further extension, the power of speech: examples are liquorice, long pepper, grapes and *vidari*.

Lekhaniya Scrapes mass from the body, reducing its juices; examples include most bitter and pungent substances like nutgrass, turmeric, barberry, *guggulu*, black pepper, powdered ginger and *triphala*.

Sandhaniya Solidifies the stools and so has an anti-laxative (though not necessarily constipating) effect; examples include *guduchi*, mango seed, *manjishtha* (*Rubia cordifolia*) and barberry.

Trptighna Literally, 'destroys satiation', which, on the level of the body, means increases appetite; on the mental level it involves the stirring up of desire. Examples: fresh ginger, *chitraka, vidanga, guduchi*, calamus, nutgrass and long pepper.

Varnya Enhances the 'colour' of the organism (including, but not limited to, the complexion and lustre of the skin and the body's aura); examples include sandalwood, vetiver, liquorice, *manjishtha* and *vidari*.

Other actions are more straightforward: herbs like ajowan, asafoetida, bayberry, calamus, cardamom, cinnamon, clove, garlic, ginger, nutmeg, cumin, dill and fennel make *vata* return to its proper direction of flow (*anuloma*); and elecampane, *talisa* (*Abies webbiana*), eye of bamboo, cardamom, *tulasi, punarnava*, long pepper, *haritaki* and asafoetida control cough, asthma and other respiratory problems. The modes of action differ from herb to herb: asafoetida and *haritaki* control cough and asthma by freeing the downward movement of *apana*, while *punarnava* does so by eliminating excess water from the body, and cardamom and long pepper act less by relieving *apana* and more by freeing the movement of prana in the chest.

Because different medicines act in different ways to produce the same result, when they are combined they often cause a synergistic effect: their total action is greater than the sum of their individual actions would be. Combinations of medicines are popular both because they require a smaller dose and because they act on more systems than many single drugs would. Not all herbs combine well, however, and care must be taken not to create combinations in which the ingredients conflict with one another in quantity, quality or action. After considering the various characteristics of various plants the ancients created a few combinations whose members support and enhance one another's effects so well that they have become Ayurvedic mainstays. *Triphala* (see pp. 220–1) is the supreme example of such a combination; others include:

Ashtavarga   A group of eight herbs that return life to the system and rejuvenate it. The herbs are named as *jivaka, kakoli, kshiraka-koli, mahameda, meda, rddhi, rshabhaka* and *vrddhi*, but their identification is a major controversy.

Dadimashtaka Churna is a powder that contains pomegranate, sugar, *Trisugandha* and *Trikatu*; it improves the appetite, enkindles the digestive fire, is *kanthya* (see p. 247), improves intestinal tone and function, and is useful in cough and fever.

Dashamula (the Ten Roots)   Used mainly to control *vata* anywhere in the body in such varied conditions as asthma, colic, toothache and difficulty in giving birth, especially when taken as a decoction, by mouth or in an enema, or as a medicinal wine. It is composed of the roots of *bilva* (*Aegle marmelos*), *kashmarya* (*Gmelina arborea*), *agnimantha* (*Premna serratifolia*), *patala* (*Stereospermum tetragonum*), *shyonaka* (*Oroxylum indicum*), *brhati* (*Solanum indicum*), *shveta brhati* (the same, but the white-fruited variety), *shalaparni* (*Desmodium gangeticum*), *prshniparni* (*Pseudarthria viscida*), and *gokshura* (*Tribulus terrestris*). Each member also has its own individual uses; for example, *brhati*'s leaf juice is used with fresh ginger juice to stop vomiting, and its fruit relieves certain skin diseases.

Panchakola   Includes the powders of ginger, long pepper fruit and its root, *chitraka* and *chavya* (a *Piper* species); it improves appetite and digestive fire, digests *ama* and is useful in distension, colic and other digestive complaints.

Trikatu (the Three Pungents)   Ginger, black pepper and long pepper, used together mainly to control conditions in which *kapha* or *ama* obstructs *vata*, especially in the respiratory tract.

Trisugandha (the Three Aromatics)   Cinnamon, cardamom and *tamalapatra*; when *nagakeshara* (*Mesua ferrea*) is added, this group becomes the *Chaturjata*. *Trisugandha* and *Chaturjata* are often used for the same purposes as *Trikatu*, but are sweeter and milder.

As time passed more and more recipes were created, many of which are still in use today. Some of the later texts offer detailed instructions;

for example, Sharngadhara specifies that in his treatise when a drug appears twice in a recipe, its quantity should be doubled; when sandalwood is mentioned in a recipe for a medicated powder, wine, oil or ghee, white sandalwood should be used, while red sandalwood is indicated in recipes for decoctions or for pastes for external application. When a plant is mentioned without specifying what part of it is to be used, the root is indicated. Many of the older texts are not so detailed, however, and their interpretation is often controversial, as traditions differ from state to state. Hence the advice that a wise doctor should alter recipes as needed.

PLANT PREPARATIONS

The choice of which substance to use and how to use it is influenced by environmental factors such as climate and season, and by the drug's appropriateness for the user's constitution, condition, age, habituation, psychological state, digestive capacity and physical strength. Tolerance must be created for some powerful drugs, such as long pepper. The dose of a medicine is never fixed, but depends entirely on the patient's condition. The various possible routes of administration depend on the disease being treated; they include all possible variations of applications on to the skin and into any body opening. Charaka even suggests that when a king or prince suffers from a 'hot' or 'cold' fever, he embrace a luscious woman whose body has been thoroughly smeared with the paste of sandalwood or *agaru* respectively.

When the recipe has been selected, fresh substances must be used. All herbs should be as juicy and full of sap as possible, since sap is the plant's *rasa* and has an innate affinity for the patient's *rasa*; it helps purify and nourish the patient's own 'juice'. No ingredient should be more than a year old except ghee (for certain uses), jaggery and honey (which improve with age), grains, long pepper and *vidanga*; *guduchi*, *kutaja*, *vasa* (*Adhatoda vasica*), *kushmanda* (*Benincasa hispida*), *shatavari* and *ashvagandha* particularly should be used fresh whenever possible.

Not all herbs are available in all places or all year round, however, and part of the reason for subjecting them to processing is to help preserve them. Most preparations, including pills and jams, remain potent for a year (unless they contain minerals, which may preserve them longer), though powders are best used within two months, and medicated ghees and oils within four months. Medicinal wines and *bhasmas* (incinerated minerals, see below) improve with age. Some of the earliest modes of preparation were a group of five methods called the *Pancha Kashaya Kalpana*: expressed juice, paste, decoction, hot infusion and cold infusion, in order from heaviest to lightest.

Expressed juice

The plant is crushed and the juice extracted through a clean cloth; this method is used for juicy plants such as aloe, *amalaki*, *brahmi*, coriander leaves, garlic, ginger, *guduchi*, holy basil (*tulasi*) leaf, lemon, lime, *neem* leaf, onion and *vasa*. If the herb is dry, its powder is added to twice its weight in water, allowed to sit for twenty-four hours and then strained. The dose is about 1 ounce, depending upon the potency of the material.

Putapaka is also considered a kind of juice. To prepare it, a two-finger-thick layer of mud is applied over a paste of the drug wrapped in leaves of banyan, *jambu*, *kashmarya* or banana and is cooked on a cow-dung fire until it is red-hot. Examples: *kutaja* with *jambu* leaf, given with honey in diarrhoea; ripe pomegranate fruit with honey, for diarrhoea; the whole plant of *kantakari* (*Solanum xanthocarpum*) for cough; dry ginger with juice of castor root for loss of appetite and for *vata* diseases; *surana* (*Amorphopallus campanulatus*) for piles.

Paste or powder

Crushing the plant with liquid produces a paste; without liquid, a powder. Ginger, garlic, onion and most leaves and roots can be prepared in this way. Sesame paste (*tahini*) is given with butter, or with paste of *nagakeshara* with butter and sugar, for bleeding piles. The usual dose of a paste or powder is to 1/5 to 2/5 ounce; powders are usually given with water.

Powders made from combinations of various drugs are extensively used in Ayurveda, *Triphala* being the epitome of such preparations. Other examples are listed below.

Hingvashtaka Churna   Its ingredients are black pepper, ginger, long pepper, *ajamoda*, rock salt, cumin, black cumin (*Nigella sativa*) and asafoetida. It is used mainly to free *apana*'s downward movement, to cure flatulence, indigestion, colic and constipation.

Jatiphaladi Churna   Nutmeg and eighteen other ingredients are taken in equal parts, with an amount of marijuana leaves equal to all the rest together. Being anti-spasmodic and astringent, it is meant mainly for diarrhoea, dysentery and conditions of malabsorption such as sprue, but has also been used to treat cough spasms, asthma, loss of appetite, consumption, migraine, mania and menstrual pain or excessive bleeding.

Mahasudarshana Churna   Contains *Triphala*, *Trikatu* and almost fifty other herbs; half of its bulk is *kirata-tikta* (*Swertia chirata*), a very bitter medicine. This powder is diaphoretic and diuretic, and is given in fevers (including malaria), enlargement of the liver and spleen, fatigue, nausea, hepatitis, gallstones and cirrhosis, and has at times been used in many other conditions, including indigestion, bronchitis, asthma, anaemia, mumps, backache, chest pain due to *ama*, inflammation of the cervix or ovaries, lymphatic leukaemia, appendicitis, optic neuritis and stye.

Saraswata Churna   Prepared by mixing together herbs that tone the nervous system, such as calamus, *shankhpushpi* and *ashvagandha*, and potentiating them with *brahmi* juice. It is a brain tonic used in mania, epilepsy, mental weakness, nervous strain and some forms of paralysis.

Sitopaladi Churna   Named for its main ingredient, rock candy, which is a known sore-throat soother, *Sitopaladi* also contains cinnamon, cardamom, long pepper and eye of bamboo. It is used mainly in colds, coughs, asthma and other respiratory complaints, such as pleurisy, in consumption and in indigestion, loss of appetite, fever and haemorrhages.

Talisadi Churna   Adds black pepper, ginger and *talisa* (*Abies webbiana*) to *Sitopaladi*'s ingredients, and is used mainly for cough and asthma, but also for enkindling the digestive fire and digesting

ama in fevers, vomiting, diarrhoea, emaciation, abdominal distension, malabsorption and anaemia.

Trikatu Churna   Usually made with equal amounts of ginger, black
pepper and long pepper, *Trikatu Churna* is used to enkindle the
digestive fire and to reduce *ama*, *kapha* and fat. It has also been
used in certain skin and urinary diseases, in asthma and to purify
the throat.

Triphala Churna   Some physicians like to mix together equal quantities of *amalaki*, *haritaki* and *bibhitaki*; others vary their proportions
according to the disease to be treated. Sharngadhara advised one
part *haritaki*, two parts *bibhitaki* and three parts *amalaki*, thus
enhancing its *kapha-* and *pitta*-reducing properties. He advised it
for use in urinary disease, swellings, inflammations and infections,
periodic fevers, skin and eye diseases, and to enkindle the digestive fire and rejuvenate the body. For use in *vata*-caused indigestion, diarrhoea or piles or other *vata* diseases, more *haritaki* might
be added.

Sometimes powders are used for external applications, such as
Dashanga Lepa, which contains such herbs as liquorice, valerian,
red sandalwood, cardamom, *jatamamsi*, turmeric, barberry, *kushta*
(*Saussurea lappa*), and *shirisha* (*Albizzia lebbeck*); it is applied to
mumps, boils, abscesses, erysipelas and neuralgia.

Decoction

One part of fresh herb (if dry, it is first added to an equal quantity
of water and left to stand for half an hour) is added to sixteen parts
by weight of water and the mixture boiled down to one-fourth.

In Kerala the decoction is strained and then boiled again until it
is reduced to one and a half times the weight of the original herb;
this is one full dose when mixed with jaggery, honey, sugar,
medicated ghee, powder or another substance. In other regions the
dose is usually about an ounce mixed with an equal quantity of
water. Decoctions are often used as vehicles for other medicines.

Clay pots are best for cooking decoctions. If they are unavailable,
then for *kapha* problems a copper pot should be used; for *pitta*
problems, a silver or bronze pot; and for *vata* problems, a gold or

iron pot. Glass pots are permissible, but aluminium pots should never be used! This method is best for roots, stems, barks and, occasionally, fruit; the plant parts are used once and then discarded.

Common decoctions (*kvatha*) include:

Dashamula Kvatha   Made of the Ten Roots (see p. 249); used for fevers, coughs, colds, neuralgia, giddiness and after childbirth.

Mahamanjishthadi Kvatha   Containing almost fifty ingredients, it is named for *manjishtha* (*Rubia cordifolia*), a blood purifier whose deep red colour once made it a dye. This decoction is used in skin diseases, gout, menstrual disorders and other blood-based ailments.

Maharasnadi Kvatha   Contains *rasna*, ginger, *bala*, castor root, cedar, calamus, *vasa*, *haritaki*, *punarnava*, *guduchi*, *gokshura*, *asvagandha*, *aragvadha*, *kantakari*, *brhati* and four other herbs; used mainly as a vehicle for the various compounds of *guggulu* in rheumatism, arthritis, sciatica, lumbago and several types of paralysis.

Punarnavadi Kvatha   Contains *punarnava*, barberry, turmeric, ginger, *haritaki*, *guduchi*, *chitraka* and *bharngi* (another controversial herb); used mainly in enlargement of the liver or spleen, oedema, ascites, inflammations and rheumatic disorders.

A related preparation is the milk decoction, in which one part herbs, eight parts milk and thirty-two parts water are boiled together until one-fifth the original volume of the milk remains. This preparation is used to strengthen the system when made with *ashvagandha*, *shatavari*, nutmeg and *brahmi*; to prevent excessively astringent medicines from disturbing the system, when made with *arjuna*; to treat chronic fevers, especially when made with *Dashamula*; and when made with *bala*, jaggery and powdered ginger, to make urine and faeces flow freely.

Hot infusion

One part plant is added to eight to ten (some say only four) parts hot water, and left to sit for at least half an hour (some say to use it immediately). This method is good for delicate plant parts that cannot take boiling, such as leaves and flowers and some aromatic herbs. A common example is liquorice root.

Cold infusion

One part plant is added to six parts of water. It is kept for twelve hours overnight and squeezed and strained the next morning. This method is good for very delicate plants and for the treatment of *pitta* conditions. Hibiscus, jasmine and sandalwood are sometimes used in this way, as are *guduchi* (for chronic fever), coriander (with sugar for thirst or burning sensations, especially of the urinary tract) and *sariva* (*Hemidesmus indicus*, 'Indian sarsaparilla') for calming *pitta*.

From these five main methods of preparation several other methods developed:

Mantha

One part of drugs is mixed with four parts of cold water and churned well until thick. A popular recipe includes dates, pomegranates, grapes (or raisins), *tintidika* (*Rhus parviflora*), tamarind, *amalaki* and *parushaka* (*Grewia asiatica*), and is given to relieve the complications of alcoholism.

Panaka

One part of herb is added to sixty-four parts of water and boiled to one-half to prepare medicated water for use in cooking gruels and meat soups, and for assuaging thirst in fevers. For fevers, commonly used herbs include white sandalwood, vetiver, nutgrass and powdered ginger. Boiling pure water to one-eighth, one-fourth or one-half of its original volume is said to make it lighter and more digestible; to improve the digestion, to relieve *kapha*, *vata*, *ama* and excess fat; to purify the bladder; and to help cure cough, respiratory distress and fever.

Arka

These distillates are prepared by boiling the herb in water and collecting the steam that it produces. Common distillates include those of mint, *ajowan*, *brahmi*, *Dashamula*, *gorakhamundi* (*Sphearanthus indicus*, a blood purifier), *manjishtha*, *punarnava*, and fennel.

Jams (*Leha, Avaleha, Modaka, Paka*)

Jams are semi-solid or solid sweetened preparations made by taking a paste or powder of the main ingredients and cooking it in milk or water, adding ghee, sugar syrup, and/or small amounts of other herbs. A jam is ready when it can be stretched into a 'string' between the fingers and when it sinks into water whole, without spreading. Many jams are used as vehicles for other medicines, but they can also be used on their own, especially as rejuvenatives and aphrodisiacs.

Common jams used in the therapy of disease include those prepared from *kutaja* or *bilva* (mainly for diarrhoea and dysentery), *surana* (*Amorphopallus campanulatus*, for piles), *vasa* or *kantakari* (both for respiratory problems), grapes or pomegranates (bleeding disorders and other *pitta* problems) and turmeric. Jam of fresh ginger is used mainly to strengthen the digestive fire, while jam of powdered ginger (*Saubhagya Shunthi Paka*) is given as a winter tonic and to treat weakness in women after childbirth. *Supari Paka*, betel-nut jam, is given to tone the uterus, before or after giving birth, and to reduce menstrual bleeding and leucorrhoea. *Agastya Haritaki Leha*, the recipe for which was said to have been revealed by the sage Agastya, strengthens the lungs and is mainly used in respiratory diseases, such as shortness of breath, cough, asthma, and consumption; and in exhaustion and piles.

The most famous of all Ayurvedic jams is *Chyvanprasha Avaleha*, which was concocted by the Ashvin twins to restore youth to the sage Chyvana. It contains forty or more herbs and is sometimes fortified with minerals, but its main ingredient is *amalaki*. It is a rejuvenator, tissue builder and general tonic, and is a remedy for debility, whether as a result of exhaustion, disease or old age; respiratory afflictions such as consumption, hoarseness, asthma and tightness of the chest; and such other varied conditions as heart disease, anaemia, gout, weakness of *shukra*, urinary complaints, constipation and weakness of the bones. It also promotes intelligence, memory, sexual desire and beauty, and prevents ageing.

Medicinal Wines (*Asava* or *Arishta*)

Arishtas are made from decoctions and *asavas* from expressed juices, both usually fermented with the flowers of *dhataki* (*Woodfordia fruticosa*). Medicinal wines are often used as vehicles for other medicines and to enkindle the digestive fire. Common *asavas* are those made of *Panchakola*, *bhallataka* (*Semecarpus anacardium*), sandalwood, grapes, *datura*, aloe, long pepper, *punarnava*, vetivert and *vasa*. Common *arishtas* are made from *babbula*, *bala*, *Dashamula*, cedar, cumin, *khadira*, *kutaja*, *musta*, *sariva* and *vidanga*. *Dashmularistha*, one of the most popular of the medicated wines, is used in indigestion, malabsorption, loss of appetite, asthma, cough, consumption, vomiting, anaemia, hepatitis, piles, skin diseases, diabetes, urinary stone, pain on urination, ascites and emaciation. It nourishes the lean, gives progeny to the childless and stimulates the production of semen, strength and lustre.

Iron or copper can be added to *Kumari Asava*, the wine of aloe, to help scrape *ama* from the liver, and iron is an important ingredient in *Lohasava*, which is given in anaemia since alcohol helps the body to absorb iron. The only medicinal wine of animal origin is *Takrarishta*, which is made of fermented buttermilk and is used in digestive disorders.

Pills

Pills became popular in Ayurveda for the same reasons that they are popular today: each one is a pre-measured dose of medicine in a convenient self-contained package that requires no or very little further preparation before taking. Many pills are made by cooking powdered herbs with jaggery or sugar, or by mixing with a liquid such as honey or with a resin such as *guggulu*. When mixed with a liquid, the process is usually termed *bhavana*; enough liquid is added to soak the powder well (Kerala), or equal parts of powder and liquid are mixed (West India). In Kerala the mixture is then dried in the sun before being made into pills; in other parts of India it is slowly ground in a mortar and pestle until it loses its liquidity.

Bhavana fulfils the definition of *samskara* as the 'lending of other properties to a substance'. *Bhavanas* can be given to enhance a herb's actions, as in the case of *Vishvabheshaja Vati*, in which ginger powder is potentiated by a *bhavana* of ginger juice, a process that is repeated three, seven or twenty-one times, or to attenuate them, as in *Amapachaka Vati*, in which a *bhavana* of aloe juice, which is cool and calming, is given to *haritaki*, *Trikatu*, *nux vomica*, asafoetida, sulphur and rock salt, all of which are hot and intense. Aloe also scrapes *ama* away from the tissues, so its use synergizes the mixture even while making it milder.

Some common pills are:

Eladi Vati Contains cardamom, cinnamon, *tamalapatra*, long pepper, liquorice, dates, raisins and sugar. When sucked, it promotes expectoration in bronchitis, cough, cold and other respiratory diseases.

Kankayana Guti Contains several hot herbs, including *bhallataka* plus the tuber known as *surana*, barley alkali, and jaggery; used mainly for abdominal pain, malabsorption, parasites and piles.

Lavangadi Vati Clove, black pepper, *bibhitaki* and *khadira*, with a *bhavana* of decoction of *babbula* bark. It is sucked to soothe the throat and promote expectoration in diseases of the throat and respiratory tract.

Samshamani Vati Essentially solidified decoction of *guduchi*, it is useful in most *pitta* diseases.

Sanjivani Guti A combination of parasite-killing herbs such as *vidanga*, aconite and *bhallataka* with ginger, long pepper, *triphala*, calamus and *guduchi*, and a *bhavana* of cow's urine. In indigestion, loss of appetite, chronic fevers in which all the *doshas* are aggravated, poisoning by various creatures, diarrhoea and dysentery, *Sanjivani* (as its name promises) 'brings the patient back to life'.

Guggulu preparations

While *guggulu* does help to hold pills together, its multifarious uses have given rise to a whole class of compounds in which its scraping and anti-inflammatory actions are directed to their targets by the additions of herbs having appropriate 'fields of action'. Because *guggulu* is used mainly in *vata* and *kapha* diseases, these compounds are usually given with *Maharasnadi* decoction as a vehicle. Almost two dozen compounds of *guggulu* are used in Ayurveda, including:

Gokshuradi Guggulu   Though *guggulu* itself has no particular effect on the urinary tract, this compound does because it contains *gokshura*; it is used in all sorts of urinary diseases and for prostatic problems.

Kaishora Guggulu   Its main ingredient other than *guggulu* is *guduchi*, which makes it effective in the treatment of *pitta*-caused afflictions.

Kanchanara Guggulu   The addition of *kanchanara* (*Bauhinia variegata*) makes this compound useful for swollen glands, particularly in the head and neck region (as in scrofula and Hodgkin's disease), and for fistulas or draining sinuses. It also scrapes fat from the body.

Lakshadi Guggulu   Mixed with red lac and other herbs, this compound is used mainly to help knit together fractured bones.

Mahayogaraja Guggulu   The only common *guggulu* compound that contains minerals, including sometimes gold, *Mahayogaraja Guggulu* is used in diseases of the nerves, such as multiple sclerosis or paralysis, in rheumatism and chronic arthritis, and occasionally in spermatorrhoea, piles, colitis, heart disease, asthma and bronchitis. For best results, it is used in conjunction with an application of *Mahanarayana* Oil or *Mahamasha* Oil to the affected part.

Punarnavadi Guggulu   Given, as *punarnava* would be, for skin disease, jaundice, oedema, ascites and inflammations.

Simhanada Guggulu   Used mainly in the acute stages of rheumatoid arthritis, but also in indigestion due to *ama*, paralysis, asthma, elephantiasis, ascites and hernia.

Triphala Guggulu   A compound of *Triphala*, *Trikatu* and *guggulu* with a *bhavana* of *Triphala* decoction, *Triphala Guggulu* removes obstructions to the channels and dries out the body. It is used in acute arthritis and rheumatism, to help control obesity, and for boils, carbuncles, abscesses, sinuses and so on.

Yogaraja Guggulu   This compound, which contains almost three dozen herbs, is used in rheumatism and rheumatoid arthritis, gout, diseases of the nerves, piles, epilepsy, urinary diseases, heart disease, anaemia and other conditions in which *vata* is aggravated; Sharngadhara claims it makes both men and women fertile. It is given with different vehicles for different purposes (e.g., with cow's urine for anaemia due to *kapha*, with honey to reduce body fat, with decoction of *guduchi* for gout).

One very useful pill that contains *guggulu* is *Chandra Prabha*; it also contains *shilajit*, a variety of herbs such as calamus, nutgrass, *guduchi*, cedar, cinnamon, cardamom, *Triphala* and *chitraka*, the five varieties of salt, and incinerated iron, topped off with a *bhavana* of *Triphala* decoction. *Chandra Prabha*'s name means 'moon shine' or 'moon glow', which refers to its ability to control 'watery' diseases such as diabetes, urinary problems and disturbances of semen (the moon rules the oceans); to regulate and regularize the menstrual cycle (which is ruled by the moon); and to purify the emotions (which are also under the moon's sway).

A partial list of diseases in which *Chandra Prabha* is administered includes albuminuria, urinary stone, urinary obstructions and the twenty types of abnormal urine (including diabetes); pruritis of the vulva, leucorrhoea and ovarian cyst; inguinal hernia, hydrocele and cysts or tumours of the male genitals; and, occasionally, colic, abdominal distension, constipation, lumbago, asthma, cough, psoriasis and other skin diseases, anaemia, jaundice, cirrhosis, piles, enlargement of the liver or spleen, diseases of the teeth or eyes, digestive weakness, loss of appetite and fever.

SNEHA

Sneha (medicated fats) may be for internal use, such as most of the medicated ghees; external use, such as many of the medicated oils; or both, such as *Kshira Bala* Oil, which is medicated with milk and *bala* root, and *Maha Sneham*, a medicated mixture of the four main fatty things: oil, ghee, bone marrow and body fat. The normal proportions for preparation of a medicated fat are one part paste of the drug being used to four parts fat to sixteen parts liquid; this varies according to the specific ingredients used and whether they are fresh or dry.

The drug–fat–water mixture is boiled until the water evaporates; then it is strained. Such fats are cooked until they make no sound when put into fire, when a drop of water makes the fat crackle, when the sound, colour and bubble size of the fat change, and when the foam subsides (in the case of a ghee) or starts to subside (in the case of an oil). In Kerala three states of 'cooked' are distinguished: soft, when the paste of the drugs is still paste-like; unctuous, when the paste has come to the consistency of a wax; and hard-greasy, when the paste has turned black, will keep a finger imprint and can be rolled between the fingers. Cooked beyond the third stage, a fat becomes ineffective; undercooked, it causes *ama* by weakening the digestive fire. Soft-cooked fats are used in Kerala for nasal medication; unctuous-cooked fats are chosen for internal use and enema; and fats cooked to the hard-greasy stage are applied to the body. Milk, yoghurt, rice gruel or other substances called for by the recipe are added to the fat at the mud-like stage (before soft-cooked, when most of the water is gone and the paste is like mud) and then the whole mixture is cooked to the appropriate stage.

Frequently in Kerala some fats, usually oils, are medicated more than once, to potentiate them and enhance their effectiveness. After one cooking the oil is strained and used with fresh water and herbs, and the process repeated as many times as desired. The lower potencies (medicated 3, 7 and 11 times) of oils are used mainly to purify the channels and regulate their flow, and the higher potencies (medicated 21, 41 and 101 times) are used mainly for rejuvenation and aphrodisiac medications. Those oils medicated 1,000 times are even better. An example is *Kshira Bala* Oil.

OILS

Hair oils are commonly medicated with *amalaki, bhrngaraja, brahmi* and hibiscus, all plants that exert beneficial effects on the brain as well as on the hair. Calamus oil, which also helps balance and concentrate the brain, is more often applied into the nose than on to the head. Oil prepared from plant alkalis has been used to treat skin eruptions and earache; *bilva* oil is used in deafness. Other oils commonly used in western India include:

Chandanbalalakshadi Oil   Applied to the chest and forehead in bronchitis, respiratory disease, fever, cough, consumption and pain.

Jatyadi Oil (which includes copper sulphate) and *Nirgundi* Oil Applied to skin diseases.

Mahamasha Oil   Usually contains goat's flesh; is used in paralysis, body pain and other *vata* diseases.

Narayana Oil   Also used in treating paralysis, body pains and other *vata* ailments, and is good for fertility.

Vishagarbha Oil, which contains poisons like oleander, *datura* and aconite and is applied to *ama*-obstructed joints to help pierce the obstruction.

In Kerala the art of medicating oil has been perfected. Some pharmacies in that state produce more than one hundred different varieties of medicated oils. A few of these are:

Anu Oil   Two of its ingredients are rain-water collected from the first downpour of the monsoon each year and goat's milk. It is mainly for use in the nose, for all diseases of the head and its organs.

Bala Oil   For fertility, to cure exhaustion, especially after giving birth, to strengthen delicate people and to cure *vata* diseases.

Dhanvantram Oil   Especially good for chronic *vata* diseases; available in all potencies.

Ganda Oil   Applied to fractures, sprains and strains to help them heal more quickly.

Kshira Bala Oil   For acute and chronic rheumatism, hemiplegia, facial paralysis and so on. The higher potencies are particularly effective.

Pinda Oil   Especially used for acute rheumatic disease when a cooling oil is needed.

GHEES

Medicated ghees are usually taken with milk. They include:

Brahmi Ghrta (with *Shankhapushpi*) For mental diseases and to promote intelligence.

Mahatiktaka Ghrta Made of many bitter herbs, and used for skin diseases.

Phala Sarpis Its main ingredient is *shatavari*, and it is used to promote fertility.

Triphala Ghrta For eye diseases, especially conjunctivitis.

Ghees made from *arjuna, ashwagandha* and *ashoka* For the heart, nervous system and female reproductive tract respectively.

MINERALS

Although minerals are part of the Ayurvedic pharmacopoeia, they must be considered separate from plant and animal substances because their introduction marks a definite change in direction for the Ayurvedic system. Charaka and Sushruta mention only a few minerals. The extensive purification and preparation methods necessary to make such substances fit for use became widely taught and used only in the wake of the spread of the Tantric religion after the beginning of the Christian era. Tantric practitioners experimented with methods for achieving physical immortality; the by-products of these experiments were adopted into Ayurveda as medicines. *Kajjali*, the black sulphide of mercury that is the basis for a wide variety of Ayurvedic medicines, is first mentioned by Vagbhata; and by the time of Sharngadhara, mineral medicines had become prominent in northern India.

There are many possible reasons why minerals displaced plants in northern India, and to some extent in eastern and western India as well. Incinerated minerals make good medicines because, by and large, they get better with age and so there is no expiry date and no danger of waste. There is no need for yearly expeditions to collect and preserve herbs, since minerals can be handed down from generation to generation. Their taste is more neutral and they are less cumbersome to administer. They are also more powerful than all but the most potent (or poisonous) of herbs, and so small doses produce large effects faster than most herbal products can. A more esoteric reason involves astrology: each of the planets has a metal and a gem associated with it (e.g., silver and pearl for the moon, and iron and blue sapphire for Saturn), the ingestion of which helps to attenuate that planet's negative effects on the individual.

Another explanation comes from historical politics. The Muslims who conquered parts of northern India brought with them their own medical system, with its strong alchemical tradition. Southern India, which was little influenced by the Muslims, has preferred to continue to rely on vegetable drugs, Kerala especially maintaining an almost purely Brahmanical tradition of medicine until recently. The breakdown of Brahmanism as a political force in northern India and its gradual supplanting as a popular religion by devotional cults and as a ritual religion by Tantra was probably mirrored by a rise in simplified folk medicines and by the development of Tantric medicine. The Siddha system of Tamil Nadu in southern India, which makes extensive use of minerals, also seems to have been strongly influenced by Tantra.

Preparing minerals

While mercury is the only mineral that can be 'brought to life' (see p. 266), metals and gems can be filled with prana after purification by mixing them with plants (to give them a touch of life) and then subjecting them to sacrifice by incineration, that touch of fire that purifies and potentiates. 'Purification' here refers primarily to purity of the qualities of the material, and only secondarily to chemical purity. A 'pure' substance may be very complex chemically, and two 'pure' substances prepared by different methods may be radically different from one another chemically, but may still perform the same actions when administered to a living being, because their characteristics, both innate and created by *samskara*, are similar.

Purification for metals other than mercury is usually a two-step process: first thin sheets of the metals are heated red-hot and quenched, three times, seven times or more each in sesame oil, buttermilk, cow's urine, sour rice gruel, decoction of *kulattha*, and sometimes latex of *arka* (*Calotropis gigantea*). Easily melting metals such as lead and tin are poured as liquids into these substances instead. Then each metal is further purified according to the requirements of the recipe to be prepared. Finally, they are 'killed', which here means made chemically unreactive, by converting them into oxides or sulphides.

The heavy metals used in modern medicine, such as the gold salts sometimes used to treat rheumatoid arthritis, are toxic and often cause serious side-effects because they are soluble; they enter the circulation and react with the tissues. Ayurvedically prepared metals and minerals are relatively or absolutely chemically inert; they exert catalytic effects on metabolic processes but do not react, or react very little, chemically with the tissues. Hence the tests for a well-prepared *bhasma* (literally, 'ash'; an incinerated metal or mineral): there should be no smoke or colour change when it is added to a flame, which demonstrates its lack of reactivity, and it should float on water and should fill the lines on the fingertip, which demonstrate its particle size.

Because they are not soluble, a *bhasma*'s particles must be tiny for them to work their way into the circulation; a well-made *bhasma* enters the system faster and stays there longer than does a herbal preparation. When administered in the traditional way, by mixing a pinch with honey and placing it under the tongue, a *bhasma* releases to the tissues a subtle form of oxygen, produced during the process of incineration, which provides an immediate 'lift', followed shortly thereafter by the effects of the mineral itself. *Bhasmas* are traditionally stored in such a way that they can continue to take on oxygen.

Mercury

Of all the inorganic substances used in Indian medicine the most important is mercury. While there is disagreement about when and from where mercury was introduced into Ayurveda, some averring that it was adopted from the Chinese and others that it was adopted from Siddha medicine, it is clear that the art of preparing mercury, called *Rasashastra* or 'the science of *rasa*', became the backbone of Tantric alchemy. *Rasa* is one of the names of mercury (another is *parada*, 'that which takes one to the opposite shore of the ocean of manifested existence') because mercury is said to possess all six tastes and, properly prepared, to promote optimal nutrition and health of all the tissues, beginning with *rasa*. Mercury became popular in medicine because it can be used in treating almost any disease; it comes close to being a true panacea because it controls all the body's juices.

Mercury is unique among minerals for another reason: it is the only mineral that can actually be 'brought to life'. Substances that once lived differ from those that have never felt the touch of the life-force; properly prepared, a plant is even more 'alive', more filled with prana, than it was while it lived. Mercury goes through an extensive purification process, after which it is alchemically 'brought to life'. It is then given *samskaras*, as if it were a small child, to mould and shape its force; then its 'appetite' is awakened and it is 'fed', usually with gold; and finally it is 'bound', made to 'swoon' and then 'slain', sacrificed to obtain access to its prana.

Mica

One of the most popular of *bhasmas* is that of mica. There are four varieties of mica – white, yellow, red and black. Only black mica is used in medicine, and it has, in turn, four varieties: when thrown into fire one type leaps like a frog, another hisses like a snake, a third separates into layers, and only the fourth, or 'adamantine', variety remains quiet, even on strong heating; only it is used in Ayurveda. After thorough purification and rubbing with various plants, mica is put into an earthenware dish, an identical dish is placed atop it, and the resulting spheroid is sealed with a cloth and a coating of clay or mud. It is then placed into a *gajaputa*, a cubical hole in the ground one metre (yard) on each side, into which 1,500 cakes of cow dung have been placed (two-thirds of them below the mica and one-third above). The dung is then ignited and allowed to burn out and cool before the dishes are opened and the mica collected. This entire process is one *puta*. Some metals use smaller pits than the *gajaputa*, and others use no pit at all but are incinerated on the earth's surface.

Mica is incinerated at least until it has lost all of its characteristic sparkle, which might take seven to twelve *putas*, but the best quality of mica *bhasma* is that which has been subjected to either 100 or 1,000 incinerations. Each *puta* further potentiates the mica, making its action subtler and subtler, very much as dilutions and succussations (shakings) are used to potentiate homeopathic medicines. Mica that has been incinerated less than 200 times works mainly on the digestive tract; the closer it gets to 1,000 *putas*, the greater its effect on the nervous system and the mind. Part of the effect of the medicine is derived from the purity and intention of its maker, of course, and the value of the higher potencies of mica is enhanced by the tremendous dedication necessary to invest the years necessary to incinerate it 1,000 times. Most Ayurvedic pharmaceutical companies today, pressured by economic constraints, use short cuts, such as electric ovens, to produce their higher potencies of mica; their results do not compare with those obtained through the original process.

Mica, which strengthens both body and mind, is given in asthma, consumption, chronic diarrhoea or dysentery, fevers, diabetes, anaemia, jaundice and enlargement of the liver or spleen. It rejuvenates the respiratory tract. When mica *bhasma* is unavailable, that of magnetic iron is used as its substitute.

Iron

Iron, which is astringent in taste, was one of the first metals to be used Ayurvedically, both as a medicine and in the preparation of medicines, some remedies absorbing iron from the iron vessels in which they were made. The *bhasmas* of magnetic iron, cast iron and steel all have different properties and uses. So, too, does *mandura*, which is prepared by pounding a ball of red-hot iron with a hammer on an anvil and then incinerating the flakes thus produced, allowing them to rust or powdering them after sprinkling them with cow's urine and then boiling them in *Triphala* decoction. Iron salts were apparently also created by smearing iron plates with tamarind, lemon and other sour substances and collecting the granules thus formed. Ten incinerations are usually sufficient to produce a standard quality iron *bhasma*, but, like mica, 100 or 1,000 incinerations are preferred.

Iron *bhasma*, particularly that of magnetic iron, can be used alone as a stimulant in debility, but it is usually combined with other substances. *Navayasa Loha*, for example, contains iron *bhasma* mixed with *Triphala*, *Trikatu*, nutgrass, *vidanga* and *chitraka*. Iron's main actions being on blood, the bowels and the nervous system (the brain absorbs more harmful minerals, like cadmium and lead, when body iron levels are low), it is used in anaemia, consumption, ascites, piles, skin diseases, loss of appetite, digestive weakness, general debility and as a heart and bowel tonic. *Dhatri Loha*, which contains iron, *amalaki* and liquorice, combats hyperacidity, colic, gastric ulcers, anaemia and jaundice. *Saptamrita Loha* is used to treat headache and nosebleeds, and other preparations of iron, such as *Pradarari Loha* (which contains various herbs as well as mica *bhasma*) are given to control leucorrhoea, excessive menstrual bleeding and other female complaints.

Mandura bhasma is diuretic and acts preferentially on the liver and spleen; it is used alone and in combinations, such as *Punarnava Mandura* and *Triphala Mandura*, to treat anaemia, oedema, jaundice, various other abdominal and digestive diseases and generalized weakness.

Iron pyrites, the sulphide of iron better known as fool's gold, is used in Ayurveda as a substitute for gold in treating anaemia, leucorrhoea, urinary diseases, skin diseases, poisoning, diabetes, disorders of the nervous system, jaundice, ascites, eye diseases, fevers, consumption and cardiac weakness, especially in compounds such as Vagbhata's *Tapyadi Loha* (in which it is combined with *shilajit*, silver *bhasma*, *mandura bhasma*, *chitraka*, *Triphala*, *Trikatu*, *vidanga* and sugar). Ferrous sulphate is made into an oil for application to ulcers, and its *bhasma*, which is milder than that of metallic iron, is given for the same purposes. *Gairika*, or red ochre, an iron-containing clay, is used mainly for external application.

Gold, silver and copper

It appears that the gold of gold *bhasma* is still metallic, existing in a state of fine subdivision without being oxidized by the *bhasma*-making process. It is not dangerous to the body since gold itself is a noble metal and does not substantially react with the tissues. Gold is sweet and bitter, but hot, unctuous and heavy, and improves the intelligence, the capacity to learn and the memory. It counteracts the effects of poisons (especially bacteria) on the body, strengthens the nerves and is a rejuvenative and aphrodisiac, acting as a sexual stimulant and increasing sexual power. It is used to increase the mental and physical appetites and to strengthen and invigorate the system, especially in debilitating diseases such as chronic fevers, consumption, neurasthenia, heart disease, anaemia and chronic digestive disturbances. Gold is also reported to arrest pigmentary degeneration of the retina.

Bhasma of iron pyrites is the approved substitute for gold *bhasma*, while gold water (take a piece of 24-carat gold in 16 fluid ounces of water and boil down to 8 fluid ounces; take one teaspoon daily) and gold tincture (immerse a piece of 24-carat gold in pure alcohol in a brown bottle and let it sit for at least one month; the dose is five to ten drops in water) can also be used. Even the wearing of gold can produce a beneficial effect. Pure gold is preferred since after amalgamation with other metals, gold's attributes change; white gold, for example, is cooler than yellow gold.

Silver is cooling though sour, and is used to cool the mind, emotions and body in conditions such as neuritis and neuralgia, inflammations of the mucous membranes, diseases of the reproductive system and lunacy. It is also aphrodisiac and is useful in conditions of debility. Even in ionic form silver is fundamentally non-toxic to human cells, more so than gold. Copper, which is bitter but hot, scrapes excess substances from the system and is used in diseases of *vata* and *kapha*, especially cough, asthma, consumption and afflictions of the liver and spleen. Copper sulphate is applied externally to cauterize skin growths or ulcers.

Other metals

Tin *bhasma* is used mainly for inflammations of the stomach, urethra and other mucous surfaces, especially when mixed with *shilajit* and mica *bhasma*. Its main uses are in diabetes, spermatorrhoea, peptic ulcer, skin diseases and, most importantly, in diseases of the genito-urinary tract. Tin has been shown to protect the testes from damage from cadmium more effectively than even zinc, especially when used as tin sulphide ('mosaic gold', or *Suvarna Raja Vangeshvara*), which shows no toxicity even at twice the normal maximum dose. Being a vasodilator, tin has also been used as a heart tonic. Tin *bhasma* is often used in concert with the *bhasmas* of zinc and lead.

Zinc carbonate (calamine) taken internally helps to dry up the excessive secretions created by inflammations, just as it does externally in the form of calamine lotion. *Bhasmas* of brass and bronze are occasionally used, and antimony sulphide is a reputed eye-lotion.

Most people are unaware that arsenic is an essential micronutrient for the human body. We rarely hear of arsenic deficiency because arsenic appears in many common foods, including corn and linseed. Arsenic oxide is used in Ayurveda as a tonic and cardiac or sexual stimulant, but it is very 'hot', so its sulphides are more commonly employed. *Manasshila* (red sulphide of arsenic, or realgar), is a febrifuge and tonic; its smoke is inhaled to stop spasms of cough or asthma, and it is applied externally to skin diseases. It appears in the asthma-fighting compound called *Shvasa Kuthara*. *Haritala* (yellow sulphide of arsenic or orpiment) is used to reduce fevers, stimulate menstrual flow and, being one of the most powerful of stimulants, to make the feeble stronger and the impotent potent. *Haritala* is used as a *bhasma* as well as in the processed and crystallized form called *Rasamanikya*, which is used in respiratory diseases. It also appears in compounds like *Brhat Kasturi Bhairava* (for chronic fevers), and both it and *Manasshila* appear in *Samirapannaga* (for relief of asthma, neuralgia, chronic fevers) and in *Smrti Sagara Rasa* (used in treating epilepsy, mania and weakness of memory).

Other minerals

Borax is used mainly to expel congestion from the respiratory tract and the female reproductive tract. It appears mainly in combination, in compounds such as *Shvasa Kuthara*, *Mahamrganka Rasa* (for cough, bronchitis, asthma), *Someshvara Rasa* (used to treat leucorrhoea, urinary diseases), *Rajah Pravartini Vati* (to induce menstruation), *Agnikumara Rasa* (to stimulate the digestive fire) and *Karpuradi Vati* (for gingivitis and pyorrhoea). Alum is used in eye diseases, saltpetre as a diuretic, black clay as an astringent, and even asbestos, it is said, was once applied to ulcers.

Various calcium compounds have also found their way into Ayurveda, including *bhasma* of gypsum, which is used as a tonic and antacid; marble, which is sometimes used as an antacid, and lime. Quicklime (calcium oxide) is used externally to burn away unwanted hair, warts or moles, and to treat ringworm. Slaked lime (calcium hydroxide) has been given in diarrhoea, dysentery and vomiting, and for ulcers and burns.

Compounds of mercury and sulphur

Mercury *bhasma* (oxide of mercury), being extremely 'hot', is of limited therapeutic utility. Mercury's chlorides and iodides are soluble and therefore undesirable, but its sulphides are insoluble even when exposed to stomach acid and are non-toxic so long as they are properly prepared and used. In fact, mercurous sulphide (black sulphide of mercury) is used in industrial processes to scavenge free mercury from the environment.

Sulphur is of four types, as students of modern chemistry will agree: yellow, white, red and black. Yellow sulphur is used in Ayurveda to prepare medicines for internal use, and white sulphur is used for those to be applied externally. Sulphur is purified by boiling it in an iron vessel with an equal amount of ghee and, when it melts, pouring it into milk. Like mercury, it is sometimes also sublimed: a small flask is placed in a large, wide-mouthed pot filled with salt, which is then heated; the sulphur or mercury is then brought to 'boiling' by the hot salt rather than direct heat and collected on the bottom of an upper pot cooled with wet cloths. Although sulphur is used in Ayurveda mainly to bind mercury, it has a starring role in *Gandhaka Rasayana*, in which it is given *bhavanas* of cow's milk, cardamom, cinnamon, *tamalapatra*, *nagake-shara*, *guduchi*, *Triphala*, dry ginger, *bhrngaraja* and fresh ginger; this remedy is used in gout, skin diseases, dental abscess, arthritis, diabetes, piles, and other conditions in which blood is polluted.

After the complicated processes by which mercury is purified, including subliming, are completed, purified sulphur is added in a ratio of one part mercury to two, four, eight or even more parts of sulphur, to ensure that none of the metal remains unreacted. The mixture is then slowly rubbed in a large mortar and pestle for at least twenty-four hours until a fine black powder of mercurous sulphide is obtained. This is *kajjali*, used as a medicine itself and as an ingredient in other medicines. *Kajjali,* like *guggulu*, is a superb *yogavahi*; it drags whatever it is mixed with down into the deepest and most inaccessible parts of the system. It also exerts a preservative effect, so pills containing *kajjali* or other mercurial compounds remain potent far longer than purely herbal pills.

When *kajjali* is incinerated, it is converted into red sulphide of mercury – mercuric sulphide – known in Ayurveda as *rasa sindura*. The most famous form of *rasa sindura* is known as *Makaradhwaja*, which has been used in Ayurveda for at least five centuries. Gold is added to mercury before it is made into *kajjali* when *Makaradhwaja* is the ultimate product; this *kajjali* is then placed in a narrow-mouthed glass bottle and gradually heated on a sand bath (that is, as in subliming, but using sand instead of salt) The bottle fills with reddish fumes as the temperature rises, and on cooling *Makaradhwaja* is found at the bottle's neck. It is a strong tonic for the heart and an aphrodisiac and rejuvenator, strengthens the nervous system, and is mainly used therapeutically in respiratory ailments and to overcome mental and physical debility. It is usually given under the tongue, like a *bhasma*, and is sometimes added to *Chyvanaprasha*. A related compound is *Purna Chandrodaya Rasa*, which strengthens all the major organs and promotes vitality and memory. Some call it the greatest of all drugs because it is so useful. *Rasa sindura* is also prepared with silver, copper, arsenic oxide or the sulphides of arsenic.

Other mixtures, like *Suvarna Raja Vangeshvara*, which contains tin and is good for most disorders of the genitals, fail to rise to the neck of the glass bottle during cooking. Still other preparations do not use the glass bottle at all, like *Suvarna Parpati*, a compound that is used mainly in colitis and malabsorption syndromes. Though *Makaradhwaja* has the same ingredients as *Suvarna Parpati*, the differences in processing cause differences in action; *Suvarna Parpati* has no effect on the sex organs, while *Makaradhwaja* does.

Some compounds are prepared only in a mortar and pestle, and others, such as *Hemagarbha* (made of *kajjali* and gold and copper *bhasmas* and used mainly in chronic lung and heart diseases) and *Ratnagarbha* (which also includes gemstones and is used for similar problems), are cooked in a closed pot suspended in a porous bag in an appropriate liquid. *Hemagarbha* is often made into a small stick, which is rubbed on a stone with honey and the resulting paste given as needed; this method ensures small particle size, thorough mixing with the vehicle and quick action.

Among the other widely used medications that contain mercury sulphide are:

Arogya Vardhini   Also contains *bhasmas* of iron, mica and copper, *Triphala*, *shilajit*, *guggulu*, *chitraka* and *katuka* (*Picrorhyza Kurroa*), and is given three *bhavanas* of *neem*-leaf juice. It is given in hepatitis and other forms of jaundice, in liver congestion or cirrhosis, in enlargement of the liver or spleen, and in anaemia, oedema, obesity, diabetes, indigestion and ascites.

Brhat Vata Chintamani   *Rasa sindura* is mixed with the *bhasmas* of gold, silver, mica, iron, coral and pearl, and four *bhavanas* of aloe juice are given. Its main use is control of extremely aggravated *vata* in paralysis, nerve disorders, mental disorders, consumption, heart disease and like conditions.

Chandrakala Rasa   A fine example of how powerfully hot substances can be attenuated by *samskara*, it also contains *bhasmas* of copper and mica attenuated with *bhavanas* of nutgrass decoction, pomegranate juice, Bermuda grass juice, *ketaki* juice (*Pandanus tectorius*, the screwpine flower), aloe juice and other *pitta*-relieving herbs. It is used to calm bleeding and burning sensations all over the body.

Maha Lakshmi Vilasa Rasa   *Rasa sindura* is mixed with aconite and with *bhasmas* of gold, silver, copper, mica, magnetic iron, steel, *mandura*, tin, lead and pearl. One *bhavana* is done with honey, the mixture is then reincinerated and a final *bhavana* is done with *chitraka* decoction. The result is mainly used for lung and heart diseases, for chronic fevers, and for digestive complaints, elephantiasis, migraines, sexual debility, delirium and pains in the joints, head and chest. It is also a rejuvenator.

Suvarna Sutashekhara   Contains *bhasmas* of gold, copper and conch shell, aconite, datura seed, *Chaturjata*, *Trikatu*, *bilva*, *kachoraka* (*Angelica glanuca*) and borax, with one or twenty-one *bhavanas* of *bhrngaraja rasa*. In spite of its many hot ingredients it is used almost exclusively in *pitta* diseases, but only when *pitta* is afflicted by *ama*. Hyperacidity, vomiting, indigestion, headache, cough, asthma, diarrhoea, dysentery, urticaria and *pitta*-caused mental disorders are some of its indications. Its active ingredients are very small in amount when so many *bhavanas* are given, but its effects are substantial because of the potentiation.

Tribhuvana Kirti Rasa   Contains aconite, *trikatu*, borax and long pepper root, with a *bhavana* each of the juices of *tulasi* leaf, ginger root and datura leaf. It is used to break high fevers in pneumonia, influenza, measles, tonsillitis, strep throat and the like.

Vasanta Kusumakara Rasa   Contains *bhasmas* of gold, silver, mica, magnetic iron, tin, lead, coral and pearl, with *bhavanas* of cow's milk, sugar-cane juice, *vasa*-leaf juice, sandalwood decoction, vetiver decoction, turmeric juice, banana stem juice, rose juice, jasmine juice and the water in which musk has been dissolved. It is used in diabetes caused by *vata*, in which it helps rebuild the tissues, and in heart and brain debility, asthma, consumption and sexual debility. It is an aphrodisiac and rejuvenative.

Adulteration of food and medicines was severely dealt with during the Classical period, but as the political situation became more chaotic, the unscrupulous saw opportunities, and widespread adulteration has now been common for centuries. Concern about purity is especially important when selecting metallic remedies, which can be quite poisonous if wrongly prepared. *Caveat emptor*.

Gemstones

Unless they are to be worn, in which case they are subjected to other methods, gems also must be purified, by various processes including quenching in aloe juice or human breast milk, before they are used in medicine. Diamond, because of its hardness, has an especially complicated process including, at various points, the use of *brhati*, *kulattha*, *kodrava*, *haritala*, donkey's urine, horse's urine, the blood of bedbugs and heat; the poisonous frog's urine is also sometimes used. Thereafter the gems are incinerated, or are immersed in alcohol for a month to potentize the alcohol (gems are not boiled in water like metals).

Gemstones have a strong effect on the mind. Most of them promote intellect and longevity; many also virilize. Diamond *bhasma*, one of the most difficult of all *bhasmas* to prepare, gives the body strength and firmness, is a strong aphrodisiac, is good for eyesight and is especially used in chronic debilitating diseases such as consumption, diabetes, cancer and old age; it is also given in impotence. Tourmaline is used as a substitute for diamond. Ruby is very hot, balances the *doshas* (unless *pitta* is already high) and enhances courage; it mainly reduces *vata* and is a tonic for the nerves and heart. Yellow topaz is used mainly to relieve *vata* and *kapha*.

Blue sapphire is reputed to be the most difficult gemstone to use properly, but when it is, it balances the three *doshas*. Emerald does the same, improves the immunity and is especially useful in treating anaemia and asthma. Lapis lazuli is cooling, promotes digestion and tissue nutrition, improves immunity and is useful in chronic debilitating diseases. Turquoise has an anti-toxic effect. Cat's-eye is cooling and, by making *vata* move in its proper direction, promotes increase in the tissues. *Gomeda* (hessonite) cures indigestion and skin diseases and improves strength. Amethyst is good for *vata* and *pitta*; it calms the nerves and the emotions. Quartz crystal is cooling and is used in treating haemorrhages, chronic fevers, burning sensations, anaemia, jaundice, asthma and debility. Wine drunk from a jade or agate cup allays palpitation of the heart.

Undoubtedly the two gems most commonly used in Ayurveda are those that come from the sea: pearl and coral. Both can be prepared as *bhasmas* but are more commonly made into *pishti*, by crushing them, rubbing them thoroughly with rose water or *ketaki* water, and drying them under the rays of the moon. These *samskaras* enhance the gems' already profound cooling effects. Pearl (whose substitute is mother-of-pearl or moonstone) is antacid, nervine and sedative; it calms overexcitability of the nerves and is used in hyperacidity, asthma, cough, consumption, haemorrhages, peptic ulcer, liver and kidney ailments, herpes and most other *pitta* diseases. Pearl is especially beneficial for growing children and pregnant women. Coral is used for basically all the same purposes. Both promote balance in all three *doshas*.

Pearl, coral and mother-of-pearl appear, together with the *bhasmas* of conch shell and cowrie shell, in the compound known as *Pravala Panchamrita*. It, too, is cooling and controls *pitta*; its main effect is on the digestive tract, especially in diseases such as diarrhoea, malabsorption, acid indigestion, gastritis, enteritis, peptic ulcer and cardiac distress. Cowrie, the main ingredient in *Lokanatha Rasa*, works mostly on the small intestine, while conch concentrates on the stomach. Conch *bhasma* is made into a pill called *Shankha Vati*, which relieves loss of appetite, colic, flatulence and abdominal distension, and promotes strong digestion.

Colours

Because good quality gemstones are expensive, sometimes their colours alone are used in medicine. Of these, red and yellow are the two 'hot' colours (just as the spleen and liver, which are 'red' and 'yellow' respectively, are two 'hot' organs). Red has a stronger effect on blood and vitality, and yellow acts more strongly on the digestion. Hue is important; many light yellows are cheerful and digestive, while stronger yellows can promote desire, enhance frustration and make the system bilious. Bilious yellow-green is the colour of jealousy. The red of blood is much more intense and violent than the red of the hibiscus flower.

Red increases metabolic activity and raises blood pressure, 'heating up' the body and stimulating the mind, but may increase *pitta*. Ruby red can increase cravings. Orange has many of red's qualities, but is more mellow. Green, especially grassy green and blue-green, tends to reduce *pitta*, calm the nerves and reduce tension. As the green gets bluer, it gets cooler, reducing blood pressure and metabolic activity. The blues may increase *vata*. While red is the colour of 'hot', passionate anger, blue-black can augment the intensity of 'cold', implacable, hate-filled rage. Overexposure to, or improper assimilation of, sky-blue can stupefy, and even white, the colour of purity, is not wholly innocuous, for when ego becomes overaware of its own supposed purity, white becomes the colour of pride.

Colours can be consumed as medicine by filling a bottle of the appropriate colour (or a clear glass bottle coated in the appropriate colour of plastic or cellophane) with water and exposing it to sunlight for several hours or several days, then drinking that water. Wearing clothes of the appropriate colour also has a significant effect; red clothes help increase digestion and cure constipation (since red enhances *pitta*), while blue clothes may decrease digestion and cause constipation (since blue increases *vata*). Red clothes make their wearer more active and aggressive, and blue clothes create greater introspection.

The effect of tint is not limited to wearing apparel; it extends to the colours of the walls of your living space, the car you drive and every other implement you use frequently; you must make sure that the shades you select keep your *doshas* in balance. Suppose you are angry and about to become violent when you step into a room whose walls are painted bright pink. That pink colour will manipulate your hormones in such a way that your heart will no longer be able to beat fast enough to permit you to explode into a rage. Should you stay in this room for too long, overexposure to pinkness will imbalance your endocrine system, producing in you the condition known as 'malillumination'.

Gold, silver and copper, which are such good medicines for *vata*, *pitta* and *kapha* respectively, can also be profitably consumed as colours. As a part of daily routine, the texts suggest staring fixedly into a golden bowl full of cow's ghee (which is golden in colour). Alternatively, you can stare at the flame of a ghee lamp or imitate those yogis who gaze fixedly at the rising sun just as it is coming up in the morning before its rays become too powerful to damage the vision. Metallic gold is, after all, said to be solidified sun-rays, and, like exposure to sunlight, exposure to it increases both sex drive and fertility, improves some forms of depression and manic-depressive psychosis, and may be helpful in schizophrenia, migraine and anorexia. Silver's beneficial effects can be collected by staring at milk in a silver bowl or at the moon (silver being solidified moon-rays), and copper's effects by gazing at, or surrounding oneself with, copper.

11

DISEASES

Ayurveda's approach to the management of illness is perhaps best illustrated by examining the application of the general principles of treatment to a few specific conditions, tracing the paths of the *doshas* through the wastes and tissues, impelled by causative factors like diet and emotions.

DIARRHOEA

Diarrhoea occurs when, due to various causes, the watery elements of the body undergo increase, invade the digestive tract, quench the digestive fire and get mixed with the faeces. *Vata* then causes them to move downward out of the body in large amounts. One hundred and eight types of diarrhoea, fifty-one of which are due to *ama*, are delineated, and can be classified into six basic categories: due to *vata*, to *pitta*, to *kapha*, to all three, to grief and to fear. In all varieties disturbance of *apana vata* loses its quality of dryness; instead of drying and solidifying the faeces as usual, it breaks them up and mixes them with water. When diarrhoea involves *ama*, disturbance of *apana* is due to obstruction to the channels; otherwise it is due to direct aggravation by the *doshas* or emotions. Whether or not *ama* is present often depends on how long it has taken for *apana* to become disturbed after the digestive fire became weak.

Unlike diarrhoea, which can be either a disease or a symptom, constipation is regarded only as a symptom and not as a disease, except when it occurs as a result of ignoring the desire to defecate. Constipation is, however, never neglected, because it causes other conditions, including sometimes diarrhoea. In India there is a national awareness of the importance of a clean bowel, and Indian

278

patients commonly complain to doctors of all systems that 'my belly just isn't cleaning itself out'. The texts are filled with laxative prescriptions, and traditional Ayurvedic physicians regularly give purgatives to their patients to make sure their wastes flow freely. One reason that *Triphala* is so highly valued in Ayurveda is that in larger doses it is a safe, mild laxative. Overuse of strong purgatives can itself cause both constipation and diarrhoea; such a condition is difficult to rectify because of the profound weakness and lack of tone that develops in the overstimulated musculature of the gut.

The premonitory symptoms of diarrhoea include pricking pains in the chest, navel, rectum, lower abdomen and flanks, weakness of the body, obstruction to free passage of intestinal gas, constipation, distension of the abdomen and indigestion. Diarrhoea due to *vata* alone is often frothy and viscid, and the patient excretes relatively small amounts with noise and pain frequently. When *pitta* is involved, the matter expelled is deep yellow, bluish or reddish from bile, and the patient feels thirst, fainting and burning sensations and may develop ulcers in the mouth. *Kapha*-modulated diarrhoea is often white and mucousy, large in amount, relatively cool and painless, and sometimes causes goose-flesh. When the heat of the tears of a grief-stricken individual disturbs *vata*, or when *vata* is directly increased by fear, liquid is expelled from the body with or without faeces, and usually without any bad smell, at least until the digestive fire becomes sufficiently weakened by the imbalanced *apana* that *ama* develops.

When grief, fear or other factors that immediately provoke *vata*, such as the jolting received by travelling over a rough road or the shock of a sudden plunge into cold water, are the causes of diarrhoea, the aim is to calm the nerves and muscles that have been overstressed with general anti-*vata* treatment plus such substances as *bilva*, nutmeg and marijuana leaves. When, however, the diarrhoea is caused by *ama*, the first treatment is to wait and watch, as it is a natural purification, which should be stopped only if dehydration occurs. If the diarrhoea is suppressed before *ama* has been eliminated from the digestive tract, the residual *ama* will further plug the channels, aggravating *apana* and worsening the problem. It is for this reason that in diarrhoea with *ama*, particularly when there is abdominal distension, heaviness and pain, it is best to give a mild laxative, especially *haritaki*, which digests *ama* while scraping it from the tissues. Such purgation also expels any excess of the *doshas* from the system and so eliminates the proximal cause of the condition. If *vata* is the main cause, enema is often indicated, sometimes with raw blood.

Even if laxatives cannot be used, permitting the diarrhoea to die away on its own drains the excess of *vata* force from the body, making recurrence of the illness less likely. When dehydration threatens, or when the patient is otherwise too weak, too young, too old or pregnant, the desire to calm *apana* must be postponed while the elimination of wastes is temporarily shut down. Ayurveda distinguishes between drugs like kaolin, pectin and atropine, which simply bind up the system, and drugs like *mocha rasa* (the gum of *Salmalia malabarica*), nutmeg, *bhallataka*, *kutaja*, ginger powder, the inner kernel of the mango seed, marijuana leaves, pomegranate, nutgrass, *nagakeshara* (*Mesua ferrea*), *chitraka*, *bilva* and cumin, which improve intestinal tone and 'holding power'. Such substances, called *grahi* in Sanskrit, are the most desirable of remedies for diarrhoea because they return the disturbed organs to normal. Properly prepared, opium can both stop up the intestines and increase their 'holding power'. Doses of *haritaki* smaller than those used for laxation also improve this 'holding power'; *Sanjivani* Pill, which contains *haritaki*, is particularly beneficial. All medications for diarrhoea should be given before food to help calm *apana*.

The best of all *grahi* substances is buttermilk (for those with whom it agrees), which is astringent, sour and sweet, and cures all three *doshas*. Like the milk from which it is prepared, it quickly increases *shukra* and, therefore, *ojas*, and, like milk, which is a secondary tissue of *rasa*, when ingested it performs *rasa*'s function, namely nutrition causing tissue exhilaration. Buttermilk with rock salt and lemon or lime juice kills *vata*; with honey or sugar, kills *pitta*; and with *Trikatu*, kills *kapha*. Once the patient has a desire for food, light food should be given, especially with buttermilk. If fresh buttermilk is not available, fresh non-fat yoghurt blended with at least equal parts of water may be used in its stead. Unblended, undiluted yoghurt has *ama*-increasing properties and should be avoided.

During acute diarrhoea with *ama* only weak tea made from

powdered ginger should be consumed until most of the *ama* is eliminated. Then, or immediately if *ama* was not present, gruel made from roasted grain (especially rice or barley) can be added, consumed with buttermilk. Once the urgency of the condition has been ·eliminated and *apana* has begun to return to normal, the digestive fire must be rekindled with appropriate herbs. The diet must be strictly limited to light, easy-to-assimilate foods until the intestinal tone returns to normal. Medicinal wines are especially useful at this stage, as they improve digestion and relax *vata*. Stimulants like caffeine must be avoided in conditions caused by a sudden *vata* increase or intense emotions, since stimulants worsen *vata* aggravation. Nutmeg can calm almost any diarrhoea.

Diarrhoea, *grahani* (a more chronic condition in which the 'holding power' of the small intestine is lost) and haemorrhoids can all cause one another. Compounds called *parpatis*, made of mercury sulphide mixed with iron, copper, mica or gold, are frequently used in *grahani* (a condition that includes, but is not limited to, sprue, malabsorption, and some dysenteries), and piles are treated internally by medicine to enkindle the digestive fire and externally by fumigation with·such substances as snakeskin, marijuana leaves and human hair. Should diarrhoea become chronic, fear of its return frequently triggers a new attack, since fear is a direct cause of the condition. Reassurance that the condition will not return so long as the dietary and activity guidelines are followed is therefore essential in such cases, lest the vicious cycle perpetuate itself. Time generally lessens grief, but the tendency to fear is innate in *vata*-type people and must be countered by general *vata*-controlling measures, such as oil and heat over the abdomen; deep, slow breathing; simple yoga postures; and meditation.

FEVER

Diarrhoea is often beneficial to the body because it forcibly expels *ama* which would otherwise find its way into the tissues. If *ama* is permitted to remain, it is certain to cause a disease such as fever, which occurs when the *doshas* enter the *Rasa* Channel, most often because of obstructions produced by *ama*. These *doshas* drag heat with them from the digestive fire, weakening it and so setting the stage for increased *ama* production. Normally, excess heat is eliminated from the tissues by sweating, but when *ama* blocks sweat and the heat is unable to exit in any other way, fever supervenes. The premonitory symptoms of fever may include fatigue, restlessness, bad taste in the mouth, discoloration of skin, watering of the eyes, alternate like and dislike for cool wind and warm sunlight, yawning, body-ache, feeling of heaviness in body, goose-flesh, lack of appetite, lethargy, lack of interest in anything and feeling cold. These symptoms vary according to the predominant *dosha* (e.g., less appetite in *kapha*, more burning sensations in *pitta*).

The disease 'fever' is defined as the condition in which there is obstruction to sweat, rise in body temperature and generalized body-ache. There are eight kinds of fever (three caused by one *dosha*, three caused by two *doshas*, one caused by all three *doshas*, and one caused by external causes), and they generally pass through three stages: unripe (*ama*), ripening and *ama*-free. Fever caused by *vata* displays chills or rigours, dryness of throat and lips, loss of sleep and other *vata* symptoms; it comes on and intensifies at irregular times. *Pitta*-type fever produces a very high temperature, loss of sleep, delirium, fainting or giddiness, sweating (an exception to the rule) and other *pitta* symptoms; it usually remains continuously high. *Kapha*-caused fever causes stiffness and ache all over the body, a mild increase in temperature, excessive sleep and other *kapha* symptoms. These symptoms combine when the *doshas* combine, and may produce unpredictable results, as in *vata–kapha* fever (influenza), during which the patient may sweat. Some authorities consider pneumonia to be *vata–pitta* fever.

Before beginning treatment, one must consider the 'gait', or direction of flow, of the heat of the fever. In an 'inward' fever the surface body temperature is not particularly high, but the heat inside produces internal burning sensations, intense thirst, delirium, breathing trouble, giddiness, joint and bone pain, and obstruction to the *doshas* and to urine, faeces and sweat. An 'outward' fever may show a very high body temperature, but the other symptoms it displays are mild and so it is easier to treat. In chicken-pox and measles Indian parents traditionally give their children milk or yoghurt mixed with jaggery, which aggravates the *doshas* and draws them from the extremities back into the digestive tract, thus helping the fever change its course from 'inward' to 'outward'. The child is also surrounded with *neem* leaves to provide a 'cooling' atmosphere.

The treatment of fever proceeds in three stages: at its onset, when *ama* is predominant, fasting is prescribed; in its middle, when *ama* is being digested, medicine to facilitate its digestion; and at its end, when *ama* has been digested, a mild, sweet, *pitta*-calming laxative to expel the accumulated hot *pitta* from the body. Even though purgation is the purification meant for *pitta*, it must not be used at the start of a fever because *ama* obstructs the channels, denying the *doshas* a free passage out of the body. Because fever is a natural protective reaction, which has been shown to perform such functions as improvement in immune function and withholding of nutrients from bacteria, it should not be artificially suppressed unless all other expedients to keep it at a moderate level, such as applying cold compresses, alcohol or ice to the forehead and belly, fail.

The duration of a fever depends upon the movement of the body's *doshas*; just as their movement from their normal locations into the tissues needs time, so also does the reverse movement. *Vata* fever arises quickly and disappears quickly, though it may recur; *pitta* fever takes a moderate amount of time; and *kapha* fever lasts longer than the other two. Fevers that manifest according to climate and season (i.e., *vata*-caused fever in the rainy season, *pitta*-caused fever in the hot season, or *kapha*-caused fever in the winter) resolve more quickly and are easier to treat than those that arise 'out of season'.

Fasting is the best treatment for the onset of a fever, because it both digests *ama* and reignites the digestive fire. If the patient's strength is low, he or she can be given gruel; otherwise, it is best to give nothing but sips of hot medicated water until all the *ama* is gone. Heated water, drinks and food are indicated in all stages of all fevers (except those in which *pitta* is extremely high), since their heat digests *ama* and hastens sweating. Sweating can also be encouraged by indirect methods, such as heavy clothes or blankets, or by sleeping in a closed warm room, but not by direct heat, since *pitta* is central to fever's pathology.

Once *ama* begins to be digested, medicated gruels of rice or mung beans with bitter herbs should be given as a light diet that will encourage both sweating and digestion of *ama*. The bitter taste calms *pitta* and so controls fever from its root. It also purifies the mouths of the channels and ignites the digestive fire. *Guduchi*, *neem* and nutglass are common bitter herbs used for this purpose. *Mahasudarshan* Powder, *Samshamani* Pill, and *Bhunimbadi* Decoction are also employed. The pungent taste, available in such herbs as ginger and holy basil, is used in fevers in which there is much *ama*. *Tribhuvana Kirta*'s poisonous ingredients, such as aconite and datura, help to create sweat when the fever is due to *kapha* or *vata*; *Sutashekhara Rasa* is given in *pitta* fevers when *ama* is present; and decoction of *Trikatu* or *Panchakola* can be used for *kapha*.

If fever becomes chronic, medicated ghee is the best medicine to counteract the dryness of the *rasa* tissue and loss of *ojas* that the abnormal heat causes; Charaka says that treating chronic fever with ghee is like pouring water on to a burning house. The *Vasanta Kalpas* (see 293) are also good, as they contain potentiated butter. The fresh leaf juice or decoction of the leaves or bark of *parijataka* (*Nyctanthes arbor-tristes*), which is one of the five wish-granting trees of heaven, is given for chronic fever, as is a mixture of *guduchi*, *neem* and black pepper.

In periodic fevers, like malaria, treatment during an attack is as for ordinary fever; between attacks one gives bitter herbs, mild laxatives, rejuvenatives and reassurance, not permitting the patient to expect the fever to return. Malaria, the premier periodic fever, is difficult to extirpate from the system, but some success has been reported with compounds of *karanja* (*Pongamia glabra*), *kirata* (*Swertia chirata*), *Evolvulus alsinoides*, *katuka* (*Picrorhyza kurroa*) and *kuberakshi*. *Alstonia scholaris*, or *saptaparna*, seems to cure malaria, and the Chinese have reported success at curing quinine-resistant malaria with an extract of Sweet Annie (*Artemisia annua*).

In fevers resulting from external causes (falling in love, planetary influences, black magic, etc.) *ama* is usually not predominant and the excess heat is eliminated by mild purgation, the use of *pitta*-controlling substances and other methods that draw heat out, such as a cold foot bath or a massage of the soles of the feet with ghee. Entertainment and other pastimes that discourage the creation of anger also help. Above all, the *doshas* must be kept free-flowing. Suppression of a fever with the help of modern drugs drives the abnormal heat deeper and deeper into the tissues instead of permitting the system to experience it and release it. When months or years later that heat can no longer be suppressed, a major inflammation arises as if from nowhere. Once fever reaches the deepest tissues, it becomes very difficult to treat; little wonder that during the Atharva-Vedic era fever was regarded as the king of all diseases.

One potential complication of neglected fever is *rakta pitta* ('*pitta* in the blood', or haemothermia). *Pitta* is particularly associated with sweat and blood. The blockage of sweating that occurs during fever prevents excess heat from exiting the body. Should this heat enter the blood, *rakta pitta* results: the blood takes on *pitta*'s liquid and fluid qualities, losing some or all of its ability to clot. Haemorrhage in the upper or lower digestive tract or through the pores of the skin is the most common symptom, and treatment proceeds along anti-*pitta* lines, especially with the help of substances such as Bermuda grass juice, aloe vera gel, *mocha rasa* (the gum of *Salmalia malabarica*), *vasa* (*Adhatoda vasica*), pearl and coral, lac, *sariva* (*Hemidesmus indicus*), *lodhra* (*Symplocos racemosus*), sandalwood and hibiscus.

The symptoms of freedom from fever are: sweating, lightness, itching of the head, ulcers in the mouth, sneezing and desire for food.

DIABETES

Diabetes is one of a group of twenty conditions, called *pramehas*, in which the quality of the urine is altered. The ten kinds produced by *kapha* are easily curable, the six *pitta* types are curable with difficulty and the four *vata* varieties are incurable but treatable. The most serious form of *prameha* is *madhumeha*, diabetes mellitus. Sushruta distinguished two varieties of *madhumeha*: one genetic (in his phrase, 'caused by *dosha* in the sperm and ovum') and therefore incurable, and the other caused by 'dietary indiscretion'.

Sushruta knew that although diabetic parents tend to give birth to diabetic children, this is not always the case. He writes that the patient of the incurable type of diabetes has a thin, rough body, eats little but is very thirsty and is restless, symptoms that are, in fact, typical of insulin-dependent diabetes mellitus (Type I); and that patients of the latter type (non-insulin-dependent diabetes mellitus, or Type II) are obese and generally indolent. Type II diabetes is, like gout and obesity, known as one of the 'diseases of affluence', which arise in people who have 'too much': too much food, too much leisure, too much comfort. Oversleeping, especially during the day, lack of exercise, laziness and overeating, especially of cold, oily, sweet, fatty things, which increase *kapha*, are said to cause the disease that we know as Type II diabetes mellitus.

The premonitory symptoms of diabetes mellitus include accumulation of tartar on the teeth, burning sensations on the palms and the soles of the feet, stickiness of the skin all over the body, thirst and a persistent sweet taste in the mouth. The characteristic symptoms are: increased frequency of urination, especially at night, delayed healing of wounds and sweetness of the urine.

Treatment depends upon whether *kapha* or *vata* is predominant. If *kapha* predominates, reduction of weight by exercise and change of the diet is often enough to control the problem. The diet should include barley, to help soak up the excess 'moisture' in the tissues; the coarser grains, like millet and sorghum, which with their high fibre prevent simpler sugars from being absorbed so quickly; bitter gourd (the best vegetable for this condition), *kulattha*, mung beans, fenugreek, garlic, and onion. If dietary change alone is insufficient, such substances as *katuka*, *shilajit*, turmeric mixed with *amalaki*, *guduchi*, *neem* leaves, *jambu* seeds, *bilva* leaves and *madhuvinashini* are given. Medicinal wine of *jambu*, *Triphala Guggulu* and *Arogya Vardhini* are also used; the single most useful medicine for *kapha*-type diabetes is *Chandra Prabha*. One popular and effective treatment involves the use of a cup made out of the wood of *asana* (*Pterocarpus marsupium*). Each night the cup is filled with water, which the diabetic drinks the next morning.

Herbs and dietary change must be accompanied by exercise if weight is to be lost. Although vigorous exercise is suggested for *kapha*, many overweight people have *vata* constitutions; for them consistent, mild exertion (such as daily brisk walking) is often sufficient, the idea being to convince the system to burn off some of its extra bulk by raising its overall level of daily activity. While therapeutic emesis (vomiting) is the purification of choice for *kapha*, it is not necessarily appropriate in *kapha*-caused diabetes unless *kapha* is clearly aggravated in the digestive tract, from where it can be extracted. If the condition is very chronic, it may take some time for the *doshas* to present themselves for removal; for this reason consistency in treatment is essential.

Insulin-dependent diabetes is an auto-immune disease in which the immune system attacks and destroys the cells in the pancreas that produce insulin. Emaciation occurs because the sweet fraction of the ingested food is thrown out of the body; it cannot be assimilated because no insulin is available to the system. The bark of *asana* has been reported to regenerate the insulin-producing cells of the pancreas, but this is usually possible only if the disease is of recent origin. It is very difficult for an insulin-dependent diabetic to go off insulin entirely. In such conditions Ayurveda proposes general measures for the control of *vata*, anti-*ama* therapy to reduce the intensity of the auto-immune reaction, and the use of mineral preparations, especially *Vasanta Kusumakara*, which helps blood-sugar levels to stabilize and permits reduction in the dose of insulin.

While insulin and modern drugs can keep a diabetic's blood sugar at or near normal levels, they cannot prevent the varied complications for which diabetes is notorious, many of which are due to deterioration of the blood vessels. Bitter remedies, dietary restrictions and yoga postures all help to prevent such complications. When they do develop, Ayurvedic techniques can assist in their management; for example, carbuncle, a sort of diabetic abscess, is dangerous to lance because of these changes in the blood vessels, and so leeches may be applied to suck the poison out.

RESPIRATORY DISTRESS

Shvasa, or dyspnoea ('respiratory distress'), is defined as 'undue awareness of breathing'. Dyspnoea on exertion means you have trouble breathing only when you exert yourself; dyspnoea without exertion means the problem exists even when you are at rest. Both are caused by the movement of *vata* in an abnormal direction as a result of *vata* alone or an obstruction by *kapha*, which, in turn, is caused by, for example, heavy, sticky, cold, *kapha*-producing food; allergic or sensitivity reactions to food, dust, mould or pollutants;

overexertion; and fear. The same sorts of cause that produce *shvasa* also produce cough, hoarseness and hiccups (whose alternative name – hiccough – indicates its close relationship to cough); these conditions are in a sense the same disease manifested in different locations.

Ayurveda distinguishes five types of respiratory distress: *maha shvasa* (in which the breathing rate is very high with loud breathing like a bull), *urdhva shvasa* (with prolonged expiration), *chhinna shvasa* (Cheyne-Stokes breathing: a high breathing rate followed by no breathing, occurring in cycles of about one minute), *tamaka shvasa* (bronchial asthma) and *kshudra shvasa* (dyspnoea on exertion). The first three conditions are grave signs often portending imminent death; their treatment is difficult. The last is treated by rest and by the same sort of compounds used to treat asthma.

Bronchial asthma is called *tamaka* (dark) *shvasa* because, says the text, 'it always worsens in darkness'. After the sun goes down, patients feel that they are drowning in the ocean of night, oppressed by a feeling of being unable to take in sufficient prana from the atmosphere. The fear generated by this sensation worsens the condition. Characteristically, the spasms are less while sitting and worse when lying down. Bronchial asthma has three subdivisions: caused by extreme *kapha*, caused by minimal *kapha* and associated with *pitta*. Because *kapha* is implicated in all types, even if only slightly, asthma is said to be 'born from the stomach', the principal seat of *kapha*.

Bronchial asthma is one of those maladies, like recurrent fevers and epilepsy, in which the patient suffers periodic 'attacks' of the disease, and treatment during an attack differs from that administered between attacks. During an attack the physician must first decide whether purification or pacification is more appropriate, by evaluating the relative strengths of patient and disease. Purification for the extreme *kapha* type can be done with emesis, or for strong patients, emesis followed by a mild laxative to ensure free downward movement of *apana*, for when *apana* is regulated, prana automatically tends to fall into line. Smoke is often inhaled after emesis; in asthma the smoke of *manasshila* (arsenic bisulphide) sprinkled on a fire is often used. For the minimal *kapha* type, either *kapha* can be increased by 'arousing' it or, since one of the roots of the Prana Channel is the digestive tract and since respiratory distress is often due to the improper upward movement of *apana*, an enema may eliminate the breathlessness.

When purification is not indicated, sips of 2 fluid ounces of strong liquorice tea given with 1 fluid ounce of Narayana Oil with chest fomentation provides some relief in most cases. Application of heat to the chest is essential, since after fomentation the phlegm will come out even by coughing; it is therefore written that in asthma 'even those who should not be fomented,' such as pregnant women, 'should be fomented, if only for a moment'. Saffron given repeatedly with honey can also provide immediate relief, especially when *kapha* is in excess. Inhalation of the smoke of powdered datura leaves cuts short almost any attack of asthma.

Between attacks treatment depends on the precise nature and intensity of the disturbance of the *doshas*. *Shvasa Kuthara* is indicated for the extreme *kapha* variety; it contains *kajjali*, aconite, borax, *manasshila*, black pepper and other herbs, and can also be given sublingually every fifteen minutes during an attack. When stronger medication is needed, one can use compounds such as *Chaturbhuja Kalpa*, which contains *rasa sindura*, *haritala*, *manasshila*, gold *bhasma* and other substances.

Other compounds include powders such as *Sitopaladi* and *Talisadi*; *bhasmas* of deer antler, mica or *arka* flowers (*Calotropis gigantea*); sixty-four times potentiated long pepper, especially for the minimal *kapha* type; jams such as *Chyvana Prasha* and *Agastya Haritaki* to return *vata*'s direction to normal; medicinal wines of *dashamula*, long pepper, datura and ephedra; and compounds of *rasa sindura*. *Hingvashtaka* powder is given when *apana* is clearly involved.

Between attacks yoga postures should be regularly practised, under careful supervision. Breathing exercises are essential and must to be tailored to the individual. All causative factors, especially cold, heavy, oily foods, should be avoided, and ginger and turmeric should be eaten in plenty. Fear is a powerful causative factor and so, as with diarrhoea and fever, regular reassurance that progress is being made is essential, that the mind be strong enough to shrug off fear when blackness descends around it and a spasm seems ready to start. Confidence-building measures, such as the practice of the martial arts, may help free the patient from fear's grip.

Related to *shvasa* is cough, which is caused by irritation from smoke or dust, consumption of dry food, entry of food into the respiratory tract, excessive exercise and suppression of the urge to sneeze. Like respiratory distress, cough is due to change in the normal *gati*, or 'gait', of *vata*, causing prana *vata* to be expelled through the nose and mouth, creating a sound like that made by a broken bronze pot. *Vata* cough is dry and paroxysmal, and leads to difficulty in breathing, chest pain, hoarseness and dryness of the mouth. *Pitta* cough has hot symptoms, such as a metallic or acrid taste in the mouth, thirst, dryness of the mouth, headache and even fever. *Kapha* cough has excess mucus, nausea, indigestion, heaviness of the limbs, loss of taste in the mouth and headache.

Sitopaladi or *Talisadi* powders and the jams of *vasa* or *kantakari* (*Solanum xanthocarpum*) are popular cough-relievers, and most of the substances used to treat *shvasa* can also be used for cough, hoarseness and hiccups. Cystic fibrosis, a condition of chronic respiratory insufficiency caused by abnormally viscid mucus, is also a form of *shvasa*. Though caused by a genetic defect, and so incurable, it often responds to the same sort of methods and substances used to treat other forms of *shvasa*.

CONSUMPTION

If fever was king in the Atharva-Veda, by the Classical era consumption had become the foremost of ailments. In Ayurveda consumption is called *raja yakshma*, meaning both the 'king of diseases' (because of its numerous symptoms and complications) and the 'disease of kings', as explained in the chapter on pathology. It is an ancient disease; the Rig-Veda contains a charm for chasing *yakshma* from all parts of the body. One reason consumption was so feared is that parents can transmit its tendency to their children as a sort of karmic *dosha* or miasma, the 'tubercular miasma' that is well known to homeopathy. *Raja yakshma* is not limited to pulmonary tuberculosis; it includes all causes that 'consume' the body. Chronic beryllium poisoning and the disease sarcoidosis produce pathological changes in the tissues almost identical to those produced by TB; though the proximate causes differ, the product is effectively one.

Neglect of other respiratory diseases can lead to consumption, whose principal causes are grouped into four categories:

Recklessness or foolhardiness 'The performing of an action without regard to your capability to perform it'; Madhava mentions as examples fighting with strong opponents, falling from heights, forcibly restraining running bulls or horses, taming or fighting with wild animals such as elephants, throwing heavy stones or logs, reading loudly, long-distance running, swimming mighty rivers, running along with horses, sudden jumping, strenuous dancing and other such violent, ill-thought-out acts.

Restraint of natural urges.

Wasting of the tissues Particularly caused by excessive orgasmic sex, but also grief, old age and excess exercise,

Improper diet Chiefly exceedingly heavy, oily and cold, *kapha*-increasing food or excessively dry, scanty, non-nutritious, *vata*-enhancing food.

All three *doshas* are involved in consumption. It can develop in two ways: the normal direction ('with the hair') and the reverse direction ('against the hair'), which refer to the direction of nutrition of the tissues. Both result in bodily drought, as Charaka writes: 'When the increased doshas led by *kapha* block the Channels of first Rasa and then the other tissues, or when the tissues beginning with shukra are depleted by such practices as excessive sex, then all the tissues become wasted and the patient dries up.'

Depletion of the tissues by *vata*-inducing causes, such as excessive sex, results in bodily drought quickly; *vata* is quick and dry, so 'juice' is lost directly. This is, however, the reverse direction of pathology, 'reverse' because the higher tissues become emaciated before the lower ones. The lower tissues suffer first and the disease develops more slowly when the pathology proceeds in the normal direction, as a result of increased *kapha*, which is slow and wet. Only after this watery element obstructs the channels and blocks *vata*'s flow does inadequate tissue nutrition develop.

The prodromal symptoms of consumption include respiratory distress, body ache, runny nose, dryness of palate, vomiting, digestive weakness, cough, increased sleep and a sort of 'toxicity' of mind and body. Some people's eyes become bright white and they crave meat and sex; others dream of being carried away by a crow, parrot, porcupine, peacock, vulture, monkey or chameleon, or see rivers without water, trees without leaves, wind, smoke or forest fires, symbolic of the storm of dryness gathering within the body.

Consumption, especially in its form as pulmonary tuberculosis, produces a wide variety of symptoms. Some of the first to appear are 'complete heating' (a sense of affliction in the shoulders and flanks), burning of the hands and feet, and fever. The fever is often high, but the patient thinks it is mild because of the distorting effects of 'complete heating' on the mind. These are followed by aversion to food, respiratory distress, cough, hoarseness, diarrhoea, blood in the sputum, a feeling of fullness in the head and irritation of the throat.

Purification is usually not called for when consumption has developed in the reverse direction, but even when *kapha* is high, no purification is permitted initially because 'the patient's strength is due to faeces alone', which is to say that only the presence of faeces in the colon restrains *apana* from becoming thoroughly disturbed, as *vata* always does when its residence becomes empty, and further drying up the system. Both constipation and diarrhoea must be prevented.

Charaka tells us that 'in consumption the patient should eat meat, drink wine and always be free of worries'. This is not the normal 'eating, drinking and being merry' that may have led to the patient's downfall in the first place; this is the judicious use of meat, medicinal wine and rest that can fan the almost extinct fire of life back into a flame. Medicinal wines are prescribed according to the pattern of symptoms present, but those of grapes and *Dashamula* are commonly used. The meat indicated is the meat of carnivores, whose digestive fires are strong enough to digest meat itself, a very heavy substance. Their meat, in a sense, digests itself.

Francis Zimmermann observes that the carnivore is at the top of the food chain, just as *shukra* is at the top of the tissue chain. Soup of the meat of carnivores is, therefore, highly concentrated 'juice', the essence of an animal whose flesh is composed of the essence of other animals whose flesh is composed of the essence of plants. Lions, tigers, panthers, jackals, hyenas and vultures were once eaten for this purpose. Now that their meat has become difficult to procure some physicians advise their patients to eat crow – a sound suggestion even symbolically, since too often the cause of the patient's plight is wilfulness, for which 'eating crow', that admission of responsibility for one's state that is a prerequisite for healing, is the cure.

Tuberculosis is still an ailment to reckon with in many parts of the world, and is rising again in the West thanks to the AIDS epidemic. AIDS is itself a consumptive disease; it 'dries up' the body, which cannot nourish its tissues without healthy *rasa*. Like classical consumption, in AIDS one must first change one's ways, relinquishing the recklessness that leads to 'volitional transgression'. Then the aim is to maintain the strength of the digestive fire, keep the channels unclogged and ensure that the tissues are pampered and well-fed.

Most substances used to treat respiratory distress can also be used to treat consumption. Mineral compounds including *Makaradhwaja* and *Purna Chandrodaya Rasa* are often used because of their ability to strongly stimulate the body's fires. *Vasanta Kusumakara* is used, as in diabetes, to nourish the tissues, and *Brhat Vata Chintamani* helps prevent *vata* from cycloning out of control. *Vasanta Kalpas* are particularly good for the fever of consumption, which dries out the tissues. These *kalpas* contain mercury sulphide, to nourish *ojas* and penetrate every cell in the body; zinc carbonate, which enhances the digestive ability of the tissues; and black pepper, which enhances digestion. To protect the tissues from dessication by black pepper, which is dry, the *Vasanta Kalpas* are potentiated with butter. Because butter may obstruct the channels, the final potentiation is done with juice of the Indian lime, which enkindles fire and rejuvenates.

Laghu Malini Vasanta is used when symptoms like fever are more pronounced; *Swarna Malini Vasanta*, which contains gold, when the Prana Channel needs support; and *Madhu Malini Vasanta*, which contains eggshell *bhasma*, to promote strength when the disease is ravaging the deeper tissues, such as flesh or *shukra*. The *Vasanta Kalpas* also prove useful in other diseases that require *kapha* or *ama* to be scraped, including fever, cough, leucorrhoea and, sometimes, diabetes and heart disease.

HEART DISEASE

Hrdroga is not limited to the modern 'heart disease' but also encompasses other conditions occurring in the region of the heart, including pressure applied to the heart by gases in the stomach or colon, which, if they persist over a long period, may affect the heart adversely. The heart is the root of the *Rasa* and Prana Channels and the seat of *ojas*, the mind, and of consciousness. There is no doubt that the seers who formulated Ayurveda were aware of the brain's importance, and these statements should be understood to mean that your consciousness resides in your heart most of the time, whether or not you are aware of it. The chief causes of heart disease are excessive thinking and worry, activities that reflect an overuse of the mind, which overworks the organ in which it resides much of the time. 'Thinking' includes both linear, mundane thinking and emotional thinking; when their free expression is inhibited, the emotions oppress the heart and weaken its muscle. This is one possible reason for the fact that many more men than women have heart attacks, since men are usually taught to hold in tears and women are usually permitted to allow them to fall freely. Men also often seem to learn to be distrustful and quick to anger, both of which damage the heart.

These mental factors interact with various physical factors to create heart disease. *Vata*-inducing causes, such as over-exercise, restraint of natural urges and overactivity aggravate *vata* and promote spasm in the circulatory system. When *pitta* is aggravated, it narrows the channels by promoting inflammation. *Kapha*-enhancing causes, such as heavy, cold, sticky food, lack of exercise and sleeping during the day, increase the body's 'moisture' and cause obstruction by clogging vessels with *ama* (when cholesterol, an essential nutrient, appears where it does not belong, it is 'undigested' and hence a form of *ama*). Inflammations of the heart have strong *pitta* involvement; disorders of heart-rate and ability to pump are caused mainly by *vata*; and congestive heart failure, often a result of an excess of 'moisture' in the system, is often caused by *kapha*. A variety of heart disease resulting from parasites is also distinguished; it may be caused by one or more of the *doshas*. High blood pressure is usually due to high *pitta*.

The general symptoms of heart disorders include discoloration of any kind (which sometimes shows lack of oxygen in the tissues), fainting, fever, cough, hiccups, respiratory distress, disturbed taste in the mouth, thirst, disturbances to the consciousness, vomiting, increase in *kapha*, pain, loss of appetite and oedema (especially over the feet, mainly in the evening). Most of these can become diseases in their own right as complications.

Treatment of heart disease begins with removal of the cause: elimination of the worrying and thinking that impede the proper flow of blood to the organ. Direct purification is usually not advised, though *apana* and the bowels must be kept moving normally. The *doshas* must also be balanced by appropriate therapy according to their degree of disturbance. Substances used in the treatment of heart disease include, according to the *dosha*, elecampane; deer antler *bhasma*; ghee medicated with *arka*; wine of aloe vera, *Dashamula* or *arjuna*; compounds containing mercury sulphide, including *Hrdayarnava Rasa*, *Suvarna Malini Vasanta* and *Hemagarbha*, and *Karaskara Kalpa*, which contains purified nux vomica, whose strychnine tones and activates the heart muscle; purified oleander root, which, like digitalis, contains an alkaloid that regulates the heart's rhythm; and long-pepper powder.

Food should be light and warm, with plenty of garlic (except for *pitta*), onions and ginger added. Old jaggery (at least seven years old) and old honey (as honey ages it becomes more medicinal) benefit the heart; one folk heart-tonic is the juice of one medium-sized onion plus one tablespoon of honey taken each morning before breakfast. Sugary sweets, over-refined foods, fat and caffeine, alcohol and other stimulants should be eliminated or significantly reduced, and a healthy daily routine including meditation, exercise and massage should be implemented.

For decades modern doctors believed that blocked arteries could not unblock themselves. Only recently have studies appeared proving clearly what Ayurveda has known for ages: that lifestyle changes can actually reverse coronary artery blockage and increase blood flow to the heart. Such dramatic improvements are accomplished not by drugs or surgical therapy, but by a comprehensive programme of health improvement. Dr Dean Ornish of the University of California in San Francisco prescribes a regimen that closely resembles the Ayurvedic one: a near-total vegetarian diet with an extremely limited fat intake, no caffeine, alcohol limited to a maximum of 2 fluid ounces daily, regular exercise and, most importantly, meditation, stretching and other relaxation practices derived from yoga. To help cope with the effects of these lifestyle changes, Dr Ornish's patients meet as a support group twice a week, a function that in India is often served by the joint or extended family. This regimen causes chest pains to disappear and arterial clogging to reverse in most patients.

Most surprisingly, Dr Ornish's study showed that the arteries often unclogged even without significant decreases in blood cholesterol levels. This finding agrees with other studies, which have shown that a lowered heart-rate tends to reduce clogging even when combined with a high-cholesterol diet, and that people who are peaceful and calm rather than tense and agitated rarely show elevations of blood cholesterol no matter what they eat. Moreover, the mental imagery associated with happiness, sadness, anger and fear can be differentiated by cardiovascular changes; the state of your consciousness thus exerts an immediate and frequently profound effect on the state of your body, especially your heart. Because all of us have images of all sorts in our minds at all times, it behooves everyone who wants to be healthy to ensure that the images they create for themselves are healthy ones. Most of us still believe that something has to be 'done' medically in order to tackle heart disease, when actually what needs to be done is to change the way we live.

THE DISEASE OF *VATA*

'Disease of *Vata*' is an umbrella term that includes most of what allopathic medicine calls musculo-skeletal diseases. There is no '*pitta* ailment' or '*kapha* malady', because when *pitta* and *kapha* combine with the tissues and wastes, they produce symptoms that differ from their own qualities, while *vata*-produced symptoms are much like *vata*'s own qualities. Disease of *Vata* is a sort of possession of the body by the demented genie of *vata*, producing contractures, curvatures, fractures, breaking pains, cutting pains, stiffness, lameness, paralysis, paresis, wasting, tremors, tics, convulsions, exaggerated reflexes, loss of sensation or function, loss of speech, loss of sleep, and obstructions to the channels by tumours and stones (urinary and other).

When *vata* penetrates the tissues, it creates characteristic symptoms: *vata* in blood can cause ulcers, boils and the like; in flesh and fat it causes exhaustion and a feeling of having been beaten with a stick; in bone and marrow, loss of strength in the body, loss of sleep, pain like that from being stabbed by a trident or spear, especially in the joints, and continual pain all over the body. The five *vatas* (prana, *apana*, *samana*, *vyana* and *udana*) can also be 'covered' by *pitta* or *kapha*, producing various symptoms.

Many of the ailments that collectively make up Disease of *Vata* can be correlated with modern diseases, including temporo-mandibular joint misalignment, proctalgia fugax (intense rectal pain), torticollis (wryneck), glossal palsy (paralysis of the tongue), sciatica (whose Sanskrit name refers to a vulture; a sciatica patient sometimes walks like a vulture because of the pain), tetanus and that facial paralysis which resembles Bell's palsy, resulting in asymmetry of the face, with a drooping angle of the mouth and pain, said to be caused by such activities as excessive laughing, talking or other facial activities, uneven sleeping postures and the carrying of headloads.

Characteristic of all forms of Disease of *Vata* is their tendency to repeatedly flare up after exposure to causative factors and then slowly die down until the next occasion. Differential diagnosis is important, because the same symptoms can be created by very different pathologies. For example, the chief symptom of 'Immobile Thigh' is suggested by its name; but in this case the immobility is due to the filling of the thigh with *ama*, *kapha* and fat. 'If the doctor foolishly treats this condition with oil massage,' says Charaka, 'it exacerbates quickly.'

The treatment of Disease of *Vata* is the treatment of *vata*. When it is caused by obstruction of the pathways, substances such as garlic, *rasna*, ginger, calamus, valerian, *Trikatu*, *Dashamula*, *Vata Vidhwamsa* and various *guggulus* are used, and external application is limited to castor oil or a few medicated oils, and dry heat. When it is a result of wasting of the tissues, *guggulu* must be used with caution, since it scrapes the tissues and dries them out and could cause further *vata* increase. Instead, the body should be strengthened, and nourishing oils and wet heat applied. *Bhallataka*, in those who can tolerate it, can be used to treat many kinds of Disease of *Vata*, as can metallic compounds such as *Brhat Vata Chintamani*. Branding is sometimes used in treating sciatica.

Because the chief characteristic of Disease of *Vata* is that it surges and ebbs, a consistent, regular lifestyle is the only permanent answer to *vata*'s innate erratic quality. Pain being a prominent symptom in most forms of *vata* disease, the combination of aversion to pain and concern that it may return inexorably promote deep-seated fear. As with other conditions in which fear is an important factor, reassurance and confidence (in oneself or one's therapist) are essential to the healing process.

CANCER

Though some members of the family of ailments that make up Disease of *Vata* can be correlated with some specific musculo-skeletal or neurological diseases in modern medicine, Disease of *Vata* cannot be equated with any single pathological category. Like Disease of *Vata*, cancer is a group of related conditions. The hallmark of cancer is the rebellion of cells against the organism's 'I-ness' (self-identity), the rebels proliferating wholly on their own, out of control due to repeated immuno-insult. All cancers involve all three *doshas*, but when a cancer arises as a result of deranged *vata*, and its presenting symptoms are identical with one of the forms of *vata* disease, it must be identified as Disease of *Vata*, even though all cancers are not Disease of *Vata*, just as Disease of *Vata* is not limited to cancer.

Dr Vasudev D. Agate is a professor of anatomy in the Ayurvedic college in which I studied. His tribulations began on 17 April 1988 at about 10:15 PM while lying on his bed. Suddenly an intense shooting pain began in the centre of the bottom of his left foot, so sharp that he first thought someone had stabbed him. No treatment could relieve his increasingly severe pain and tenderness. Blood tests showed almost ten times more white blood cells than normal, of which 19 per cent were 'blast' cells (immature forms). This report was confirmed by a second test, and then a bone-marrow biopsy was performed. On 2 May the bone-marrow report suggested a diagnosis of an advanced stage of acute myeloblastic leukaemia (AML), a disease in which, even with chemotherapy, most patients do not survive much longer than a year. Given that Dr Agate's blast cells had increased to 67 per cent by 3 May, the specialists gave him between eight days and two months to live, and said that he might depart in as little as twenty-four hours. They offered him expensive experimental treatments, but unofficially, doctor to doctor, they told him not to bother, just to go home and try to be comfortable until the end came.

With this death sentence from the experts, Dr Agate gave in to extreme emotional upset and continuous weeping. On 3 May Vaidya B. P. Nanal, Poona's most eminent Ayurvedic physician, visited Dr Agate's home and spent four hours taking a case history. This showed that what seemed to be a disease of sudden onset had, in fact, provided ample indications of its intentions. In March Dr Agate's wife had had an unusual and foreboding omen, and from 2 April onwards Dr Agate had suffered from pains in strange locations, such as the centre of the forearm and the centre of the palm. He and his wife, who is also a doctor, thought these must be due to over-exertion. Ayurvedic medicine stopped the pain temporarily, and on the morning of 17 April Dr Agate had said, 'I won't exert myself at all today. I'll rest all day long and see what happens.'

Vaidya Nanal has preserved records on Dr Agate since 1967, showing a 'very delicate' *vata–pitta* constitution, poor nutrition of the marrow tissue (as shown by a detached retina he had had after sports, and an episode of sudden, temporary blindness), poor nutrition of blood (his blood haemoglobin had never been above 7.5 gm/100ml, about half of normal, and he had a pronounced tendency to nosebleeds and other minor haemorrhages, especially during the summer months), and a pronounced habit of eating every sort of junk food.

Vaidya Nanal ignored the blood reports, the bone-marrow tests and the allopathic diagnosis, preferring to look at the case purely with Ayurvedic eyes. When *vata* penetrates the bone or marrow tissues, the result is intense pain in the bones and joints, which flits from joint to joint and muscle to muscle, loss of strength in the muscles, loss of sleep and constant pain in the body. These symptoms, and the history of poor nutrition of the tissues, made the diagnosis clear: Disease of *Vata*, namely, *vata*-in-bone-and-marrow, with secondary loss of *ojas* (a symptom of which is extreme fear). The prognosis, Vaidya Nanal thought, was not good: 'If he keeps to the regimen, all will go well, but this is only physical treatment; he also needs the proper mental attitude, and right now he is in a state of terror; even if his power of discrimination is working satisfactorily, *ahamkara* may create a problem.'

Vaidya Nanal has preserved twenty years of cases of cancer patients who had been completely cured of their cancers with Ayurvedic treatment following chemotherapy, surgery or radiation. Here, however, there was no question of allopathic therapy, so Ayurveda alone would have to suffice. The main aim would be to calm *vata* and purify blood. Dr Agate stopped all treatment from other doctors (except for homeopathic cell salts) and began Vaidya Nanal's treatment on 7 May at 7 AM. First was a powder containing *bhasmas* of silver and tourmaline, mixed with *ashvagandha*, *sariva*, purified sulphur, pearl extract, purified nux vomica and other ingredients, taken with *Dhatri Leha* (a medicated jam made of *amalaki*), after which he ate two almonds that had been soaked overnight, and then milk medicated with *ashvagandha* and other herbs. After half an hour he took two pills of *Arogya Vardhini* and two pills of a turmeric preparation with three teaspoons of ghee. 'Most scientists', says Dr Agate, 'say not to take fat in cancer, but I took a lot.'

At noon and in the evening he took two more *Arogya Vardhini* and two more turmeric pills, and at night a heaped teaspoonful of *Gandharva Haritaki* (a preparation of *haritaki* in castor oil) with a decoction of herbs including *sariva*. In addition, three times a day *Bala Narayana* Oil was gently applied to his whole body for half an hour, followed by a fifteen-minute application of warm water to induce mild sweating; oil and heat are crucial for control of *vata*. The oil had to be applied very slowly and without pressure, as otherwise he would shout with pain.

Cancer seems to develop in a particular organ because of that organ's psychological significance. While that organ is sometimes a good place to begin therapy, it is not a good place to remain, because real health involves the whole organism. Removing the malignancy from the affected body part must be coupled with making that part return to harmony with the whole organism, lest the disease recur elsewhere later. None of Vaidya Nanal's medicine was given with the intention of killing the aberrant blood cells, which, after all, were only the symptoms of the problem, the indicators that allowed us to know that the bone marrow was not healthy. Instead of trying to smash non-functional tissues, Ayurveda coaxes them to begin working again by rekindling their digestive fires and nourishing them. Violence enhances cellular fear; nourishment, cellular confidence.

Dr Agate's pain gradually disappeared within ten days of commencing this treatment, and he began to be able to walk around in his room. After fifteen days he could walk to the bathroom; after three weeks, he walked on his own, without any support. After a month he was able to bathe with his own hands. The migratory pain in his joints was more persistent, but it totally disappeared within three months, as did his constant low-grade fever.

After a month and a half of therapy, Vaidya Nanal changed the medicine by adding gold *bhasma* and removing sulphur, nux vomica and pearl, and by substituting *Laghu Malini Vasanta* for the turmeric pills. Also, finding that his patient had had severe constipation for at least the past twenty years, he added an enema of 4 fluid ounces of sesame oil, given at night. Told to hold the oil as long as possible, at least fifteen minutes, Dr Agate dedicatedly held the oil inside all night long, and did so every night for three months until November, when it was changed to alternate nights. By January he was getting a good bowel movement only on the days when there was no enema; and when he took the enema, his bowels would not empty properly. Vaidya Nanal then told him, 'Now you no longer need the enema; when a treatment starts to give you a result contrary to what you had expected, you must change it.'

The nosebleeds that had troubled Dr Agate persistently throughout his life troubled him a lot during this treatment. Nosebleed is actually quite common in leukaemia, and patients often die due to this or other haemorrhage. May is in the middle of Poona's summer, and each May evening under the influence of summer-induced *pitta*, his nose would bleed from about 7 PM. until 1 or 2 AM, causing him and his family extreme concern. Vaidya Nanal directed him to soak cotton with Bermuda-grass juice and pack his nose with it for the whole night and, if necessary, the next day. After this treatment, the bleeding stopped intermittently for two or three days, and after about five days, it stopped for good; it has not returned. 'Beside its well-known haemostatic effect,' says Dr Agate, 'we in India believe that Bermuda grass is good for removing obstacles, since it is beloved of Ganesha, the god who removes obstacles.'

The blast cells in Dr Agate's blood started returning to normal after about six months, but Vaidya Nanal never even bothered to look at the blood reports; they played no part in his evaluation of his patient. One day in November during a routine visit Vaidya Nanal's face displayed a very serious mien, and he told Dr Agate, 'You are responding well, but as long as there is fear in your mind, there will be a problem. I am working on your body only, but we must remove the fear. You must now start repeating the Gayatri mantra.'

The Gayatri mantra is the premier Vedic mantra, an invocation to the sun. Dr Agate was at this time somewhat agnostic and had little faith in mantras, but he had tremendous faith in Vaidya Nanal, who had pulled him back from the very door of death, and so he began to repeat the Gayatri mantra 108 times a day, with inhalation, retention of breath and exhalation at specific syllables. It did not take long for the result to show itself: his fear disappeared, replaced by an overwhelming confidence. Now he repeats Gayatri all day long, whenever he has free time, more than 1,000 times daily.

When a mantra is repeated, it creates an image, perceived or not, within the mind of its repeater. By repeating the Gayatri mantra, Dr Agate created an image of the sun within his consciousness. The sun is a powerful, noble, health-giving, disease-destroying being whose rays dispel fear and weakness from the heart, and this image of the sun, coupled with the vibrations of the mantra, transmitted these positive qualities into Dr Agate's often-negative mind and revolutionized it. Mental imagery, especially visualization, is so powerful that 'seeing' can truly become believing, which is why it must be used with great care. Every thought inexorably exerts its effect on the body; in imagery the end does not justify the means, the end *is* the means. Visualizing violence, such as attacks against cancer cells, reinforces violence; cancer cells are, after all, the body's own, and to attack them is to attack the body. There is already too much violence in the world; we need to visualize benign, constructive presences and with their help create benignness in our own lives.

It cannot be too strongly emphasized that the Gayatri mantra is no more a 'cure for cancer' than is gold or silver *bhasma*, *ashvagandha*, *amalaki* or any other herb or mineral. 'Cancer' is an allopathic disease, and *'vata*-in-bone-and-marrow' is an Ayurvedic condition. Vaidya Nanal stresses that not only does he use different medicines for different people, even in the same condition, but that he would also have suggested a different mantra for a different sort of patient. Therapy must be tailored to the precise needs of the individual being treated.

Dr Agate began going to the Ayurvedic college again in July 1988, and resumed his normal schedule of lecturing from mid-August. He continued to oil and heat himself thrice daily for about a year and a half, and now does it only daily because the pain has totally disappeared. The skin rash that he had since almost the start of his illness has improved but has yet to fully disappear, and he still has other minor symptoms, such as occasional bleeding gums and dry cough, but overall, in mid-1991, he has been back to near normal for more than two years.

When he did not quickly die, the cancer experts decided, 'We must have made an error in diagnosis; it must be pseudo-leukaemia.' But re-checking all the blood slides convinced them that the first diagnosis had been right. Then they said, 'Well, it must be in remission. Be prepared, it will return.' Vaidya Nanal replied, 'I never diagnosed cancer, so I have no opinion on whether or not it is in remission. Our way of thinking is totally different from the allopathic approach.'

Cancer might as well be called 'giving up', since it is a disease in which your 'I-ness' 'gives up' its responsibilities and permits a new centre of self-awareness to arise within your organism. Dr Agate's organism 'gave up' because of a combination of physical and mental factors. Sometimes extreme physical damage, as by radiation, chemicals or chronic hepatitis B infection, is alone sufficient to induce surrender even in the most positive, well-adjusted, bipolar individual by convincing the body's cells that continued life is impossible. Sometimes otherwise healthy bodies are consumed when their minds lose their 'reason for living'. Usually, though, all three Sheaths (of Food, Prana and Mind) are attacked by causative factors when 'I' decides to throw in the towel, and all three sheaths require treatment if 'I' is to reclaim its birthright. Most important, however, is treatment of the mind, because cancer is an assault on the deepest level of your 'you-ness', your existence as an individual, and only healing of that individuality can remove the malignancy from all your parts.

You have to sit down and talk to yourself, no matter how silly it may seem; have a meeting of the members of the board of directors of your being, and let mind, body and spirit take some drastic steps to change things. If, like Mary, you choose to personify your 'shadow self' and 'give it a talking to', you had best be sure you will be able to 'send it packing' when you are through with it. And you must send it packing with love, not hate, unless you want to retain that hate within you, ready to whelp another shadow-being when conditions become ripe. If you do not feel strong enough to deal with your 'shadow self' on your own, you should find something (like the sun) or someone who can induct that image into your being, and let he, she or it do the work.

Diarrhoea, one of the shallower disturbances to one's identity, and cancer, one of the most profound, both share *prajnaparadha* as their prime cause. 'Physical treatment for physical diseases' is an Ayurvedic motto, but physical treatment alone is rarely sufficient to extirpate all traces of disease from a being because it cannot oust 'volitional transgression' from the mind. Only that health improvement plan that redresses imbalances on all levels of an organism qualifies as true Ayurvedic therapy.

12

REJUVENATION AND VIRILIZATION

In Sanskrit rejuvenation is *rasayana*, literally 'the path of juice', a process of replenishment of the quality and the quantity of the body's fluids. Ageing means loss of juice; just as old leaves dry out and blow away, bodies become shorter, smaller and stringier as they age. Joints dry out and leak; plasma volume decreases, as does total body weight; mass is lost from the bones by osteoporosis. Sharngadhara notes that with each passing decade the body loses, one by one, childhood, growth, lustre and complexion, intelligence, skin health, strength of sight, virility, valour, discrimination, the use of the sense organs of action, the use of the other senses and, finally, if one reaches the goal of 120 years of age, one's life itself. *Rasayana* is meant to enhance health and *ojas*, produce top-quality bodily tissues, eliminate senility and other diseases of old age, lengthen life and enhance memory, intelligence, youth, lustre, sweetness of voice, strength of body and senses, and beauty.

Though healthy *rasa* tissue is essential to produce healthy blood and other tissues, the *rasa* of *rasayana* reflects more the concentrated hormonal essences, like *ojas*, and that mysterious secretion of the pineal called *amrta*, the nectar of immortality. Some seekers spend their entire lives searching for *amrta*, either from their own internal supplies or from external sources. Tantric alchemy was founded on attempts to convert mercury, which is esoterically the semen of Shiva, the god of transformation and death, into *amrta*. Recall that mercury, the only common metal that is liquid at room temperature (and therefore predominantly composed of the water element), is also called *rasa*. It is said that by the judicious use of rejuvenating herbs one can prolong one's life by four to five hundred years, but if one knows how to properly prepare and use mercury, one can go on indefinitely.

Those of us who do not even know how to go about looking for *amrta* must make use of other substances and hope for the best. Most of us are not physically prepared to become immortal anyway; we need rejuvenators just to help us maintain what health we have. *Rasayana* is also used by some doctors in India to protect tissues against iatrotrauma (that is, damage caused by other treatment, such as the use of anti-tubercular drugs or chemotherapy). Some yogis use a different approach, actively 'drying out' their bodies with tobacco and marijuana, reducing their diets and controlling prana's movement in order to reduce the production of their physical juices and allocate most of their resources into the production of *ojas*. This practice replaces their dependency on the external *rasas* of the world with dependency on the internal *rasa* of God-consciousness. *Rasayana* requires a clear idea of the desired result if the 'juice' imbibed is to reach the desired location in the organism.

REGENERATION

Charaka describes in detail the *rasayana* of old: on an auspicious day after the performance of various rituals, to the sound of priests intoning hymns, the patient entered a hut into which neither light nor wind from outside could come, and remained there in peaceful meditation for four to six weeks while the rejuvenating substances did their work. During this period the subject's hair, teeth and nails all fell out and regrew, and he shed his skin and regrew it. Some decades back Pandit Madan Mohan Malaviya, the father of Benaras Hindu University, was given such a treatment by Tapasviji Maharaj, a yogi who lived more than 160 years, but the Pandit, who could not endure all the restrictions, emerged before completion of the full course of treatment and so obtained only moderate results. Indeed, very few modern people could sit in the dark with nothing to occupy their minds for even a few days, even for rejuvenation.

So far as modern medicine knows, while tissues like the tonsils and the spleen can regrow from a few remaining cells, the only true physical regeneration occurs during the healing of a fractured bone via the reawakening of some of its marrow cells, which again become embryonic. Lower animals are more fortunate: salamanders can regrow legs and tails in unusual ways, rat forearms can regenerate after amputation, and the heart of a living newt can be made to repair itself within six hours after as much of half of it has been cut away. One common requirement for such regeneration is that the animal be young; even in humans, a fingertip that is accidentally chopped off will always regrow within three months as long as the child is less than eleven years old. Actual regeneration of body parts through *rasayana* therapy thus seems like a distinct if distant possibility. Until such time as processes for true regeneration are developed or rediscovered, we will have to remain satisfied with *feeling* like we have become young again, instead of actually returning to crib or cradle.

PEACE AND AGITATION

Modern scientists have confirmed a truth that has been long known and practised by yogis: there are two ways in which life can be extended, namely by eating the absolute minimum necessary and by lowering the body temperature. A good start to lowering your body temperature is to lower your mental temperature. Passion of any sort is hot, and heat destroys *ojas*, so a fiery temperament weakens your immunity, decreasing your odds for extended survival. A cool head preserves *ojas* and enhances longevity; in the words of Vagbhata, 'Those who speak the truth, who never become angry, who lead a spiritually pure life and are always serene are considered to be rejuvenated daily.'

Charaka speaks of two types of *rasayana*: with substances and without. The substance-free variety, called the 'behavioural *rasayana*', is the type described by Vagbhata; other restrictions include avoidance of all intoxicants, especially alcohol; the elimination of all physical or mental conflict and all other negative emotions; and the daily consumption (with proper digestion and assimilation) of foods of the sweet taste, mainly cow's milk and cow's ghee with honey. A full series of *panchakarma* purification procedures must be performed before beginning this discipline, which must be strictly followed if it is to work.

Long ago the Ayurvedic sages consulted Indra, the king of the gods, to obtain rejuvenatives for 'dwellers in towns and villages'. Even then urban life and longevity seem to have been mutually exclusive; how much more so today? Most of us city-dwellers must augment our discipline with a rejuvenating substance. Still, it is ideal to consume such substances away from home, where external discipline can be imposed to shore up one's own weaknesses of will. During such a retreat one must eliminate salt from the diet, regulate sleep, desist from sex and travel, enjoy only mild exercise and avoid loud speech, violent behaviour and other *vata*-provoking activities. The retreat should be scheduled for the most salubrious time of year (in India this extends roughly from mid-September to mid-March) when the juices of the environment are ample, proper in taste and free-flowing. When the juice of a rejuvenating substance waters the seed of discipline sown in the field of a purified body during the proper season, a good crop of regeneration is assured.

The Tibetans also prescribe *rasayana* during retreat after external and internal purification, 'internal bathing' being done with medicines made with cow's urine, which has the special ability to clean the *rasa* and blood tissues. Dr Donden explains that the body must be cleaned before either virilization or rejuvenation, otherwise it is like trying to dye a dirty cloth; the dye will not take wherever there is dirt. Tibetan *rasayanas* also require patients to visualize the descent of *amrta* into their being, to enhance the substance's regenerating effect.

A retreat provides a restful opportunity to re-examine one's life and to alter its direction if necessary, giving people permission to do things they would not be able to do otherwise. Retreats allow people sufficient relief from internal pressures to provide perspectives on how to meet their requirements in life by means other than illness. In Kerala Ayurvedic 'nursing homes', which encourage their inmates to undergo treatment for a month at a time, sometimes provide the only free time away from the responsibilities of family, studies or work that a person may be able to legitimately demand, a freedom that is itself highly therapeutic.

SUBSTANCES

Rasayana's results depend greatly on preparation, both the substance's preparation and your preparation for taking it. *Rasayana* medicines prepared by Tibetan physicians possess three levels of potency: the medicinal ingredients, the power of the mantras used in their preparation and the personal power of the monk who prepared them. Most Ayurvedic rejuvenators were once carefully prepared with mantras as well; the *Shatavari* Oil recipe propounded by Krsna Atreya directs the collector of the roots to face north at the time of collection in a worshipful mood, repeating the 'uprooting mantra' while digging in the ground with a pointed stick of *khadira* wood in order to collect the roots that have grown in the northern direction. There is a separate mantra, the 'drinking mantra', to be repeated while using the oil.

Later, when physicians developed a preference for preparations that relied less on the magic of the preparation ritual and more on the drug's own efficacy, simplified recipes became available. Sharngadhara provides two separate ways to prepare *Lokanatha Rasa*: one a simplified version, which is used mainly to treat *grahani*, and the other, which, 'given with the correct vehicle, can cure all diseases'. Restrictions for this second version include: eat off a bronze plate, taking only sweet foods and consuming nothing sour, avoiding everything whose name begins with the syllable '*ka*'; consume the remedy during the first two hours of the morning during an auspicious *nakshatra* (lunar constellation) and weekday while the moon is waxing; worship Lokanatha ('Lord of the World', an epithet of Shiva); feed unmarried young women; and offer donations. A similar procedure was also followed with remedies like *Mrganka Rasa* and *Hemagarbha Rasa*.

Many rejuvenating substances are repeatedly processed to potentiate their effects. Some Tibetan *rasayanas* are called 'essence-extract' medicines: you boil down various substances, add milk and boil down again, then add butter and boil down again. Finally, you add sugar and dried honey and the pill is rolled. These pills are consumed as part of a ritual practised for two to three months, the main part of which is the visualization of yourself as a deity and of the medicine as the deity melting into light and changing into *amrta*. *Bhavana* is a common 'essence-extract' procedure in Ayurveda, as is the repeated cooking of *Kshira Bala* Oil or Mica *Bhasma*. Another method instructs that various substances can be added to a growing marijuana plant (which is a *rasayana*), including mercury, medicinal wine or meat soup; then the plant's essence is extracted and repeatedly fed to a mango tree. The mangoes thus produced are very potent; they were much favoured by the Mughal emperors.

Generally, *rasayanas* are given first thing in the morning to take advantage of a well-rested digestive tract. Some *rasayanas* are heavy and cannot be used if *ama* is present in the body; examples include almonds, dates, liquorice, lotus seeds, milk, *shatavari* and many of the tubers. Others are hot and strengthen digestion, such as *chitraka* and *bhallataka*, but do not nourish the tissues themselves and so must be combined with other substances. Medicated jams such as *Chyvana-prasha* and those of *asvagandha*, almond, *brahmi*, *kushmanda* (winter melon) and *musali* (*Curculigo orchioides*, probably) are popular because they contain nutritive substances along with the rejuvenator. Some *rasayanas*, such as garlic, long pepper, *bhallataka* and *shilajit*, are so powerful that they must be consumed in gradually increasing doses so that your system becomes gradually habituated (*satmya*) to them. Once you have reached your level of maximum tolerance, you then slowly reduce the dose to zero.

Many substances used to treat diseases of particular organs can be used to rejuvenate those organs, including *shilajit* or *gokshura* for the urinary tract, *punarnava* for the liver and lymph system, and *ashva-gandha* for the nervous system. Calamus, *jatamamsi*, *shankhapushpi*, *bhrngaraja* and other herbs that enhance a weak intelligence can further sharpen an already sharp intellect. Some *rasayanas*, including *ashwagandha*, calamus, garlic, *guggulu* and *haritaki*, are especially good for *vata*; others, such as aloe, *amalaki*, *brahmi*, saffron and *shatavari*, are ideal for *pitta*; and still others, like *bibhitaki*, elecampane, *guggulu* and long pepper, work best on *kapha*. *Rasayanas* can also be classified by the tissue they most affect, such as mica for *rasa*, iron for blood, *ashvagandha* for flesh, *shilajit* for fat, coral or conch for bone, calamus for marrow, and *ashvagandha* or *shatavari* for *shukra*.

Almost all mineral medicines can be used as rejuvenators, especially those containing gold. Charaka listed *guduchi*, *haritaki*, *amalaki*, pearl, *shatavari*, *mandukaparni* and *punarnava* among his all-time favourite rejuvenators. Perhaps *amalaki* is the best of all.

VIRILIZATION

Rejuvenation and virilization are often considered together because they are both concerned with preservation and maintenance of 'juice'. Sex being one of the greatest expenditures of 'juice', virilization (the science of aphrodisiacs) is also a juice-repletion procedure. Sharngadhara advised the use of *rasayanas* and *vajikaranas* (virilizers; literally, 'makers of stallions') so that a man could enjoy many women without concern over his loss of semen. This attitude probably reflects the prevailing sentiments of his age, in which kings and nobles spent most of their spare time in their harems. The main reason Charaka offered for virilization was to ensure the production of healthy, intelligent, well-motivated children by ensuring healthy bodies and full sexual ecstasy at conception, the time when the child's constitution is fixed. For this reason he advised full bodily purification before virilization treatment.

'Any article that is sweet, unctuous, life-promoting, nourishing, heavy and pleasing to the mind', says Charaka, 'is to be regarded as virilific.' Virilization includes both nourishment and excitation of the sexual organs and is more important for men, who must create and maintain an erection and who lose more *shukra* than women do during the sex act. Because it is the ego that, identifying itself with the penis, sets in motion the train of events that leads to erection, a man's 'face' or sense of personal identity is very important to his sexual health. Health and virility are causally linked.

One presumes that virilization is named after horses instead of sparrows, pigeons or some other exceptionally sexually active animal because the horse is an ancient Vedic fertility symbol, and possibly also because of the size of the horse's penis. Concern over penis dimension has apparently existed ever since men began to court women, for Sharngadhara lambasts the 'fools who use unnatural methods', especially a paste of poisonous insects, to increase the size of the penis, a practice that can cause rashes, pustules, ulcers, abscesses and gangrene. Some also apply, to increase hardness rather than size, a special oil medicated with arsenic trioxide, which is also potentially dangerous; the wise apply only oils medicated with mild rejuvenating herbs like bala, *shatavari* or liquorice, *Ashvagandhadi* Oil, or simple almond oil.

Virilization is also important for that one woman in ten who ejaculates during orgasm and needs to replace her lost juice, and for those individuals who have unhealthy semen or menstrual blood. In *vata* increase semen becomes greyish and has an astringent taste; in *pitta* increase it is yellowish, sour and gives off a rotten odour; in excess of *kapha* it is greyish-white, sweet, very sticky and cool; and in impurity of blood it has a putrid, decomposing odour. Healthy semen is white, heavy and sweet, with a taste like honey, and (like healthy menstrual blood) can easily be washed off if it falls on a piece of cloth.

Since both rejuvenation and virilization deal with 'juice', the same substances are often useful for both. Aphrodisiacs for men may be divided into those that promote the production of semen, such as milk, ghee, onion, *vidari*, *shatavari*, *musali*, *gokshura*, liquorice and the semen of various animals; those that purify and strengthen semen, like *kushtha*, bayberry, cuttlefish bone, sugar cane, and vetiver; those that promote the fertility of semen, such as *brahmi*, *shatavari*, Bermuda grass, *amalaki*, *guduchi*, *katuka* and *bala*; those that increase excitability, such as *akarakarabha* (*Anacyclus pyrethrum*), saffron, clove, garlic, long pepper and, to a certain extent, asafoetida (thanks to its powerful downward action); and those that strengthen the nerves and discourage premature ejaculation, such as *ashwagandha*, sandalwood, nutmeg, *bhang*, *jatamamsi* and valerian.

Krauncha Paka, made from *kapikacchu* (*Mucuna pruriens*), which contains L-dopa, is a favourite Ayurvedic aphrodisiac jam; L-dopa strongly stimulates the sex drive in many men treated with it for Parkinsonism. *Musali Paka* and *Musali Churna* are given with milk and ghee to increase sexual vigour, as is *Ashvagandhadi Churna* and one variety of *Shatavari Churna*, which when given with cow's milk at bedtime, says Sharngadhara, makes a man insatiable with women. Each author has his own favourite recipes. Lolimraj, for example, maintains that the man who knows the proper way to prepare and use liquorice can enjoy sex many times a night for as long as he likes.

Phala Ghrta is another compound with two recipes: a simple variety for treating female reproductive diseases and promoting female fertility, and another variety, good for the fertility of both men and women, in which the herbs, including the juice of the roots of the mysterious *lakshmana*, are cooked on an auspicious day with the ghee and milk of a cow of a single colour who has a living calf. Strange and exotic aphrodisiacs include *nakraretas* (which seems to mean crocodile semen) and the flesh of the white snow frog, which is reportedly the main ingredient in Tibetan virilizers.

Virilizing medicines are not limited to oral use. Recipes for virilizing enemas are also to be found in the texts, especially those prepared by the essence-extract process; Charaka comments that the virilizing enema should be cooked 100 or 1,000 times to make it more efficient 'if a man is affluent enough'. After the enema is ready, 'then, having duly worshipped the god Shiva, the preparation should be placed on the back of an elephant and a white umbrella held over it to the accompaniment of Vedic chants, blowing of conches and the beating of drums', and it should be administered as an enema 'to the accompaniment of the sounds of auspicious words, benedictions, prayers, and divine worship', for external prosperity and internal 'prosperity' (of *rasa* and *shukra*) are related.

Virilization is, therefore, not merely a matter of swallowing potions and pills; it is a state of affluence of body. Some years back a physician of my acquaintance virilized a prince with the help of ten roosters. He fed the roosters a rich diet mixed with *bhasmas* for several days, then sacrificed one of them and added its flesh to the food of the others. This continued until only one rooster remained to be sacrificed. Its flesh, filled with *bhasmas* and other aphrodisiac substances, such as musk, was cooked to perfection with onions and other virilizing vegetables. Served to the prince, it worked efficiently and quickly because of his surroundings: incense and fragrances, rich raiment and furnishings, mood music, and the sight and touch of gorgeous, nubile young women. This is the virilization meant for enjoyment.

KUNDALINI

Vajikarana is also used, both in Buddhist and Hindu Tantra, for spiritual purposes: using the sexual energy to awaken the sleeping *kundalini* energy at the base of the spine and make it rise in a controlled fashion to consummate its own internal sexual union with its upper polarity in the brain. As a being develops, *kundalini* projects into matter; 'awakening' *kundalini* involves disengaging it from its external identifications and returning it to identification with pure consciousness. As it releases its hold, the energy it had used to hold on to the body is liberated as heat, just as the energy stored in a piece of wood by photosynthesis is released as heat when you ignite it. The awakening of *kundalini* is an incineration (hopefully slow and controlled) of one's own limited personality; in this sense *kundalini* yoga is a permanent form of stress release. So long as its return is not obstructed in any way, there is no cause for alarm, but when it encounters a blockage to its free passage, it may destroy the microcosm.

In the myth of the destruction of Daksha's sacrifice, on which occasion many diseases first appeared in the world, Daksha (which means 'dextrous, adept') attempted to perform a sacrifice without inviting Shiva, the embodiment of consciousness. A sacrifice is the establishing of a relationship with the cosmos by the offering of one's energy (heat). Daksha tried to perform his sacrifice without properly acknowledging the role of the unseen but ever-present universal consciousness, which is the basis of all existence. Shiva's wife, Sati ('the True One'), insisted upon attending the sacrifice, over Shiva's objections, but when she arrived, Daksha, her father, ignored her and insulted her husband. Overwhelmed with emotion, she incinerated herself with a fire she created from within. When Shiva learned of her action, he was overcome with rage (*raga*) and created a being who destroyed the sacrifice and decapitated Daksha. Sati was later reborn as Parvati ('Daughter of the Mountain') and eventually, after much penance, was reunited with Shiva.

This allegory can be interpreted as a cautionary tale on the birth, growth, maturity and decline of human cultures and societies: so long as they maintain a harmonious relationship with the universe, they persist, but when they plunge into selfish jingoism, they decline. It is also an explanation of life in the microcosm, with Daksha representing the limited personality; Sati, the *kundalini shakti*; and Shiva, her opposite polarity. An individual ego is led away from identification with pure consciousness by the allure of mani- fested existence. During the process of manifestation into flesh the ego selfishly identifies with the basket of limitations (the elements, tastes and so on) essential for existence, the soul's pure, true form (Sati) becomes separated from her husband (Shiva, pure conscious- ness) and is 'reborn' at the bottom of the chain of mountains, which is the spinal cord.

The experience of manifesting a being on the physical plane

liberates a quantity of unbalanced heat, which manifests first as desire and then as disease in body and mind. Charaka tells us, 'All living beings come into the world with fever on them and likewise with fever on them they die. It is the great delusion; enveloped by it, creatures do not recall any action done in their previous lives. It is fever alone that in the end takes away the life breath of all living beings.' The force that eventually drags you away from existence is present the moment you enter the world. It is this heat of desire that can both cure and cause disease, depending upon whether or not it is properly harnessed. Expression of rage engenders disease, while control of passion eliminates it; Shiva under the sobriquet of Rudra is both feared for his anger and adored as the first of all physicians.

The act of fleeing from Daksha's sacrifice caused *gulma* ('phantom tumour', a type of abdominal swelling) in some beings; the consumption of sacrificial materials caused leprosy (and other skin diseases) and diabetes; fear, grief and shock gave rise to insanity; epilepsy developed in those exposed to the impure touch of the attacking spirits; the being who killed Daksha became fever in the world; and *rakta pitta* developed from the excessive heat of fever. These maladies are seven of the eight major diseases listed in Charaka's section on diagnosis as being due to greed, malice and anger, the eighth being consumption, which is due to Daksha's curse of his son-in-law, the moon. Awakening *kundalini* without first entering into right relationship with consciousness creates disease by liberating more energy than the system can digest.

SPIRITUAL MEDICINE

Myths are created to preserve and propagate esoteric knowledge from generation to generation while hiding it from the uninitiated. The myth of mercury as Shiva's semen and sulphur as his wife Parvati's menstrual blood reflects both a physical reality – mercury can be used to purify and increase semen, and, properly prepared, sulphur is a good medicine for blood purification – and an astral reality: mercury and sulphur can be used, if one knows the method, to awaken *kundalini* and help it rejoin Shiva. The fact that the majority of doctors and patients who use these and other esoterically significant substances know nothing of these hidden significances or how to make use of them simply shows what an efficient concealer of reality a myth can be.

There is thus more to Atharva-Vedic medicine than meets the modern eye; its concentration on ethereal, symbolic medications probably reflects a concern for the health of practitioners who had entered realms of reality that appear only symbolically on our mundane plane of existence. Only a strong ego can fortify the system to protect it from all onslaughts, and when *kundalini* is busy disengaging itself from the body, ego-*ahamkara* is no longer sure of its own definition. What we call '*kundalini* awakening' has other labels applied to it in other spiritual paths, but all involve the same process. Spiritual medicine is not medicine to somehow make you more moral or altruistic; it is rather meant to preserve your life while your entire being undergoes a revolution of consciousness. As your spiritual development progresses, your ability to cure yourself with physical medicine alone diminishes, and other, more shamanic methods of treatment become necessary.

Shamans are sometimes confused with schizophrenics because of their ability to maintain a version of reality separate from the one the rest of us cooperate to create. While a shaman wilfully enters and leaves altered states and maintains his or her ability to function in society, a schizophrenic is a helpless victim of alternative reality who cannot function normally. Traditional psychology views any deviation from the 'norm' of our consensus reality as pathological, a position that led commentators to theorize that Swami Vivekananda's guru, the great saint Ramakrishna Paramahamsa, had 'epilepsy' because he would slip in and out of spiritual trances all day long. Many different shamanic traditions exist in India, but the most important is certainly Tantra, the successor of the Atharva-Veda, which was likely the successor of some previous tradition.

Through visualization Tantra harnesses the energy released as *kundalini* disengages from the body. Those engaged in such visualizations must be even more cautious than other visualizers. Madame Alexandra David-Neel, who lived in Tibet for many years, once used her powers of visualization to bring a phantom monk into being. Though he was but a shade, he was visible to other people and took on an independent existence of his own. Because her motives were not absolutely 'pure' – she had acted on a whim to see if it were possible – the monk eventually became inimical to her and began to behave threateningly, much as a cancer does, which is also a personal creation. It took her much time and effort to 'unthink' him.

The seers of the Vedas differ from us in the important respect that their *kundalinis* are fully awakened and under their full control, and whatever they visualize quickly comes into being. A doctor is a dim reflection on the physical plane of such a seer; while a physician treats individuals, seers treat nations, planets and even the entire cosmos.

AFTERWORD

The city of Benaras has been continuously inhabited longer than any other city in the world, and so more than any other city it epitomizes urban life. On the surface today's Benaras is dirty and crowded, but beneath its veneer of squalor beats a heart livelier than any other.

Perhaps India's holiest city, Benaras is the residence of Lord Shiva, the deity who presides over death and transformation. Each morning along the banks of the River Ganga thousands of pilgrims mingle with the city's own priests, yogis, gurus and disciples, all performing their own particular transformational rituals to maintain their personal relationships with the universe. In the midst of India's chaos, which is at its most chaotic in Benaras, a ceaseless striving for order remains, an eternal search for what is constant, coherent and true amid change that is as perpetual as the Ganga's flow.

In one of Benaras' by-lanes lives a friend of mine whom I call Tauji (meaning elder brother, though he is old enough to be my father). For many years Tauji performed marriages and other rituals of passage. Now that he is semi-retired, his sons and grandsons have assumed these duties and he has more time to spend with his two beloved cows, who live on the ground floor of his house. When I visit him, he serves me fresh milk from these cows, and we sit near them and chat. Sometimes we talk about health, about the different herbal mixtures he concocts according to season to strengthen digestion, the powders he uses to treat his cows and the potions he takes to solve his own health problems. We talk about the kinds of leaves that are best for poultices, the benefits of drinking Ganga water and the wonders of pure ghee. Sometimes he asks me for advice, and sometimes he gives me advice. Tauji has

Ayurvedic physicians for relatives; his knowledge of medicine comes from this family tradition and from his own personal obervation.

Tauji's life is an Ayurvedic life and, even though he is not himself a doctor, his achievements can be likened to those described in this passage from Charaka:

Whatever endeavour an Ayurvedic practitioner makes toward the relief of the ailments affecting those who walk the path of righteousness, those who propagate righteousness, and his family, relatives and seniors, and in whatever measure he meditates on, expounds or practises the spiritual truths enshrined in this science of life – all this constitutes the higher virtue (*dharma*) of his life.

Whatever store of wealth or patronage he is able to secure . . . and whatever relief from distress he is able to extend to those who have sought his protection – all this constitutes the wealth of his life.

Whatever renown comes his way, . . . whatever honours and services he commands, and whatever measure of health he is able to confer on those whom he loves – all this constitutes the satisfaction of a medical man's life.

There are Taujis all over India for whom Ayurveda is a daily reality. That Vedic faith in 'the true, the harmonious, the vast' which has maintained Benaras for more than sixty centuries is the same innately unshakeable faith that preserves Ayurveda wherever people long to live a righteous life. We are all going to die; of this there is no doubt. The only doubt is whether or not we will waste our lives. While we live we are stewards of life itself, and we have a chance to make a difference to ourselves, our families, our communities and our world, a chance to promote art, grace and culture, to refine the manifestation of consciousness on Earth and weaken the barbarity of selfishness, to give civilization a little extra breathing room. The ultimate purpose of Ayurveda, the Veda of Life, is to protect and strengthen life itself. If when you leave our world, you leave it even slightly better than it was when you entered it, you will have made life more liveable for those who will follow you, and yours will have been a life well lived.

BIBLIOGRAPHY

Becker, Robert O. and Selden, Gary, *The Body Electric*, New York, William Morrow, 1985.

Bhagavat Sinh Jee, H. H., Maharaja of Gondal, *Aryan Medical Science: A Short History*, Delhi, Rare Reprints, 1981.

Bhattacharya, Deborah, *Paglami: Ethnopsychiatric Knowledge in Bengal*, New York, Syracuse University Press, 1986.

Bhishagratna, K. L., *Sushruta Samhita*, Varanasi, Chowkhamba, 1968.

Chattopadhyaya, Debiprasad, *Science and Society in Ancient India*, Calcutta, Research India Publications, 1977.

Chopra, R. N., *et al.*, *Glossary of Indian Medicinal Plants*, New Delhi, Council of Scientific & Industrial Research, 1956.

Chopra, Col. Sir R. N., *et al.*, *Indigenous Drugs of India*, 2nd edn., reprinted, Calcutta, Academic Publishers, 1982.

Comba, Antonella, 'Caraka Samhita, Sarirasthana I and Vaishesika Philosophy', in G. J. Meulenbeld and D. Wujastyk (eds.), *Studies in Indian Medical History*, Groningen, 1987, pp. 43–61.

Dahanukar, Sharadini and Thatte, Urmila, *Ayurveda Revisited*, London, Sangam Books, 1989.

Dash, Bhagwan, *Ayurvedic Treatment for Common Diseases*, Delhi Diary, 1974.

Dash, Bhagwan, *Fundamentals of Ayurvedic Medicine*, Delhi, Bansal & Co., 1978.

Devaraj, T. L., *The Panchakarma Treatment of Ayurveda*, Bangalore, Dhanvantari Oriental Publications, 1980.

Donden, Dr Yeshi, *Health Through Balance: An Introduction to Tibetan Medicine*, Ithaca, NY, Snow Lion Publications, 1986.

Filliozat, J., *The Classical Doctrine of Indian Medicine*, Delhi, Munshiram Manoharlal, 1964.

Foss, Laurence and Rothenberg, Kenneth, *The Second Medical Revolution: From Biomedicine to Infomedicine*, Boston, Mass, Shambala, 1987.

Bibliography

Gandhi, Maneka, *Brahma's Hair*, New Delhi, Rupa & Co., 1989.

Harman, Willis, *Global Mind Change*, Indianapolis, Knowledge Systems, 1988.

Heyn, Birgit, *Ayurvedic Medicine*, trans. D. Louch, Wellingborough, Northants, Thorsons, 1987.

Jolly, Julius, *Indian Medicine*, trans. Kashikar, New Delhi, Munshiram Manoharlal, 1977.

Kakar, Sudhir, *The Inner World: A Psycho-Analytical Study of Childhood and Society in India*, 2nd edn, New Delhi, OUP, 1989.

Kakar, Sudhir, *Shamans, Mystics and Doctors*, New Delhi, OUP, 1990.

Kutumbiah, Dr P., *Ancient Indian Medicine*, Madras, Orient Longmans, 1962.

Lad, Vasant, *Ayurveda: The Science of Self-healing*, 2nd edn, Santa Fe, Lotus Press, 1985.

Lad, Vasant and Frawley, David, *The Yoga of Herbs: An Ayurvedic Guide to Herbal Medicine*, Santa Fe, Lotus Press, 1986.

Leslie, Charles (ed.), *Asian Medical Systems: A Comparative Study*, Berkeley, University of California Press, 1976.

McCutcheon, Marc, *The Compass in Your Nose and Other Astounding Facts about Humans*, JP Tarcher, 1989.

Mehta, P. M. (ed.), *Charaka Samhita*, Jamnagar, Gujarat, Gulab Kunverba Society, 1949.

Meulenbeld, G. J. and Wujastyk, D. (eds.), *Studies in Indian Medical History*, Groningen, 1987.

Mitra, Jyotir, *A Critical Appraisal of Ayurvedic Material in Buddhist Literature*, Varanasi, Jyotiralok Prakashan, 1985.

Mooss, N. S., *Single Drug Remedies*, Kottayam, Kerala, Vaidyasarathy Press, 1977.

Mooss, N. S. (ed. and trans.), *Vagbhata's Astanga Hrdaya Samhita, Kalpasthana*, Kottayam, Kerala, Vaidyasarathy Press, 1984.

Mooss, Vayaskara N. S., *Ayurvedic Flora Medica*, Kottayam, Kerala Vaidyasarathy Press, 1978.

Mukhopadhyaya, Girindranath, *History of Indian Medicine*, New Delhi, Oriental Books Reprint Corporation, 1974.

Murthy, Prof. K. R. Srikanta (trans.), *Madhava Nidanam*, Varanasi, Chaukhambha, 1987.

Nordstrom, Carolyn R., 'Ayurveda: A Multilectic Interpretation', *Social Science and Medicine*, vol. 28, no. 9, pp. 963–70.

Nordstrom, Carolyn R., 'Exploring Pluralism: The Many Faces of Ayurveda', *Social Science and Medicine*, vol. 27, no. 5, 1988, pp. 479–89.

Ornish, Dean, *Dr Dean Ornish's Programme for Reversing Heart Disease*, New York, Random House, 1990.

Powles, John, 'On the Limitations of Modern Medicine', in *Science, Medicine and Man*, vol. 1, London, Pergamon Press, 1973.

Pugh, Judy, 'Astrological Counseling in Contemporary India', *Culture, Medicine and Psychiatry*, vol. 7, no. 3, 1983, pp. 279–99.

Ray, Sir Praphulla Chandra, *A History of Hindu Chemistry*, Calcutta, Chatterjee & Co., 1925.

Ray, P. and Gupta, H. N., *Charaka Samhita: A Scientific Synopsis*, New Delhi, National Institute of Sciences of India, 1965.

Rele, V. G., *The Vedic Gods as Figures of Biology*, Bombay, D. B. Taraporevala, 1931.

Seal, Dr Brajendranath, *The Positive Sciences of the Ancient Hindus*, Delhi, Motilal Banarsidas, 1958.

Sharma, Pandit Shiv, *Realms of Ayurveda*, Arnold-Heinemann, 1979.

Sharma, P. V., *Fruits and Vegetables in Ancient India*, Varanasi, Chaukhambha Orientalia, 1979.

Siegel, Bernie S., *Love, Medicine and Miracles*, Harper & Row, 1986.

Svoboda, Robert E., *Prakruti: Your Ayurvedic Constitution*, Albuquerque, Geocom, 1988.

Tedlock, Dennis (trans.), *Popul Vuh: The Mayan Book of the Dawn of Life*, New York, Touchstone/Simon & Schuster, 1985.

Weiss, Mitchell, *et al.*, 'Traditional concepts of mental disorder among Indian psychiatric patients: Preliminary report of work in progress', *Social Science and Medicine*, vol. 23, no. 4, 1986, pp. 379–86.

Wise, T. A., *The Hindu System of Medicine*, Delhi, Mittal, 1986.

Zarrilli, Phillip B., 'Three Bodies of Practice in a Traditional South Indian Martial Art', *Social Science and Medicine*, vol. 28, no. 12, 1989, pp. 1289–309.

Zimmer, H. R., *Hindu Medicine*, Baltimore, Johns Hopkins Press, 1948.

Zimmermann, Francis, *The Jungle and the Aroma of Meats: An Ecological Theme in Hindu Medicine*, Berkeley, University of California Press, 1987.

USEFUL ADDRESSES

For further information on Ayurveda, please contact:

The Ayurvedic Institute
P.O. Box 23445
Albuquerque, New Mexico 87192–1445
USA

For Ayurvedic products unavailable elsewhere, please contact:

Kanak
P.O. Box 13653
Albuquerque, New Mexico 87192–3653
USA

INDEX

325

PENGUIN

ARKANA

NEW AGE BOOKS FOR MIND, BODY & SPIRIT

With over 200 titles currently in print, Arkana is the leading name in quality books for mind, body and spirit. Arkana encompasses the spirituality of both East and West, ancient and new. A vast range of interests is covered, including Psychology and Transformation, Health, Science and Mysticism, Women's Spirituality, Zen, Western Traditions and Astrology.

If you would like a catalogue of Arkana books, please write to:

Sales Department – Arkana
Penguin Books USA Inc.
375 Hudson Street
New York, NY 10014

Arkana Marketing Department
Penguin Books Ltd
27 Wrights Lane
London W8 5TZ

NEW AGE BOOKS FOR MIND, BODY & SPIRIT

A SELECTION OF TITLES

Neal's Yard Natural Remedies
Susan Curtis, Romy Fraser and Irene Kohler

Natural remedies for common ailments from the pioneering Neal's Yard Apothecary Shop. An invaluable resource for everyone wishing to take responsibility for their own health, enabling you to make your own choice from homeopathy, aromatherapy and herbalism.

Zen in the Art of Archery   Eugen Herrigel

Few in the West have strived as hard as Eugen Herrigel to learn Zen from a Master. His classic text gives an unsparing account of his initiation into the 'Great Doctrine' of archery. Baffled by its teachings – that art must become artless, that the archer must aim at himself – he gradually began to glimpse the depth of wisdom behind the paradoxes. While many Western writers on Zen serve up second-hand slogans, Herrigel's hard-won insights are his own discoveries.

The Absent Father: Crisis and Creativity   Alix Pirani

Freud used Oedipus to explain human nature; but Alix Pirani believes that the myth of Danae and Perseus has most to teach an age that offers 'new responsibilities for women and challenging questions for men'. It is a myth that can help us face the darker side of our personalities and break the patterns inherited from our parents.

Power of the Witch   Laurie Cabot

In fascinating detail, Laurie Cabot describes the techniques and rituals involved in charging tools, brewing magical potions and casting vigorous, tantalizing spells. Intriguing and accessible, this taboo-shattering guide will educate and enlighten even the most sceptical reader in the ways of an ancient faith that has much to offer today's world.

Water and Sexuality   Michel Odent

Taking as his starting point his world-famous work on underwater childbirth at Pithiviers, Michel Odent considers the meaning and importance of water as a symbol.

PENGUIN

ARKANA

NEW AGE BOOKS FOR MIND, BODY & SPIRIT

A SELECTION OF TITLES

The Revised Waite's Compendium of Natal Astrology
Alan Candlish

This completely revised edition retains the basic structure of Waite's classic work while making major improvements to accuracy and readability. With a new computer-generated Ephemeris, complete for the years 1900 to 2010, and a Table of Houses that now allows astrologers to choose between seven house systems, it provides all the information on houses, signs and planets the astrologer needs to draw up and interpret a full natal chart.

Aromatherapy for Everyone   Robert Tisserand

The therapeutic value of essential oils was recognized as far back as Ancient Egyptian times. Today there is an upsurge in the use of these fragrant and medicinal oils to soothe and heal both mind and body. Here is a comprehensive guide to every aspect of aromatherapy by the man whose name is synonymous with its practice and teaching.

Tao Te Ching   The Richard Wilhelm Edition

Encompassing philosophical speculation and mystical reflection, the *Tao Te Ching* has been translated more often than any other book except the Bible, and more analysed than any other Chinese classic. Richard Wilhelm's acclaimed 1910 translation is here made available in English.

The Book of the Dead   E. A. Wallis Budge

Intended to give the deceased immortality, the Ancient Egyptian *Book of the Dead* was a vital piece of 'luggage' on the soul's journey to the other world, providing for every need: victory over enemies, the procurement of friendship and – ultimately – entry into the kingdom of Osiris.

Astrology: A Key to Personality   Jeff Mayo

Astrology: A Key to Personality is designed to help you find out who you *really* are. A book for beginners wanting simple instructions on how to interpret a chart, as well as for old hands seeking fresh perspectives, it offers a unique system of self-discovery.

PENGUIN

ARKANA

NEW AGE BOOKS FOR MIND, BODY & SPIRIT

A SELECTION OF TITLES

Weavers of Wisdom: Women Mystics of the Twentieth Century
Anne Bancroft

Throughout history women have sought answers to eternal questions about existence and beyond – yet most gurus, philosophers and religious leaders have been men. Through exploring the teachings of fifteen women mystics – each with her own approach to what she calls 'the truth that goes beyond the ordinary' – Anne Bancroft gives a rare, cohesive and fascinating insight into the diversity of female approaches to mysticism.

Dynamics of the Unconscious: Seminars in Psychological Astrology II
Liz Greene and Howard Sasportas

The authors of *The Development of the Personality* team up again to show how the dynamics of depth psychology interact with your birth chart. They shed new light on the psychology and astrology of aggression and depression – the darker elements of the adult personality that we must confront if we are to grow to find the wisdom within.

The Myth of the Eternal Return: Cosmos and History   Mircea Eliade

'A luminous, profound, and extremely stimulating work . . . Eliade's thesis is that ancient man envisaged events not as constituting a linear, progressive history, but simply as so many creative repetitions of primordial archetypes . . . This is an essay which everyone interested in the history of religion and in the mentality of ancient man will have to read. It is difficult to speak too highly of it' – Theodore H. Gaster in *Review of Religion*

The Hidden Tradition in Europe   Yuri Stoyanov

Christianity has always defined itself through fierce opposition to powerful 'heresies'; yet it is only recently that we have begun to retrieve these remarkable, underground traditions, buried beneath the contempt of the Church. In this superb piece of scholarly detective work Yuri Stoyanov illuminates unsuspected religious and political undercurrents lying beneath the surface of official history.

ARKANA

NEW AGE BOOKS FOR MIND, BODY & SPIRIT

A SELECTION OF TITLES

A Course in Miracles
The Course, Workbook for Students and Manual for Teachers

Hailed as 'one of the most remarkable systems of spiritual truth available today', *A Course in Miracles* is a self-study course designed to shift our perceptions, heal our minds and change our behaviour, teaching us to experience miracles – 'natural expressions of love' – rather than problems generated by fear in our lives.

Fire in the Heart Kyriacos C. Markides

A sequel to *The Magus of Strovolus* and *Homage to the Sun*, *Fire in the Heart* centres on Daskalos, the Cypriot healer and miracle-worker and his successor-designate Kostas. The author, who has witnessed much that is startling in his years with the two magi, believes humanity may today be on the verge of a revolution in consciousness 'more profound than the Renaissance and the Enlightenment combined'.

The Western Way Caitlín and John Matthews

The Native Tradition and *The Hermetic Tradition* are now published together in one volume. The perennial wisdom of the Western Way has woven its bright and beckoning thread through religion, folklore and magic, ever reminding us of our connection with the earth mysteries of our ancestors and the mysticism of the Gnostic traditions.

Shamanism: Archaic Techniques of Ecstasy Mircea Eliade

Throughout Siberia and Central Asia, religious life traditionally centres around the figure of the shaman: magician and medicine man, healer and miracle-doer, priest and poet. 'Has become the standard work on the subject and justifies its claim to be the first book to study the phenomenon over a wide field and in a properly religious context' – *The Times Literary Supplement*

PENGUIN

ARKANA

NEW AGE BOOKS FOR MIND, BODY & SPIRIT

A SELECTION OF TITLES

Head Off Stress: Beyond the Bottom Line
D. E. Harding

Learning to head off stress takes no time at all and is impossible to forget – all it requires is that we dare take a fresh look at ourselves. This infallible and revolutionary guide from the author of *On Having No Head* – whose work C. S. Lewis described as 'highest genius' – shows how.

The Participatory Mind   Henryk Skolimowski

In a Grand Theory of participatory mind that builds on the insights of such thinkers as Teilhard de Chardin and Bergson as well as contemporaries Dobzhansky and Bateson, Skolimowski points to a new order, one brought about by a Western mind returning to, then reintegrating, the spiritual. This quest for fresh perspectives, as we approach the twenty-first century, has now become 'the hallmark of our times'.

The Magus of Strovolos: The Extraordinary World of a Spiritual Healer   Kyriacos C. Markides

This vivid account introduces us to the rich and intricate world of Daskalos, the Magus of Strovolos – a true healer who draws upon a seemingly limitless mixture of esoteric teachings, psychology, reincarnation, demonology, cosmology and mysticism, from both East and West. 'This is a really marvellous book . . . one of the most extraordinary accounts of a "magical" personality since Ouspensky's account of Gurdjieff' – Colin Wilson

The Great Year   Nicholas Campion

The Great Year raises important questions concerning the nature and function of political prophecy in late twentieth-century society, whether it be the ideological fringes of the New Age Movement, mainstream political ideology or the extremes of Stalinism and Fascism. Are we, as some contemporary writers think, coming to the End of History? Or is the belief in Millenarianism and the imminent dawning of a New Age nothing more than a collective delusion?

PENGUIN

ARKANA

NEW AGE BOOKS FOR MIND, BODY & SPIRIT

A SELECTION OF TITLES

Working on Yourself Alone: Inner Dreambody Work
Arnold Mindell

Western psychotherapy and Eastern meditation are two contrasting ways of learning more about one's self. The first depends heavily on the powers of the therapist. *Process-oriented* meditation, however, can be used by the individual as a means of resolving conflicts and increasing awareness from within. Using meditation, dream work and yoga, this remarkable book offers techniques that you can develop on your own, allowing the growth of an individual method.

The Moment of Astrology   Geoffrey Cornelius

'This is an extraordinary book ... I believe that within the astrological tradition it is the most important since the great flowering of European astrology more than three hundred years ago ... Quietly but deeply subversive, this is a book for lovers of wisdom' – from the Foreword by Patrick Curry

Homage to the Sun: The Wisdom of the Magus of Strovolos
Kyriacos C. Markides

Homage to the Sun continues the adventure into the mysterious and extraordinary world of the spiritual teacher and healer Daskalos, the 'Magus of Strovolos'. The logical foundations of Daskalos's world of other dimensions are revealed to us – invisible masters, past-life memories and guardian angels, all explained by the Magus with great lucidity and scientific precision.

The Eagle's Gift   Carlos Castaneda

In the sixth book in his astounding journey into sorcery, Castaneda returns to Mexico. Entering once more a world of unknown terrors, hallucinatory visions and dazzling insights, he discovers that he is to replace the Yaqui Indian don Juan as leader of the apprentice sorcerers – and learns of the significance of the Eagle.

PENGUIN

ARKANA

NEW AGE BOOKS FOR MIND, BODY & SPIRIT

A SELECTION OF TITLES

Being Intimate: A Guide to Successful Relationships
John Amodeo and Kris Wentworth

This invaluable guide aims to enrich one of the most important – yet often problematic – aspects of our lives: intimate relationships and friendships. 'A clear and practical guide to realization and communication of authentic feelings, and thus an excellent pathway towards lasting intimacy and love' – George Leonard

Coma: The Dreambody Near Death   Arnold Mindell

What happens to us when we are close to death? Far from being the horrific experience many assume it must be, coma can be a time of ecstasy, understanding and remarkable transformation, preparing us for what lies ahead whether we live or die.

The Act of Creation   Arthur Koestler

This second book in Koestler's classic trio of works on the human mind (which opened with *The Sleepwalkers* and concludes with *The Ghost in the Machine*) advances the theory that all creative activities – the conscious and unconscious processes underlying artistic originality, scientific discovery and comic inspiration – share a basic pattern, which Koestler expounds and explores with all his usual clarity and brilliance.

Secrets of the Soil   Peter Tompkins and Christopher Bird

In this long-awaited sequel to their bestselling *The Secret Life of Plants* Peter Tompkins and Christopher Bird explore the revolutionary methods of biodynamic agriculture introduced by the scientist–philosopher–mystic Rudolf Steiner. They show how Steiner's astonishing 'homeopathic' fertilizers and growing techniques have been used to revitalize previously barren areas and to achieve amazing feats of productivity.

PENGUIN

ARKANA

NEW AGE BOOKS FOR MIND, BODY & SPIRIT

A SELECTION OF TITLES

The Dreambody in Relationships Arnold Mindell

All of us communicate on several levels at once, and Mindell shows how much of our silent language conflicts with overt behaviour. He argues that bringing all the hidden parts of ourselves to awareness as they affect us is important for the well-being not only of our relationships but also of the community – indeed, the world – in which we live.

The Sacred Yew Anand Chetan and Diana Brueton

Recently it has been discovered that the yew can live for many thousands of years. *The Sacred Yew* is the inspiring story of one man's crusade to preserve this revered yet threatened tree and explain its importance to all our lives.

Be As You Are Sri Ramana Maharshi

'The ultimate truth is so simple.' This is the message of Sri Ramana Maharshi, one of India's most revered spiritual masters whose teachings, forty years after his death, are speaking to growing audiences worldwide. 'That sense of presence, of the direct communication of the truth so far as it can be put into words, is there on every page' – *Parabola*

In Search of the Miraculous: Fragments of an Unknown Teaching P. D. Ouspensky

Ouspensky's renowned, vivid and characteristically honest account of his work with Gurdjieff from 1915 to 1918. 'Undoubtedly a *tour de force*. To put entirely new and very complex cosmology and psychology into fewer than 400 pages, and to do this with a simplicity and vividness that makes the book accessible to any educated reader, is in itself something of an achievement' – *The Times Literary Supplement*

PENGUIN

ARKANA

NEW AGE BOOKS FOR MIND, BODY & SPIRIT

A SELECTION OF TITLES

When the Iron Eagle Flies: Buddhism for the West Ayya Khema

'One of humanity's greatest jewels'. Such are the teachings of the Buddha, unfolded here simply, free of jargon. This practical guide to meaning through awareness contains a wealth of exercises and advice to help the reader on his or her way.

The Second Ring of Power Carlos Casteneda

Carlos Castaneda's journey into the world of sorcery has captivated millions. In this fifth book, he introduces the reader to Dona Soledad, whose mission is to test Castaneda by a series of terrifying tricks. Thus Castaneda is initiated into experiences so intense, so profoundly disturbing, as to be an assault on reason and on every preconceived notion of life . . .

Dialogues with Scientists and Sages: The Search for Unity
Renée Weber

In their own words, contemporary scientists and mystics – from the Dalai Lama to Stephen Hawking – share with us their richly diverse views on space, time, matter, energy, life, consciousness, creation and our place in the scheme of things. Through the immediacy of verbatim dialogue, we encounter scientists who endorse mysticism, and those who oppose it; mystics who dismiss science, and those who embrace it.

The Way of the Sufi Idries Shah

Sufism, the mystical aspect of Islam, has had a dynamic and lasting effect on the literature of that religion. Its teachings, often elusive and subtle, aim at the perfecting and completing of the human mind. In this wide-ranging anthology of Sufi writing Idries Shah offers a broad selection of poetry, contemplations, letters, lectures and teaching stories that together form an illuminating introduction to this unique body of thought.

PENGUIN

ARKANA

NEW AGE BOOKS FOR MIND, BODY & SPIRIT

A SELECTION OF TITLES

Herbal Medicine for Everyone   Michael McIntyre

'The doctor treats but nature heals.' With an increasing consciousness of ecology and a move towards holistic treatment, the value of herbal medicine is now being fully recognized. Discussing the history and principles of herbal medicine and its application to a wide range of diseases and ailments, this illuminating book will prove a source of great wisdom.

The Tarot   Alfred Douglas

The puzzle of the original meaning and purpose of the Tarot has never been fully resolved. An expert in occult symbolism, Alfred Douglas explores the traditions, myths and religions associated with the cards, investigates their historical, mystical and psychological importance and shows how to use them for divination.

Views from the Real World   G. I. Gurdjieff

Only through self-observation and self-exploration, Gurdjieff asserted, could man develop his consciousness. To this end he evolved exercises through which awareness could be heightened and enlightenment attained. *Views from the Real World* contains his talks and lectures on this theme as he travelled from city to city with his pupils. What emerges is his immensely human approach to self-improvement.

Riding the Horse Backwards   Arnold and Amy Mindell

Arnold Mindell is the originator of perhaps the most inspiring 'school' of healing we have in the West now, process work, and in this running narrative of one of his workshops, which he gave with Amy Mindell at the Esalen community in the United States, we're taken to the heart of the magic.